Occupational Medicine: Evaluation and Management of Common Health Problems in the Workplace

Occupational Medicine: Evaluation and Management of Common Health Problems in the Workplace

Editor: Kirk Anderson

FOSTER ACADEMICS
www.fosteracademics.com

www.fosteracademics.com

FOSTER ACADEMICS

Cataloging-in-Publication Data

Occupational medicine : evaluation and management of common health problems in the workplace / edited by Kirk Anderson.
p. cm.
Includes bibliographical references and index.
ISBN 978-1-63242-794-6
1. Medicine, Industrial. 2. Medicine, Industrial--Evaluation. 3. Medicine, Industrial--Management. 4. Industrial hygiene--Management. I. Anderson, Kirk.
RC963 .O23 2019
613.62--dc23

Foster Academics,
118-35 Queens Blvd., Suite 400,
Forest Hills, NY 11375, USA

ISBN 978-1-63242-794-6 (Hardback)

Printed and bound in China.

Contents

Preface

The world is advancing at a fast pace like never before. Therefore, the need is to keep up with the latest developments. This book was an idea that came to fruition when the specialists in the area realized the need to coordinate together and document essential themes in the subject. That's when I was requested to be the editor. Editing this book has been an honour as it brings together diverse authors researching on different streams of the field. The book collates essential materials contributed by veterans in the area which can be utilized by students and researchers alike.

Occupational medicine is a field of medicine which deals with the maintenance of health in the workplace. It studies the prevention of injuries and diseases in the workplace, along with their treatment. Maintenance and increase in the productivity, and social adjustment in the workplace are the main objectives of occupational medicine. The chronic ailments caused due to work or occupational activity are called occupational diseases. Some occupational lung diseases include occupational asthma, chronic obstructive pulmonary disease, bronchiolitis obliterans and lung cancer. Contact dermatitis and urticaria, are two of the most common types of occupational skin diseases. Preventive methods for such diseases include personal protection of the workers, irritant replacement or removal, etc. This book includes some of the vital pieces of work being conducted across the world, on various topics related to the evaluation and management of common health problems in the workplace. It studies, analyzes and upholds the pillars of occupational medicine and its utmost significance in modern times. For all those who are interested in this field, this book can prove to be an essential guide.

Each chapter is a sole-standing publication that reflects each author´s interpretation. Thus, the book displays a multi-facetted picture of our current understanding of application, resources and aspects of the field. I would like to thank the contributors of this book and my family for their endless support.

Editor

1

Use of alcohol and drugs by employees in selected business areas in Norway: a study using oral fluid testing and questionnaires

Hilde Marie Erøy Edvardsen[1], Inger Synnøve Moan[2], Asbjørg S. Christophersen[1] and Hallvard Gjerde[1*]

Abstract

Background: Alcohol or drug use and associated hangover may reduce workplace safety and productivity and also cause sickness absence. The aims of this study were to examine (i) the use of alcohol and drugs, and (ii) reduced efficiency at work and absence due to such use among employees.

Methods: Forty-four companies were invited; half of them agreed to participate. Employees filled in a questionnaire and provided a sample of oral fluid, which was analysed for alcohol, 12 psychoactive medicinal drugs and 6 illicit drugs. Participation was voluntary and anonymous.

Results: Two thousand four hundred thirty-seven employees in eight business areas agreed to participate (92 % of those invited). By combining questionnaires and oral fluid testing, we found that 5.2 % had used psychoactive medication during the last couple of days, 1.4 % had used illicit drugs, 17.0 % had used alcohol during the last 24 h but only one person (0.04 %) was positive for alcohol in oral fluid. About 25 % reported reduced efficiency at work, and 5 % reported absence from work due to alcohol use during the past 12 months. The use of illicit drugs and binge drinking resulting in reduced efficiency and absence was most common among restaurant and bar workers and more common among men than women, whereas use of psychoactive medication was most common among healthcare, transportation and storage workers.

Conclusion: Impairment at work due to alcohol or drugs was rare, whereas reduced efficiency due to drinking was reported by a fairly large proportion. There were marked differences between some business areas, and across gender.

Keywords: Alcohol drinking, Illicit drugs, Prescription drugs, Workplace, Prevalence

Background

Use of alcohol or drugs and associated hangover effects may reduce workplace safety and productivity [1–3] and also cause sickness absence [4, 5]. Little is known about the use of alcohol and drugs that may affect safety and efficacy at work in Norway. A study published in 2004 found that 4 % reported having been under the influence of alcohol or drugs at work and 4 % had been absent from work because of alcohol and drug use [6]. Of the participants, 2.6 % reported having used illegal drugs and 18 % prescribed drugs during the past 12 months.

While few studies have addressed the prevalence of both alcohol and drug use and the consequences of such use in a work setting, the alcohol use-sickness absence association have been addressed in a number of studies. A recent review of 28 studies applying individual-level survey data to study a total of 48 associations between various measures of alcohol use and sickness absence, showed that there is strong empirical evidence for an association between alcohol use and both short- and long-term sickness absence [7]. One of the studies included in that review was conducted among young employees in Norway, where 8.1 % reported that they had been absent from work due to alcohol use the past 12 months [8]. This study found that the proportion of young male employees who reported having alcohol-related sickness absence was nearly twofold that of women, i.e., 10.5 and

* Correspondence: hallvard.gjerde@fhi.no
[1]Norwegian Institute of Public Health, P. O. Box 4404, Nydalen NO-0403 Oslo, Norway
Full list of author information is available at the end of the article

5.7 %, respectively. This finding is consistent with results in other studies [7]. However, less is known about gender differences with respect to drug use and consequences of such use in a workplace setting.

Results from workplace drug testing (WDT) in Norway for the period 2000–2006 showed that 2.9 % of the analysed samples were positive for drugs; only 1.0 % for illicit drugs [9]. However, WDT is used only within few business areas in Norway, primarily in shipping, oil industry and transportation, and it is likely that random workplace drug testing reduces the incidence of drug use among employees. Therefore, WDT findings do not accurately reflect the incidence of drug use among Norwegian employees in general.

The use of alcohol and drugs varies between countries and different business areas. American studies found that heavy alcohol use and illicit drug use was most prevalent among employees within the construction industry, arts, entertainment, recreation, mining, accommodation and food services and least prevalent among healthcare, social assistance and educational services [10, 11]. Differences between business areas have previously not been studied in Norway.

Research on the use of alcohol or drugs in relation to work has in most cases been performed using questionnaires or interviews. However, the use of alcohol and drugs is commonly under-reported [12–14]. A number of studies have found that analysis of biological samples may provide more accurate data than self-reports on alcohol and drug use during the last days or months [15–17]. However, drug testing cannot reveal alcohol and drug using habits and consequences of such use, so a combination of drug testing and questionnaires or interviews provides more data than using a single method alone [18–21].

The aims of this study were: (i) to examine the use of alcohol and drugs using a combination of self-report through questionnaires and testing of oral fluid (mixed saliva), and (ii) self-reported sickness absence and reduced efficiency or hangover at work due to such use among employees in eight business areas in Norway, and across gender.

Methods

We first performed a pilot study that included 526 employees during 2008–2009 [22], and a follow-up study with 1911 employees was conducted during 2011–2014. We present the total findings from both studies in this article.

Ethics

The study was approved by the Regional Committee for Medical and Health Research Ethics. The dataset was completely anonymous.

Consent

Oral informed consent was obtained from the participants for publication of reports.

Study design and setting

The recruitment of companies was performed during 2008–2013. Forty-four companies and business chains were invited to participate, and a general call for participation was published in magazines and on websites. In total, 21 companies agreed to participate, and the Norwegian Public Roads Administration agreed to let us recruit truck drivers at control stations for heavy traffic; thus, altogether 22 businesses participated.

Information about the upcoming study was distributed to all employees except truck drivers several weeks before the recruitment of employees was performed. The date for recruitment was not announced. First, the study days were selected for each company; then, either a random selection or all employees who were present in the building were contacted. Occupational drivers were recruited at a heavy vehicle checking station during scheduled controls.

For all companies except one, and for all occupational drivers, each employee was approached individually by one project assistant from the Norwegian Institute of Public Health (NIPH) and asked to participate. Written and verbal information about the project was given, and oral informed consent was obtained from all participants. Those who agreed to participate filled in a questionnaire in an area shielded from view and provided an oral fluid specimen. The questionnaire and the sample of oral fluid were placed in an unlabelled envelope that was closed and sealed and collected by a project assistant within approximately an hour.

For one company, an envelope containing the questionnaire and sampling device for oral fluid, including instructions for use, was given to random employees when entering the company facilities in the morning. The employees were asked to deliver the questionnaire and the oral fluid sample in closed and sealed, unlabelled envelopes at specified sites before noon.

The recruitment of employees was completed in 2014. In total, 2639 employees were invited and 2437 agreed to participate (92 %). The included business areas were healthcare (917 employees), finance (457 employees), manufacturing (254 employees), transportation/storage (233 employees), restaurants/bars (131 employees), public administration (211 employees), media (152 employees; questionnaires only), and research institutes (82 employees). Participation rates and socio-demographic characteristics for business areas with two or more companies and more than 100 participating employees are presented in Table 1. Data for employees in public administration,

Table 1 Employee participation rates, age and gender of all participants ($N = 2437$) across business areas

	Healthcare	Finance	Industry	Transportation and storage	Restaurants and bars	Other	Total
No. of participants	917	457	254	233	131	445	2437
Participation rate, %	98.3	96.4	91.0	95.9	92.9	78.2	92.3
Gender, % (n)							
Women	79.5 (729)	47.9 (219)	19.3 (49)	6.4 (15)	47.3 (62)	54.6 (243)	54.0 (1317)
Men	18.5 (170)	49.0 (224)	77.2 (196)	77.7 (181)	51.1 (67)	38.9 (173)	41.5 (1011)
Not reported	2.0 (18)	3.1 (14)	3.5 (9)	15.9 (37)	1.5 (2)	6.5 (29)	4.5 (109)
Age distribution, % (n)							
<30 years	14.7 (135)	9.4 (43)	11.8 (30)	23.2 (54)	78.6 (103)	14.6 (65)	17.6 (430)
30–39 years	26.8 (246)	28.2 (129)	15.0 (38)	18.0 (42)	16.8 (22)	28.1 (125)	24.7 (602)
40–49 years	26.7 (245)	24.7 (113)	30.7 (78)	22.7 (53)	3.1 (4)	22.9 (102)	24.4 (595)
50–59 years	22.0 (202)	28.0 (128)	28.7 (73)	21.5 (50)	0.0 (0)	21.6 (96)	22.8 (549)
60+ years	8.2 (75)	8.5 (39)	11.0 (28)	7.3 (17)	0.8 (1)	11.0 (49)	8.6 (209)
Not reported	1.5 (14)	1.1 (5)	2.8 (7)	7.3 (17)	0.8 (1)	1.8 (8)	2.1 (52)

media and research are presented in the column named "Other".

Data collection

For most of the companies, the data collection was performed during weekdays only. Oral fluid was collected using Statsure Saliva Sampler™ (Statsure Diagnostic Systems, Framingham MA, USA). The time required for sample collection and filling in the questionnaire was about 5 min.

The samples of oral fluid were frozen within one day after collection and thawed once before the analysis. Alcohol was analysed by an automated enzymatic method [23]. Medicinal and illicit drugs were analysed by liquid chromatography-tandem mass spectroscopy; two similar analytical methods were used during the project period [24, 25]. The analysed compounds and cut-off concentrations (above which a sample was regarded as positive) are presented in Table 2.

Two versions of the questionnaire were used. The questionnaire used for the pilot study in five businesses within transportation/storage, public administration, media and research did not include questions on drug use during the last 12 months; this question was added based on a request from one of the participating companies and was used for 17 businesses included after the pilot study had been finished.

Statistical methods

Possible differences between the prevalence of medicinal or illicit drugs in oral fluid samples from different business areas were initially assessed using Pearson's chi-square test for categorical data.

Adjusted odds ratios (OR) with 95 % confidence intervals (95 % CI) were calculated using multivariate unconditional logistic regression using SPSS Statistics Version 22 (IBM Corporation, Armonk, NY). Drug findings or self-reported data were included as dependent variable (with 2 categories; 0 = negative; 1 = positive). Independent variables were gender, age group (5 categories) and business areas (6 categories).

Results

The participation rate among invited businesses was 50.0 %. Among the employees in the participating businesses the average participation rate was 92.3 %; when using the regular recruitment procedure 95.6 % (range 80.0–100.0 %) and 67.8 % when the participation when employees were asked to deliver the envelope with questionnaire and oral fluid sample on specified sites.

Oral fluid

Positive alcohol and drug findings are presented in Table 2 and summarized in relation to business area and gender in Table 3. Only one employee (0.04 %) was positive for alcohol; this might be due to alcohol drinking the day before or due to a small alcohol intake during the working day, e.g. at lunch. Few employees were positive for illicit drugs (0.9 %) compared to medicinal drugs (3.0 %). The most frequently detected substances were the sleeping agent zopiclone (1.9 %), the sedative diazepam (0.7 %), cannabis (0.7 %), the analgesic substance codeine (0.3 %) and methamphetamine (0.1 %). The medicinal drugs that were found can in most cases be detected in oral fluid for more than 12 h after using a single dose, perhaps more than 24 h in some cases; amphetamine, cannabis (THC) and the cocaine metabolite benzoylecgonine may also be detected for more than 12 h, rarely longer than 48 h, whereas cocaine can be detected for less than 12 h after use [26].

Table 2 Substances analysed in oral fluid, cut-off concentrations and prevalence above cut-off concentrations

Compound	Description	Cut-off[c] ng/mL	Prevalence % (n)
6-Acetylmorphine	Metabolite of heroin	1.3	0.0 (0)
Alcohol		0.10 g/L	0.04 (1)
Alprazolam	Benzodiazepine; anxiolytic	0.62	0.0 (0)
7-Aminoclonazepam	Metabolite of clonazepam	0.71	0.0 (0)
7-Aminoflunitrazepam	Metabolite of flunitrazepam	0.17	0.0 (0)
7-Aminonitrazepam	Metabolite of nitrazepam	0.63	0.0 (0)
Amphetamine	Stimulant[a]	24	0.09 (2)
Benzoylecgonine	Metabolite of cocaine	9.8	0.04 (1)
Clonazepam	Benzodiazepine; anticonvulsant, anxiolytic	0.63	0.0 (0)
Cocaine	Stimulant[b]	1.8	0.04 (1)
Codeine	Opioid analgesic, antitussive	7.5	0.3 (6)
Diazepam	Benzodiazepine; anxiolytic, anticonvulsant, sedative	0.40	0.7 (16)
Flunitrazepam	Benzodiazepine; anxiolytic	0.31	0.0 (0)
3,4-Methylenedioxy-methamphetamine (MDMA)	Psychedelic hallucinogenic drug[b]	26	0.0 (0)
Methadone	Opioid used mainly for opioid dependence, but also for analgesia	11	0.0 (0)
Methamphetamine	Stimulant[b]	15	0.1 (3)
Morphine	Opioid analgesic, also metabolite of codeine and heroin	7.1	0.2 (4)
Nitrazepam	Benzodiazepine; anxiolytic	0.56	0.0 (0)
Nordiazepam	Metabolite of diazepam	0.68	0.3 (6)
Oxazepam	Benzodiazepine; anxiolytic, anticonvulsant, and metabolite of diazepam	4.9	0.04 (1)
Δ9-Tetrahydrocannabinol (THC)	Cannabis[a]	0.63	0.7 (16)
Zolpidem	Short acting hypnotic	1.2	0.09 (2)
Zopiclone	Short acting hypnotic	1.6	1.9 (43)

[a]Mostly used illegally in Norway
[b]Illegal in Norway
[c]Concentrations in neat oral fluid above which the analytical findings were regarded as positive

Medicinal drugs were detected more frequently (p <0.001) and illicit drugs less frequently (p <0.001) in samples of oral fluid from healthcare workers than in samples from employees in other business areas.

Illicit drugs were detected more frequently (p <0.001) in samples from restaurant/bar workers than in samples from employees in other business areas.

Of the 16 employees who were found to be positive for cannabis, the THC concentrations were above 2 ng/mL in native oral fluid (calculated using sample weight) in 14 cases; this concentration has been proposed as limit in the USA when oral fluid samples are used in workplace drug testing [27]. Four had concentrations between 25 and 300 ng/mL, suggesting cannabis smoking within a few hours before sampling. For two of the three employees who were positive for methamphetamine, concentrations were higher than the proposed limit of 50 ng/mL in the USA [27]. The concentrations were more than 1000 ng/mL, suggesting intake of moderate doses within the last 24 h or large doses 1–3 days ago. Those two individuals had combined methamphetamine with diazepam, which is a commonly used drug combination among problematic drug users. For five of the 43 employees who were positive for the sleeping agent zopiclone, the concentrations were above 50 ng/mL. Those high concentrations suggest that the medication might have been taken less than 6 h before sample collection. One of the diazepam users had 34 ng/mL in oral fluid, which indicates very recent drug intake or high concentration in blood. The other drug findings were of low concentrations that were unlikely to affect safety and efficacy.

Questionnaires

The results from the questionnaire are presented in Table 3. Self-reported use of psychoactive medication was fairly similar across business areas (ranging from 3.5 to 5.3 %). However, large differences were observed for

Table 3 Self-reported alcohol and drug use and results from testing of oral fluid samples

	Healthcare	Finance	Manufacturing	Transportation and storage	Restaurants and bars	Other	Men	Women	Total
Oral fluid samples, % (n)	98.8 (906)	98.2 (449)	99.2 (252)	99.6 (232)	99.2 (130)	65.6 (292)	unk.[a] (928)	unk.[a] (1226)	92.8 (2261)
Questionnaires, % (n)	100.0 (917)	100.0 (457)	100.0 (254)	97.0 (226)	100.0 (131)	100.0 (445)	unk.[a] (1011)	unk.[a] (1317)	99.7 (2430)
Psychoactive medication, % (n)									
A: Detected in oral fluid	4.6 (42)	1.1 (5)	2.0 (5)	3.0 (7)	2.3 (3)	1.7 (5)	2.3 (21)	3.7 (45)	3.0 (67)
B: Self-reported use last 48 h	4.5 (41)	3.7 (17)	3.5 (9)	5.3 (12)	3.8 (5)	3.8 (17)	4.3 (43)	3.9 (52)	4.2 (101)
Either A or B	6.0 (55)	4.2 (19)	4.7 (12)	7.3 (17)	5.3 (7)	3.8 (17)	5.1 (52)	5.2 (69)	5.2 (127)
Self-reported non-therapeutic use last 12 months	0.7 (6)	0.7 (3)	1.2 (3)	nc	1.5 (2)	nc	nc	nc	nc
Illicit drugs, % (n)									
A: Detected in oral fluid	0.0 (0)	0.4 (2)	0.8 (2)	3.0 (7)	6.9 (9)	0.0 (0)	1.7 (16)	0.3 (4)	0.9 (20)
B: Self-reported last 48 h	0.0 (0)	1.1 (5)	0.0 (0)	0.9 (2)	11.5 (15)	0.0 (0)	1.3 (13)	0.7 (9)	0.9 (22)
Either A or B	0.0 (0)	1.3 (6)	0.8 (2)	3.9 (9)	12.2 (16)	0.0 (0)	2.3 (23)	0.8 (10)	1.4 (33)
Self-reported use last 12 m	1.9 (17)	3.7 (17)	1.6 (4)	nc	28.2 (37)	nc	nc	nc	nc
Alcohol, % (n)									
A: Detected in oral fluid	0.0 (0)	0.2 (1)	0.0 (0)	0.0 (0)	0.0 (0)	0.0 (0)	0.1 (1)	0.0 (0)	0.0 (1)
B: Self-reported use last 24 h	13.4 (123)	12.3 (56)	9.8 (25)	12.4 (28)	45.0 (59)	27.2 (121)	19.2 (194)	15.3 (201)	17.0 (412)
Either A or B	13.4 (123)	12.5 (57)	9.8 (25)	12.4 (28)	45.0 (59)	27.2 (121)	19.3 (195)	15.3 (201)	17.0 (413)
Drinking habits and consequences, % (n)									
Binge drinking (≥6 units) at least once a month	11.8 (108)	25.6 (117)	23.6 (60)	22.6 (51)	58.0 (76)	27.0 (120)	30.4 (307)	15.7 (207)	21.9 (532)
Reduced efficiency or hangover at work during previous 12 m	12.2 (112)	39.8 (182)	5.5 (14)	9.7 (22)	65.6 (86)	40.9 (182)	27.8 (281)	22.4 (295)	24.6 (598)
Absence from work due to drinking during previous 12 m	0.9 (8)	9.4 (43)	1.2 (3)	3.5 (8)	20.6 (27)	8.8 (39)	7.2 (73)	3.9 (51)	5.3 (128)

[a]Gender was not reported by 109 participants
nc: Data was not collected for all groups of participants

self-reported use of illicit drugs. The proportion who reported using illicit drugs during the last 48 h among restaurant/bar workers was 11.5 % compared to 1 % or less in other business areas.

Employees in four business areas were asked about the use of illicit drugs and the non-therapeutic use of psychoactive medication (recreational use to get intoxicated or high) during last 12 months. More than 25 % of the restaurant/bar workers reported illicit drug use, less than 4 % in other business areas. Less than 2 % reported recreational use of psychoactive medication.

Self-reported alcohol use during the last 24 h, binge drinking, reduced efficiency or hangover and absence from work due to drinking was also most frequently reported by restaurant/bar workers, and was also fairly frequently reported by finance workers and workers in the group called "Other", which included media, research and public administration employees.

Comparing oral fluid and questionnaires

Some under-reporting of drug use was observed when comparing drug findings in oral fluid and self-reported drug use. Of those who were positive for illicit drugs in oral fluid ($n = 20$), 45.0 % reported using illicit drugs during the last 48 h; whereas among those who were positive for medicinal drugs ($n = 67$), 61.2 % reported intake during the last 48 h.

When adding drug findings in oral fluid to self-reported drug used during the last 48 h, the number of medicinal drug users increased by about a quarter and the number of illicit drug users increased by about the half when compared to self-reported use only. When including either analytical findings or self-reported use, recent use of psychoactive medication was most prevalent among transportation and storage workers, whereas recent use of illicit drugs was most prevalent among restaurant/bar workers.

Differences across business areas

The data presented in Table 3 suggest that there were marked differences between business areas. However, there were also significant differences between genders and age groups, making evaluation of the prevalence data more complicated. In order to study differences between business areas while adjusting for differences in the distributions of age and genders, we performed logistic regression analysis using drug findings or self-reported data as dependent variable, and business area, age and gender as covariates. The regression analyses for the detection of medicinal or illicit drugs in samples of oral fluid and self-reported inefficiency or absence due to drinking are presented in Table 4.

Due to the fact that illicit drugs were detected among employees in only some business areas and only one person above 40 years of age, the restaurant business were compared with non-restaurant business employees in total, and the employees were disaggregated into three age groups. Employees in the restaurant business had high odds ratio for being positive for illicit drugs ($p = 0.002$) when adjusting for gender and age group, compared to employees in other business areas.

Employees within the finance business and the group of businesses called "other" had significantly lower odds for being positive for medicinal drugs than healthcare employees. If comparing healthcare workers with employees within non-healthcare businesses in total, they were found to have higher odds ratios for being positive for medicinal drugs ($p = 0.001$) compared to other business areas (results not shown).

When compared with employees in the healthcare business, employees in the finance, restaurant and "other" businesses had significantly higher odds ratios for reporting reduced efficiency or hangover at work at least once during the previous 12 months ($p < 0.001$) and sickness absence ($p < 0.001$) due to drinking. Highest odds ratios were found for restaurant/bar workers.

Gender differences

The results presented in Table 3 show that illicit drugs were detected more frequently among male employees than females, and self-reported binge drinking, reduced efficiency or hangover at work and sickness absence from work due to drinking was also more frequent among males.

Logistic regression analysis was performed adjusting for age group and the six business areas (Table 4). Female employees had statistically significantly lower odds ratios compared to men to report reduced efficiency or hangover at work during previous 12 months ($p < 0.001$) and absence from work due to drinking during previous 12 months ($p = 0.010$). The difference observed between the genders for the detection of medicinal drugs in samples of oral fluid when adjusting for age group and business area were not statistically significant. However, the odds ratio for detection of illicit drugs was statistically significantly lower for females than males when adjusting for age group and business area when disaggregated into restaurant and non-restaurant businesses ($p = 0.004$).

Discussion

In this study, we combined the use of questionnaires and oral fluid testing to compare alcohol and drug use, as well as sickness absence and reduced efficiency due to such use, across eight business areas in Norway, and across gender.

Table 4 Logistic regression analysis

	Univariate analysis			Multivariate analysis		
	OR	95 % CI	*p*	OR	95 % CI	*p*
Detection of illicit drugs in oral fluid						
Non-restaurant/bar employees (referent)						
Restaurant/bar	13.70	5.57–33.69	<0.001	5.00	1.82–13.72	0.002
Females	0.19	0.06–0.57	0.003	0.19	0.06–0.59	0.004
Age < 30 years (referent)						
Age 30–39 years	0.51	0.20–1.28	0.151	0.77	0.28–2.15	0.622
Age 40+ years	0.03	0.00–0.21	0.001	0.05	0.01–0.43	0.006
Detection of medicinal drugs in oral fluid						
Healthcare employees (referent)						
Finance	0.23	0.09–0.59	0.002	0.24	0.09–0.63	0.003
Manufacturing	0.34	0.12–0.95	0.040	0.35	0.11–1.05	0.062
Transportation/storage	0.76	0.34–1.73	0.516	0.92	0.35–2.41	0.872
Restaurant/bar	0.48	0.15–1.57	0.224	0.77	0.20–2.93	0.700
Other lines of business	0.39	0.15–1.00	0.050	0.39	0.15–1.00	0.050
Females	1.66	0.98–2.81	0.058	1.27	0.67–2.42	0.462
Age < 30 years (referent)						
Age 30–39 years	0.71	0.28–1.79	0.464	0.79	0.29–2.11	0.632
Age 40–49 years	1.32	0.58–2.98	0.512	1.50	0.61–3.68	0.375
Age 50–59 years	1.83	0.83–4.05	0.134	2.18	0.91–5.22	0.082
Age 60+ years	2.37	0.95–5.94	0.066	2.83	1.05–7.63	0.040
Reported reduced efficiency or hangover at work last 12 months due to drinking						
Healthcare employees (referent)						
Finance	4.82	3.66–6.35	<0.001	5.10	3.79–6.87	<0.001
Manufacturing	0.37	0.20–0.68	0.001	0.31	0.16–0.58	<0.001
Transportation/storage	0.74	0.44–1.25	0.265	0.45	0.26–0.79	0.006
Restaurant/bar	14.18	9.35–21.52	<0.001	5.75	3.66–9.05	<0.001
Other lines of business	4.85	3.67–6.42	<0.001	4.96	3.69–6.67	<0.001
Females	0.75	0.62–0.90	0.003	0.63	0.50–0.79	<0.001
Age < 30 years (referent)						
Age 30–39 years	0.47	0.36–0.61	<0.001	0.41	0.30–0.56	<0.001
Age 40–49 years	0.30	0.23–0.40	<0.001	0.31	0.22–0.43	<0.001
Age 50–59 years	0.20	0.15–0.27	<0.001	0.18	0.13–0.26	<0.001
Age 60+ years	0.16	0.10–0.26	<0.001	0.13	0.08–0.22	<0.001
Reported sickness absence last 12 months due to drinking						
Healthcare employees (referent)						
Finance	11.93	5.55–25.60	<0.001	11.04	5.06–24.07	<0.001
Manufacturing	0.92	0.19–4.36	0.916	0.80	0.17–3.86	0.778
Transportation/storage	4.22	1.51–11.79	0.006	2.73	0.94–7.97	0.066
Restaurant/bar	29.22	12.93–66.02	<0.001	13.76	5.78–32.77	<0.001
Other lines of business	10.92	5.04–23.67	<0.001	9.92	4.54–21.69	<0.001
Females	0.52	0.36–0.75	0.001	0.59	0.39–0.88	0.010
Age < 30 years (referent)						
Age 30–39 years	0.68	0.44–1.05	0.080	0.75	0.45–1.24	0.259
Age 40–49 years	0.23	0.13–0.42	<0.001	0.31	0.16–0.59	<0.001
Age 50–59 years	0.22	0.12–0.41	<0.001	0.28	0.14–0.55	<0.001
Age 60+ years	0.13	0.04–0.42	0.001	0.14	0.04–0.48	0.002

More detailed results from one business area (healthcare) have been published in an separate article [28]. In this article we present the total findings from the pilot and main studies, which included 2437 employees from eight business areas. Data from the pilot study are included to enable the comparison between all included business areas; this has not been reported for the pilot study previously.

Few employees were impaired by alcohol or drugs at the time of collection of oral fluid. One employee had concentration of alcohol of about 0.2 g/L in oral fluid (the concentration in blood is about the same as in oral fluid), which either may be caused by drinking one glass of beer or wine within the last hour, or residual alcohol after heavy drinking the day before. For drugs, it is impossible to accurately estimate concentrations in blood based on concentrations in oral fluid due to large individual variation [29]. However, about 10 persons (0.4 %) had drug concentrations in oral fluid that might be associated with recent drug use that may affect the performance at work.

In a U. S. survey, 8.1 % reported workplace use of alcohol during the last 12 months, 0.99 % reported weekly use, 0.78 % reported alcohol-related impairment weekly, and 9.23 % reported being hungover at work during the last 12 months [30]. In Europe, the situation varies a lot between different countries; in some countries the use of alcohol during the working day has been very common. The proportion of workers who consumed alcohol during the working day was reportedly 11 % in Austria, 14 % in Denmark, 8.2 % in Poland; whereas in the Netherlands, 4 % of the workers who drank alcohol sometimes drank before going to work or at work [31]. Thus, the use of alcohol in relation to work seemed to be very much less common in our study than in some European countries.

In a study based on data from a U.S. National Survey performed in 2002–2003, a total of 14.1 % of the workforce reported having used illicit drugs during the last 12 months, 3.6 % at least once a week, and 1.25 % reported use 6–7 days a week [32]. Thus, the use of illicit drugs was significantly more common among employees in the USA than in Norway. There is little information about drug use in relation to work for other European countries [31]. However, there is large variation in the use of illicit drugs in general between European countries [33].

The results show large differences between some business areas. Restaurant/bar workers reported more often alcohol use during the last 24 h. This is partly due to the fact that for those businesses the data collection included weekends, when approximately 70 % of drinking situations occur [34]. A larger proportion of restaurant/bar workers also reported binge drinking during the past 12 months compared to employees in other business areas as well as being less efficient at work and absence from work due to alcohol use during the last 12 months. Drug use during the last 48 h was also more common among restaurant/bar workers.

The findings among restaurant/bar employees are partly related to the large proportion of employees below 30 years of age, who are expected to use more alcohol and illicit drugs than older age groups. However, when adjusting for age and gender distributions, significantly more drug use and alcohol-related hangover and absence were found among restaurant/bar employees than among employees in most other business areas. Also the fact that they are working in an environment with high availability of alcohol and work-related norms that are supportive of after-work drinking and hangover at work may have influenced their drinking habits [35].

Also previous studies have found high alcohol consumption or high prevalence of hazardous drinking among restaurant workers, both in Scandinavia and elsewhere [10, 35–38]. Previous American studies have also found that restaurant workers more often reported use of illicit drugs than employees in many other business areas [10, 11].

The proportion of workers within finance and the "Other" category (i.e., media, research and public administration employees) who reported reduced efficiency and sickness absence due to alcohol was also fairly high.

It has previously been reported that problematic alcohol and drug use may be common among health professionals [39], particularly because of their easy access to prescription medication. In our study, binge drinking, reduced efficiency and drinking-related absence was less common among healthcare workers than the other business areas. However, the use of psychoactive medication, both self-reported use and findings in samples of oral fluid, was higher among health professionals. Moreover, we found that use of psychoactive medication was more common among employees within transportation and storage than in other business areas.

Studies in the USA have found that in addition to hotel, restaurant and bar workers, employees within construction, building and grounds maintenance, arts, entertainment, sports and media businesses had higher odds ratios for illicit drug use and illicit drug impairment [10, 11, 32, 40] as well as working under the influence of alcohol and hangover at work [30]. An Australian study found that alcohol use at work was most common among hospitality, construction and financial services, whereas working under the influence of alcohol was most common among hospitality employees; in total, more than 5 % of the Australian workers admitted to having worked under the influence of alcohol and almost 2 % under the influence of drugs [41]. Another Australian study found that the risk of workers frequently drinking at levels associated with short-term harm was lowest in the education industry and significantly higher in the hospitality, agriculture, manufacturing and construction industries [42]. Alcohol-related absenteeism was also most common among hospitality and manufacturing employees in Australia [43]. Our study did not include the same business areas, but our findings are similar for employees within restaurant/bar and finance industries.

Finally, this study showed that the proportion who reported alcohol-related sickness absence was about twice as large as for men compared to women, a finding which is consistent with results from previous studies [8, 43], whereas reduced efficiency or absence due to drinking was reported about 60–70 % more often among men. A plausible explanation of this finding is that men drink more frequently than women and that they more often drink to intoxication than women, in all societies surveyed [44].

Limitations

The participating employees do not represent a random selection from the total working population or the included business areas. There might have been geographical differences between urban and rural areas as well as between different parts of the country regarding the use of alcohol and drugs. Geographical areas could not be used as covariates in the statistical analysis due to low number of companies within each business area.

It is possible that some employees who had recently used alcohol or drugs refused to participate in the study because this information is regarded as sensitive. As shown above and previously [22, 34], underreporting of alcohol and drug use on the questionnaires also occurred in spite of the fact that the project team members told that the study was anonymous.

A positive drug finding in oral fluid most likely represents drug intake during the last 48 h. However, use of some drugs more than 48 h ago might also give a positive result, particularly repeated use more than a couple of days before sample collection. On the other hand, a negative oral fluid sample does not prove that drugs were not taken during the last 48 h; intake of a single dose of cannabis, cocaine or medication will in most cases cause positive oral fluid sample for less than 24 h.

One of the companies within the finance sector required that the recruitment of employees should occur in the large entrance hall. This made it possible for some employees to deliberately avoid being asked to participate; thus, the selection of participants in this company might have been somewhat biased. For all other companies, it was not possible to avoid being asked for participation.

Conclusions

Overall, a small proportion of employees were positive for alcohol or drugs in samples of oral fluid but a significant proportion of the employees reported absence or hangover at work due to drinking. Of the studies business areas, restaurant/bar workers most often reported frequent binge drinking, reduced efficiency or absence from work due to drinking. Many of them also reported use of illicit drugs. Thus, the restaurant workers comprise a high-risk group regarding alcohol and drug use. Employees within the finance industry often reported reduced efficiency or absence because of drinking. Larger proportions of male than female workers reported binge-drinking each month, reduced efficiency or hangover at work or absence from work due to drinking during the past 12 months.

Competing interests

The authors declare that they have no competing interests.

Authors' contributions

All authors participated in designing the study and assessing the data. HMEE had the main responsibility for planning and coordinating the acquisition of data. HMEE and HG had the main responsibility for drafting the manuscript. All co-authors contributed in revising the manuscript critically for intellectual content. All authors read and approved the manuscript.

Acknowledgements

Thanks to Dr. Per Trygve Normann (NIPH), Professor Dr. Jørg Mørland (NIPH), Kjetil Frøyland (AKAN), Arne Røed Simonsen (NSR) and J. Michaél Walsh (The Walsh Group, Bethesda, MD, USA) who participated in the initiation of this study. Thanks to those who recruited employees and collected samples of oral fluid, and to Hana Adamusova and the personnel at the Division of Forensic Sciences of NIPH who analysed alcohol or drugs in oral fluid samples, and to Ritva Karinen who controlled all analytical test results.

Funding

This research was funded by the Norwegian Ministry of Health and Care Services, The Norwegian Institute of Public Health, and by a grant from the Norwegian Research Council (grant no. 185517/V50).

Author details

[1]Norwegian Institute of Public Health, P. O. Box 4404, Nydalen NO-0403 Oslo, Norway. [2]Norwegian Institute for Alcohol and Drug Research (SIRUS), P. O. Box 565, Sentrum NO-0105 Oslo, Norway.

References

1. Raes E, Verstraete A. Effects of drugs on human performance. In: Verstraete A, editor. Workplace drug testing, vol. 1. London, UK: Pharmaceutical Press; 2011. p. 35–69.
2. Ashe C, Nealy C. Substance abuse in the workplace. J Business Econ Res. 2005;3(9):51–5.
3. Wiese JG, Shlipak MG, Browner WS. The alcohol hangover. Ann Intern Med. 2000;132(11):897–902. doi:10.7326/0003-4819-132-11-200006060-00008.
4. Johansson E, Bockerman P, Uutela A. Alcohol consumption and sickness absence: evidence from microdata. Eur J Public Health. 2009;19(1):19–22. doi:10.1093/eurpub/ckn116.
5. McFarlin SK, Fals-Stewart W. Workplace absenteeism and alcohol use: a sequential analysis. Psychol Addict Behav. 2002;16(1):17–21. doi:10.1037/0893-164X.16.1.17.
6. Nesvåg S, Lie T. Rusmiddelbruk blant ansatte i norsk privat arbeidsliv [Alcohol and drug use mong employees in the private business sector in Norway]. Nordisk Alkohol Nark. 2004;21(2):91–109.
7. Schou L, Moan IS. Alcohol use-sickness absence association and the moderating role of gender and socioeconomic status: A literature review. Drug Alcohol Rev. 2015; doi:10.1111/dar.12278.
8. Schou LA, Storvoll EE, Moan IS. Alcohol-related sickness absence among young employees: gender differences and the prevention paradox. Eur J Public Health. 2014;24(3):480–5. doi:10.1093/eurpub/cku035.

9. Lund HME, Bogstrand ST, Christophersen AS. Results of workplace drug testing in Norway. Norsk Epidemiologi. 2011;21(1):55–9. http://www.ntnu.no/ojs/index.php/norepid/article/view/1426/1280. Accessed 29 Oct 2015.
10. Larson SL, Eyerman J, Foster MS, Gfroerer JC. Worker substance use and workplace policies and programs (DHHS Publication No. SMA 07-4273, Analytic Series A-29). Rockville, MD: Substance Abuse and Mental Health Services Administration; 2007.
11. Zhang Z, Snizek WS. Occupation, job characteristics, and the use of alcohol and other drugs. Soc Behav Personal. 2003;31(4):395–412.
12. Del Boca FK, Darkes J. The validity of self-reports of alcohol consumption: state of the science and challenges for research. Addiction. 2003;98 Suppl 2:1–12. doi:10.1046/j.1359-6357.2003.00586.x.
13. Harrison L, Hughes A. The validity of self-reported drug use: improving the accuracy of survey estimates. NIDA Research Monograph no. 167. Rockville MD: National Institute on Drug Abuse; 1997.
14. Rosay AB, Najaka SS, Herz DC. Differences in the validity of self-reporting drug use across five factors: gender, race, age, type of drug, and offense seriousness. J Quant Criminol. 2007;23:41–58. doi:10.3886/ICPSR02706.v1.
15. Musshoff F, Driever F, Lachenmeier K, Lachenmeier DW, Banger M, Madea B. Results of hair analyses for drugs of abuse and comparison with self-reports and urine tests. Forensic Sci Int. 2006;156(2-3):118–23. doi:10.1016/j.forsciint.2004.07.024.
16. Johnson MB, Voas RA, Miller BA, Holder HD. Predicting drug use at electronic music dance events: self-reports and biological measurement. Eval Rev. 2009; 33(3):211–25. doi:10.1177/0193841x09333253.
17. Delaney-Black V, Chiodo LM, Hannigan JH, Greenwald MK, Janisse J, Patterson G, et al. Just say "I don't": lack of concordance between teen report and biological measures of drug use. Pediatrics. 2010;126(5):887–93. doi:10.1542/peds.2009-3059.
18. Cook RF, Bernstein AD, Andrews CM. Assessing drug use in the workplace: a comparison of self-report, urinalysis, and hair analysis. NIDA Res Monogr. 1997;167:247–72.
19. Bharucha-Reid R, McCann D, Schork MA, Foxman B, Bass A, Fraser W, et al. A comparison of self-reported drug use with a urine drug screen in a working population. Exp Clin Psychopharmacol. 1995;3(3):280–6. doi:10.1037/1064-1297.4.2.150.
20. Hersch RK, McPherson TL, Cook RF. Substance use in the construction industry: a comparison of assessment methods. Subst Use Misuse. 2002; 37(11):1331–58. doi:10.1081/JA-120014081.
21. Fendrich M, Johnson TP, Wislar JS, Hubbell A, Spiehler V. The utility of drug testing in epidemiological research: results from a general population survey. Addiction. 2004;99(2):197–208. doi:10.1111/j.1360-0443.2003.00632.x.
22. Gjerde H, Christophersen AS, Moan IS, Yttredal B, Walsh JM, Normann PT, et al. Use of alcohol and drugs by Norwegian employees: a pilot study using questionnaires and analysis of oral fluid. J Occup Med Toxicol. 2010;5:13. doi:10.1186/1745-6673-5-13.
23. Kristoffersen L, Smith-Kielland A. An automated alcohol dehydrogenase method for ethanol quantification in urine and whole blood. J Anal Toxicol. 2005;29(5):387–9. doi:10.1093/jat/29.5.387.
24. Øiestad EL, Johansen U, Christophersen AS. Drug screening of preserved oral fluid by liquid chromatography-tandem mass spectrometry. Clin Chem. 2007;53(2):300–9. doi:10.1373/clinchem.2006.074237.
25. Øiestad EL, Vindenes V, Enger A, Johansen U, Hjelmeland K, Christophersen A. Elimination times for drugs of abuse in oral fluid from patients with high and repeated intake - case examples. Abstract O27. In: Lemos NP, Gordon AM, Isenschmid DS, Spiehler VR, Huestis MA, Marinetti L, Gerostamoulos D, Ropero-Miller J, Stout PR, editors. Program and abstracts of the joint meeting of the society of forensic toxicologists and the international association of forensic toxicologists, 25-30 september 2011, San Francisco, CA. San Francisco, CA: SOFT & TIAFT; 2011.
26. Verstraete AG. Detection times of drugs of abuse in blood, urine, and oral fluid. Ther Drug Monit. 2004;26(2):200–5.
27. Substance Abuse and Mental Health Service Administration. Proposed revisions to mandatory guidelines for federal workplace drug testing programs. Fed Regist. 2004;69(71):19673–732.
28. Edvardsen HM, Karinen R, Moan IS, Øiestad EL, Christophersen AS, Gjerde H. Use of alcohol and drugs among health professionals in Norway: a study using data from questionnaires and samples of oral fluid. J Occup Med Toxicol. 2014;9(1):8. doi:10.1186/1745-6673-9-8.
29. Langel K, Gjerde H, Favretto D, Lillsunde P, Øiestad EL, Ferrara SD, et al. Comparison of drug concentrations between whole blood and oral fluid. Drug Test Anal. 2014;6(5):461–71. doi:10.1002/dta.1532.
30. Frone MR. Prevalence and distribution of alcohol use and impairment in the workplace: a U.S. national survey. J Stud Alcohol. 2006;67(1):147–56. doi: 10.15288/jsa.2006.67.147.
31. Corral A, Durán J, Isusi I. Use of alcohol and drugs at the workplace. Dublin, Ireland; 2012.
32. Frone MR. Prevalence and distribution of illicit drug use in the workforce and in the workplace: findings and implications from a U.S. national survey. J Appl Psychol. 2006;91(4):856–69. doi:10.1037/0021-9010.91.4.856.
33. European Monitoring Centre for Drugs and Drug Addiction. European drug report 2015 - Trends and developments. Lisbon, Portugal: European Monitoring Centre for Drugs and Drug Addiction.
34. Horverak Ø, Bye EK. Det norske drikkemønsteret. En studie basert på intervjudata fra 1973 til 2004 [The Norwegian drinking pattern. A study based on interviews 1973-2004]. Report no. 2/2007. Oslo, Norway: Norwegian Institute for Alcohol and Drug Research (SIRUS); 2007.
35. Moore RS, Ames GM, Duke MR, Cunradi CB. Food service employee alcohol use, hangovers and norms during and after work hours. J Subst Use. 2012; 17(3):269–76. doi:10.3109/14659891.2011.580414.
36. Norström T, Sundin E, Müller D, Leifman H. Hazardous drinking among restaurant workers. Scand J Public Health. 2012;40(7):591–5. doi:10.1177/1403494812456634.
37. Moore RS, Cunradi CB, Duke MR, Ames GM. Dimensions of problem drinking among young adult restaurant workers. Am J Drug Alcohol Abuse. 2009;35(5):329–33. doi:10.1080/00952990903075042.
38. Kjærheim K, Mykletun R, Aasland OG, Haldorsen T, Andersen A. Heavy drinking in the restaurant business: the role of social modelling and structural factors of the work-place. Addiction. 1995;90(11):1487–95. doi:10.1046/j.1360-0443.1995.901114877.x.
39. Baldisseri MR. Impaired healthcare professional. Crit Care Med. 2007;35(2 Suppl):S106–16. doi:10.1097/01.ccm.0000252918.87746.96.
40. Substance Abuse and Mental Services Administration. The NSDUH report: worker substance use, by industry category. Rockville, MD: Substance Abuse and Mental Services Administration; 2007.
41. Pidd K, Roche AM, Buisman-Pijlman F. Intoxicated workers: findings from a national Australian survey. Addiction. 2011;106(9):1623–33. doi:10.1111/j.1360-0443.2011.03462.x.
42. Berry JG, Pidd K, Roche AM, Harrison JE. Prevalence and patterns of alcohol use in the Australian workforce: findings from the 2001 National Drug Strategy Household Survey. Addiction. 2007;102(9):1399–410. doi:10.1111/j.1360-0443.2007.01893.x.
43. Roche AM, Pidd K, Berry JG, Harrison JE. Workers' drinking patterns: the impact on absenteeism in the Australian work-place. Addiction. 2008;103(5):738–48. doi:10.1111/j.1360-0443.2008.02154.x.
44. World Health Organization. Global status report on alcohol and health 2014. Geneva, Switzerland: World Health Organization; 2014.

2

Correlates of employment status in individuals with asthma: a cross-sectional survey

Saara Taponen[1,3*], Lauri Lehtimäki[2,3], Kirsi Karvala[4], Ritva Luukkonen[5] and Jukka Uitti[3,4]

Abstract

Background: This study aims to elucidate factors that among adults with asthma are associated with working full-time.

Methods: This cross-sectional survey of 2613 working-age adults with asthma included questions on asthma history, symptoms and use of asthma medication, socioeconomic factors and health behavior. Full-time workers were compared to groups according to employment status: unemployed, work disability and retired due to age.

Results: Adults with asthma working full time were younger and more often nonmanual workers, experienced less asthma symptoms, used less asthma medication and smoked less than subjects with work disability. After adjusting for age, gender, smoking and professional status, having frequent symptoms of asthma during last month was associated with an increase in the risk of unemployment (OR 2.3, 95% CI 1.3–4.2) and with an increase in the risk of work disability (OR 4.4, 95% CI 2.3–8.2).

Conclusions: Among adults with asthma, full-time work was associated with younger age, less symptomatic asthma despite of less medication, nonmanual work and less smoking. Having more severe symptoms of asthma was associated with undesirable employment status such as unemployment or work disability. Possibilities to change from manual to nonmanual work may be important in preventing work disability and early exit from work.

Keywords: Asthma symptoms, Asthma, Work ability, Work

Background

Asthma is a common chronic disease among working age adults with prevalence in Finland as high as nearly 10% [1] and globally, around 4.5% [2]. Work disability of adults with respiratory conditions such as asthma is continuously a major concern due to its significant economic burden [3]. Unemployment rate among individuals with asthma is high, sick leave from work is more common among individuals with asthma than without asthma [4] and return to work takes more time from individuals with asthma especially among blue-collar workers. In cases of occupational asthma, job loss seems to be even more likely with less education [5]. In one prospective study, adults with severe asthma were 31% less likely to be currently employed [6].

Respiratory work disability has been defined in many ways, e.g. as job changes due to respiratory problems, sickness absences, or in its most serious form, complete cessation of employment due to respiratory problems [7]. In general, work disability is associated with working conditions, socioeconomic factors such as lower level education, and health behavior such as smoking [8]. Based on earlier studies, workplace exposure to dusts or other impurities is associated with work-related respiratory symptoms and disability [9] and among asthmatics, increased respiratory sickness absence [10], work disability [6] and exacerbation of asthma symptoms [11]. In individuals with asthma, higher educational attainment indeed seems protective whereas a history of smoking associates with a greater risk of work disability [6, 12].

* Correspondence: saara.taponen@finla.fi
[1]Finla Occupational Health, Satakunnankatu 18 B, 33210 Tampere, Finland
[3]Faculty of Medicine and Life Sciences, University of Tampere, 33014 Tampere, Finland
Full list of author information is available at the end of the article

Severity of asthma strongly predicts work disability among adults with asthma [6, 12, 13]. Severity of asthma also decreases the quality of life of asthma patients, as also do lower education, presence of stressful events and a poor control of asthma [14]. A survey study in the U.S. compared the employment status of subjects with work-related and non-work-related asthma and factors associated with unemployment. The results showed that those who were unable to work were more likely to have more frequent asthma symptoms, very poorly controlled asthma and increased health care utilization than their counterparts [15]. Comorbidity plays a major role as was shown in a prospective population-based study by Hakola et al. where the risk of all-cause long-term work disability increased in the presence of asthma [16].

Based on these studies it is apparent that subjects with asthma may have more difficulties in working life than subjects with no asthma. However, some adults with asthma cope well in working life while others face problems. Identifying the factors that support full-time work and holding on to a job among adults with asthma is crucial in order to support their working careers. These factors likely predict how adults with asthma cope in working life, i.e. who succeed to continue as full-time workers and who drift away from active working life due to e.g. sickness absence, disability pension, early retirement or unemployment.

The aim of this study was to investigate which characteristics of asthma are associated with employment status. Using full-time work as an indicator of coping well in working life, we assessed how asthma symptoms, use of asthma medication and socioeconomic factors are related to employment status among adults with asthma in a general population.

Methods

This cross-sectional survey study recruited all asthma patients (n = 2613) aged 20–65 years and living in the city of Tampere (total population 190,000), Finland. The cases were identified from the Medication Reimbursement Register of the Finnish Social Insurance Institution. All those who had been granted special reimbursement rights for asthma medication until the end of 1997 and were alive in October 2000 were selected. To be granted reimbursement rights by the Finnish Social Insurance Institution, the disease must fulfill the diagnostic and severity criteria of asthma, including objective data of reversible/variable bronchial obstruction and a need for regular treatment with inhaled glucocorticoids for at least 6 months after the diagnosis. Among those granted special reimbursement rights for asthma medication, the reliability of the asthma diagnosis is high [11]. The questionnaire was sent in October 2000 and the response rate was 79%. Ninety eight subjects were excluded from the analyses because it was double-checked that the respondents indeed have asthma diagnosed by a physician (some may have had asthma-COPD overlap) or because the employment status information was missing. For this study, the respondents were divided into five groups according to their working life status. There were 967 subjects working full-time, 197 unemployed subjects, 334 subjects with work disability (including all-cause sickness absence, disability pension, and disability pension applied but not yet granted) and 159 subjects retired due to age (in Finland, age-related pension starts at age of approximately 60–68 years depending on occupation and personal preferences). The fifth group consisting of subjects outside of full-time work for other reasons (e.g. housewives, students, part-time workers, maternity leave, etc.) were excluded from this study (n = 309).

Questionnaire

The self-administered questionnaire included questions on asthma history, asthma symptoms and use of asthma medication, professional status, smoking, and leisure time activities. Additional file 1: Appendix 1 lists the specific questions of the postal questionnaire that were used in this study.

Statistical analyses

In our study, we were especially interested in whether the full-time workers differ from the subjects in other three groups (unemployed, those with work disability and those retired). Our data set consisted of both continuous and categorical variables. When comparing the differences between groups we applied ANOVA with Dunnet's post-test (variances were not equal between the groups) for a continued variable age and Chi-squared tests for categorical variables.

After these preliminary studies we built logistic regression models using either unemployed vs. full-time work or work disability vs. full-time work as an outcome variable. Different asthma symptoms and information of asthma medication were used as independent variables one at a time. Our model building strategy was as follows. At first we estimated crude models and then adjusted models with age, gender, smoking, and professional status. The odds ratios with 95% confidence intervals only for the highest levels ("worst" vs. "none") have been presented in Table 3. A p-value of <.05 was considered statistically significant. All analyses were carried out using SPSS (version 23) program.

Results

Table 1 shows the characteristics of subjects in four different groups divided according to their status in working life.

Table 1 Characteristics according to working life status

	Full-time work (1) *n* = 967	Unemployed (2) *n* = 197	Work disability (3) *n* = 334	Retired (4) *n* = 159	*p*-value 1 vs. 2	*p*-value 1 vs. 3	*p*-value 1 vs. 4
Age, mean years (SD)	44.1 (10.2)	46.2 (11.0)	57.9 (8.2)	62.9 (3.8)	0.064	<.001	<.001
Gender					0.007	0.346	0.028
Women	568 (58.7)	136 (69.0)	206 (61.7)	108 (67.9)			
Men	399 (41.3)	61 (31.0)	128 (38.3)	51 (32.1)			
Smoking status					0.004	0.002	<.001
Never smoker	432 (45.0)	70 (36.1)	132 (40.0)	92 (58.2)			
Ex-smoker	217 (22.6)	40 (20.6)	98 (29.7)	38 (24.1)			
Current smoker	155 (16.1)	52 (26.8)	66 (20.0)	20 (12.7)			
Occasional smoker	157 (16.3)	32 (16.5)	34 (10.3)	8 (5.1)			
Professional status					<.001	<.001	0.001
Self-employed	98 (10.2)	10 (5.2)	25 (8.0)	7 (4.6)			
Upper level nonmanual worker	199 (20.7)	11 (5.8)	21 (6.7)	24 (15.9)			
Lower level nonmanual worker	284 (29.5)	50 (26.2)	59 (18.8)	35 (23.2)			
Manual worker	353 (36.7)	113 (59.2)	195 (62.1)	79 (52.3)			
Working from home, student, other	28 (2.9)	7 (3.7)	14 (4.5)	6 (4.0)			
Physical exercise frequency					0.133	<.001	0.007
Not at all	50 (5.2)	14 (7.3)	33 (10.1)	6 (3.8)			
Less than once a week	224 (23.3)	38 (19.7)	60 (18.3)	24 (15.3)			
1–2 times a week	423 (44.0)	75 (38.9)	125 (38.2)	64 (40.8)			
> = 3 times a week	265 (27.5)	66 (34.2)	109 (33.3)	63 (40.1)			

Data is presented as n (%) unless otherwise stated

The groups consisting of subjects working full time and of those unemployed were youngest and those with work disability and those retired were oldest. There were more women than men in all groups but the proportion of women was greatest among the unemployed and the retired.

Smoking and physical exercise

The smoking habits of full-time workers were overall lighter than in the work disability group. Among the unemployed, the proportion of current smokers was greatest and of never-smokers smallest of all groups. The proportion of ex-smokers was greatest in the work disability group. Smoking in general was less common in the retired group: there were less current smokers and occasional smokers and more never-smokers in the retired group than in the full-time work group. The groups were quite similar according to physical exercise frequency. Full-time workers reported less often no exercise at all than subjects with work disability.

Professional status

There were more upper level (20.7 vs. 6.7%) and lower level (29.5 vs. 18.8%) nonmanual workers and less manual workers (36.7 vs. 62.1%) in the full-time working group compared to the work disability group, respectively. Compared to the unemployed group, there were more upper level nonmanual workers and less manual workers in the full-time working group. Also in the retired group, there were more manual workers (52.3 vs. 36.7%) and less nonmanual workers 39.1 vs. 50.2%) than in the full-time working group.

Asthma symptoms and medication

Table 2 shows the occurrence and frequency of asthma symptoms and the use of asthma medication in different employment status groups.

Full-time workers experienced altogether least asthma symptoms: year-round symptoms, daily symptoms and wake-ups at night were less common among full time workers than among other groups, of whom persons with work disability seemed to be the most symptomatic. For example, 10.7% of full time workers vs. 45.0% of those with work disabilities experienced asthma symptoms daily or almost daily during the last month. While having less symptoms of asthma, full-time workers used less medication for asthma than subjects with work disability. Use of peroral corticoids was more common among persons with work disability than among full-time workers.

Table 3 shows the associations between asthma symptoms and employment status (unemployed vs. full-time

Table 2 Asthma symptoms in groups according to employment status

		Full-time work *n* = 870–960	Unemployed *n* = 193	Work disability *n* = 309–327	Retired *n* = 153	*p*-value 1 vs. 2	*p*-value 1 vs. 3	*p*-value 1 vs. 4
Occurrence of asthma symptoms during last year	Persistently	257 (26.8)	73 (37.8)	189 (57.8)	69 (45.1)	0.003	<.001	<.001
	Seasonally	162 (16.9)	34 (17.6)	55 (16.8)	26 (17.0)			
	Occasionally	450 (46.9)	78 (40.4)	66 (20.2)	42 (27.5)			
	None	91 (9.5)	8 (4.1)	17 (5.2)	16 (10.5)			
Frequency of asthma symptoms during last month	Daily or almost daily	93 (10.7)	39 (21.3)	139 (45.0)	38 (27.7)	<.001	<.001	<.001
	3–5 times a week	71 (8.2)	14 (7.7)	38 (12.3)	12 (8.8)			
	1–2 times a week	176 (20.2)	45 (24.6)	44 (14.2)	26 (19.0)			
	Less than once a week	336 (38.6)	58 (31.7)	58 (18.8)	40 (29.2)			
	None	194 (22.3)	27 (14.8)	30 (9.7)	21 (15.3)			
Frequency of asthma symptoms during last year	Daily or almost daily	121 (14.6)	46 (27.2)	113 (42.3)	37 (30.3)	<.001	<.001	<.001
	3–5 times a week	84 (10.1)	23 (13.6)	44 (16.5)	16 (13.1)			
	1–2 times a week	187 (22.6)	41 (24.3)	46 (17.2)	23 (18.9)			
	Less than once a week	415 (50.1)	57 (33.7)	58 (21.7)	40 (32.8)			
	None	22 (2.7)	2 (1.2)	6 (2.2)	6 (4.9)			
Nightly wake-ups because of asthma symptoms during last month	> = 3 times a month	162 (18.4)	72 (39.1)	170 (55.4)	49 (34.8)	<.001	<.001	<.001
	<3 times a month	191 (21.7)	34 (18.5)	50 (16.3)	31 (22.0)			
	None	526 (59.8)	78 (42.4)	87 (28.3)	61 (43.3)			
Nightly wake-ups because of asthma symptoms during last year	> = 3 times a month	151 (17.8)	61 (35.3)	129 (46.2)	34 (27.4)	<.001	<.001	0.004
	<3 times a month	396 (46.7)	69 (39.9)	99 (35.5)	62 (50.0)			
	None	301 (35.5)	43 (24.9)	51 (18.3)	28 (22.6)			
Use of asthma medication during last year	No	105 (10.9)	13 (6.6)	19 (5.7)	12 (7.6)	0.066	<.001	0.010
	Irregularly	190 (19.7)	39 (19.9)	38 (11.5)	18 (11.4)			
	Seasonally (e.g. springtime)	113 (11.7)	15 (7.7)	23 (6.9)	15 (9.5)			
	Continuosly daily or almost daily	556 (57.7)	129 (65.8)	251 (75.8)	113 (71.5)			
Subjects having used peroral corticoids because of asthma during last year		225 (23.5)	53 (27.3)	143 (43.7)	41 (26.6)	0.258	<.001	0.401

Data is presented as n (%)

work and work disability vs. full-time work) in adults with asthma. Even after adjusting for age, gender, smoking and professional status, having more frequent asthma symptoms during last month or nightly wake-ups because of asthma was associated to undesirable employment status such as unemployment or work disability. Occurrence of persistent asthma symptoms was associated with unemployment and use of peroral corticosteroids was associated with work disability.

Discussion

We found that among individuals with asthma, full-time work is associated with younger age, less symptomatic asthma despite of less asthma medication, nonmanual work and less smoking. Having frequent asthma symptoms or nightly wake-ups because of asthma is associated with less desirable employment status such as unemployment and work disability, even after adjusting for age, gender, smoking and professional status. Full-time work was interpreted as an indicator of successful coping in working life while all-cause sickness absence, disability pension applied or granted, unemployment or early retirement were interpreted as less desirable employment status, drifting away from working life, in this study. All subjects had clinically diagnosed asthma and the study covered all working-age adults with asthma in the city of Tampere, Finland, being well representative on population level.

Younger age was associated with full-time work. It may be independent of asthma, as younger people may be overall healthier without comorbidities. With just one health condition such as asthma, it may be easier to find ways to cope well at work compared to having multiple health issues. On the other hand, the tasks may differ between younger and older asthmatics as working life has changed and educational level is higher among younger people. Asthma may also be of different

Table 3 Associations between different asthma symptoms[a] and employment status. Crude logistic regression models and models adjusted for age, gender, smoking and professional status

		Unemployed vs. full-time work		Work disability vs. full-time work	
		Crude OR (95% CI)	Adjusted OR (95% CI)	Crude OR (95% CI)	Adjusted OR (95% CI)
Occurrence of asthma symptoms during last year	Persistently vs. none	3.2 (1.5–7.0)	2.4 (1.1–5.3)	3.9 (2.3–6.8)	1.6 (0.8–3.3)
Frequency of asthma symptoms during last month	Daily or almost daily vs. none	3.0 (1.7–5.2)	2.3 (1.3–4.2)	9.7 (6.1–15.4)	4.4 (2.3–8.2)
Frequency of asthma symptoms during last year	Daily or almost daily vs. none	4.2 (0.9–18.5)	3.0 (0.7–14.1)	3.4 (1.3–8.8)	1.8 (0.5–6.0)
Nightly wake-ups because of asthma symptoms during last month	> = 3 times a month vs. none	3.0 (2.1–4.3)	2.5 (1.7–3.8)	6.3 (4.6–8.7)	3.2 (2.1–4.8)
Nightly wake-ups because of asthma symptoms during last year	> = 3 times a month vs. none	2.6 (1.7–3.9)	2.4 (1.5–3.7)	4.4 (3.1–6.3)	2.6 (1.6–4.3)
Use of asthma medication during last year	Continuosly daily or almost daily vs. none	1.9 (1.0–3.4)	1.5 (0.8–2.9)	2.5 (1.5–4.2)	1.0 (0.5–2.0)
Subjects having used peroral corticoids because of asthma during last year		1.2 (0.9–1.7)	1.0 (0.7–1.5)	2.5 (1.9–3.3)	1.5 (1.1–2.2)

[a]Logistic regression analyses included calculations of odds ratios for less severe symptoms vs. no symptoms (e.g. seasonally vs. none and occasionally vs. none but data is shown only on worst symptoms vs. none

phenotypes in these age groups and therefore respond differently to current therapies [17].

We found that those who were working full time experienced less asthma symptoms altogether and also during leisure time than other groups. Also, when adjusted for age, gender, smoking and professional status, our results showed that having frequent asthma symptoms or nightly wake-ups because of asthma is associated with unemployment and work disability. This indicates that coping in working life may be more strongly affected by the severity of asthma rather than specific factors that may aggravate asthma symptoms at work. This supports earlier findings of severity of asthma predicting work disability [6, 12, 13], although one follow-up study of 111 workers with asthma concluded that adaptation to functional limitations played a major role in changes in sick leave in workers with asthma whereas lung function characteristics or disease history hardly played a role [18]. Some occupations such as cooks, gardeners, hairdressers and agricultural laborers still may be identified as "breath-taking jobs", needing special attention for preventive measures [19]. This however does not explain why adults with asthma overall have disruptions in their working life, including respiratory sickness absences and all-cause long-term work disability [7, 10, 16]. A study from the U.S. compared the employment status of subjects with work-related and non-work-related asthma and found that being unable to work was associated with more frequent asthma symptoms and a very poorly controlled asthma [15]. Our results suggest the same phenomena showing associations between frequent symptoms or nightly wake-ups and undesirable employment status. In the U.S. study, asthma was self-reported whereas in our study, all subjects were reliably diagnosed for asthma. It is possible that in general, working environments have improved as indoor air factors and their effects on health have been recognized [20] and thereby on population level inherent severity of asthma is a more important factor in coping in working life than occupational exposures. It is noticeable that although workers who were working full time had less symptoms of asthma and their professional status was nonmanual, they did not use more regular asthma medication. On the contrary, they used less medication, which indicates that less desirable employment status is not associated to insufficient medical treatment of asthma.

Our study shows that individuals with asthma doing nonmanual work cope better in working life than those doing manual work. This may partially be explained by a cleaner work environment. We have found earlier, in line with other studies, that exposure to impurities such as dusts, chemicals or poor indoor air quality increases aggravation of asthma symptoms at work as does physically strenuous work [11, 21].

Although not always the case in individual level, educational levels are generally lower among workers doing manual work than nonmanual. Earlier studies have shown that lower education may increase the number of sickness absence days as much as 2.5-fold [8] and it has also been shown among asthmatics that lower level education increases the risk of work disability [6, 12]. Adaptation to functional limitations may play a major role in work ability [18] and the possibilities to adapt, adjust and have influence on one's working environment are probably better among nonmanual workers.

There were more nonmanual workers in the full-time working group and the retired group compared to the groups with work disability and the unemployed, of whom about 60% of persons were manual workers. In these groups, a severe asthma and possible other health issues may affect their resilience in working life negatively. Asthma is the primary cause of disability pension in Finland in only less than 0,4% of disability pensions granted [22] whereas morbidity in musculoskeletal conditions and mental problems are leading causes of work disability [23]. A weakness of our study is the lack of information on co-morbidities and their possible effect on work ability.

The unemployed group was closest to full-time workers according to age and like full-time workers, they were younger than those with work disability and the retired. However, the unemployed group experienced more asthma symptoms, current smoking was more common and professional status was more likely to be manual than nonmanual worker than among full-time workers. In general, manual workers represent lower level education than nonmanual workers. Earlier studies have shown that unemployment among asthmatics is associated with not only lower education but also more severe asthma [5, 6]. It may be that the motivation to hold on to a manual job and perform well at work is decreased due to having more asthma symptoms.

Smoking aggravates asthma symptoms and decreases the effect of medication [24]. An 8-year follow-up study showed that improvements in working conditions and reducing smoking especially in the lower educational groups are likely to reduce the educational differences in sickness absence [8]. Eisner et al. showed that past smoking was associated with complete work disability but among the currently employed, smoking status was not associated with partial work disability [6]. In this study, the proportion of never-smokers and occasional smokers was greatest in the full-time working group and there were more ex-smokers in the work disability group than among full-time workers. It may be that with increasing asthma symptoms and decreasing quality of life due to symptoms, the motivation to quit smoking arises.

It could be assumed that physical exercise levels would be lower among those having most asthma symptoms compared to those having less symptoms. In our study however, there was no significant difference between the groups in physical exercise frequency. It may be that those who are active in working life have less time for physical exercise.

The strength of our study is that it is very well representative on population level. We recruited all working-age adults with asthma in Tampere city with established asthma and special reimbursement and diagnosis based on lung function criteria. Also, the response rate was high (79%). However, as a questionnaire-based study this lacks information on clinical measures and details of treatments on individual level. As a limitation of the study, we had data on all-cause sickness absence and lacked asthma-specific data. Also, there are limitations in the cross-sectional study design. As in all questionnaire-based studies, selection bias is possible and we do not know whether those who answered this questionnaire have e.g. more severe asthma or vice versa. The healthy worker effect, meaning e.g. that sicker individuals may be excluded from being hired or once hired, they may may seek transfer to less exposed jobs or leave work [25], may have contributed to selection bias in our study.

Our material was collected in year 2000 and some aspects in asthma treatment or working life may have changed. In Finland, our national asthma guidelines and asthma program have stressed active treatment with inhaled corticosteroids (ICS) since early 1990's [26] and the use of ICS has not changed significantly since the collection of our data. Long-acting beta2-agonists (LABA) were introduced in mid- 1990's but the use of this class of drugs has probably increased after year 2000 since the introduction of fixed ICS-LABA combinations. Finland has for long had a high level of social security and insurance system that has not significantly changed during the last decades and therefore our results from 2000 are still valid. The economic structure in Finland is typical for countries in western Europe and has not changed fundamentally after the year 2000.

Conclusions

Among individuals with asthma, full-time workers are on average younger, more frequently nonmanual workers, they smoke less and have less asthma symptoms both at work and at leisure time despite of using less asthma medication. Even after adjusting for age, gender, smoking and professional status, logistic regression analyses show that having frequent asthma symptoms or nightly wake-ups because of asthma is associated with less desirable employment status such as unemployment and work disability. This suggests that in addition to following conventional procedures such as guideline-based asthma medication, smoking cessation and reduction of exposure to asthma triggers, it may be of great importance to support possibilities to change from manual to nonmanual work in preventing work disability and early exit from work.

Acknowledgements
Not applicable.

Funding
The Finnish Work Environment Fund.

Authors' contributions
ST was the main author of the manuscript and contributed by analyzing and interpreting the data. LL and KK contributed by planning the study design, analyzing and interpreting data and writing the manuscript. Ritva Luukkonen contributed by planning and performing the statistical analyses and planning the design of this study. JU contributed as the leader of the study group, by planning the study design, analyzing and interpreting data and writing the manuscript. All authors read and approved the final manuscript.

Competing interests
The authors declare that they have no competing interests.

Author details
[1]Finla Occupational Health, Satakunnankatu 18 B, 33210 Tampere, Finland. [2]Allergy Centre, Tampere University Hospital, PO Box 2000, 33521 Tampere, Finland. [3]Faculty of Medicine and Life Sciences, University of Tampere, 33014 Tampere, Finland. [4]Finnish Institute of Occupational Health, PO Box 40, 00251 Helsinki, Finland. [5]Clinicum, Faculty of Medicine, University of Helsinki, PO Box 63, 00014 Helsinki, Finland.

References

1. Pallasaho P, Juusela M, Lindqvist A, Sovijarvi A, Lundback B, Ronmark E. Allergic rhinoconjunctivitis doubles the risk for incident asthma–results from a population study in Helsinki, Finland. Respir Med. 2011;105(10):1449–56.
2. To T, Stanojevic S, Moores G, Gershon AS, Bateman ED, Cruz AA, Boulet LP. Global asthma prevalence in adults: findings from the cross-sectional world health survey. BMC Public Health. 2012;12:204–2458. 12-204
3. Ehteshami-Afshar S, FitzGerald JM, Doyle-Waters MM, Sadatsafavi M. The global economic burden of asthma and chronic obstructive pulmonary disease. Int J Tuberc Lung Dis. 2016;20(1):11–23.
4. Hansen CL, Baelum J, Skadhauge L, Thomsen G, Omland O, Thilsing T, Dahl S, Sigsgaard T, Sherson D. Consequences of asthma on job absenteeism and job retention. Scand J Public Health. 2012;40(4):377–84.
5. Peters J, Pickvance S, Wilford J, Macdonald E, Blank L. Predictors of delayed return to work or job loss with respiratory ill-health: a systematic review. J Occup Rehabil. 2007;17(2):317–26.
6. Eisner MD, Yelin EH, Katz PP, Lactao G, Iribarren C, Blanc PD. Risk factors for work disability in severe adult asthma. Am J Med. 2006;119(10):884–91.
7. Toren K, Zock JP, Kogevinas M, Plana E, Sunyer J, Radon K, Jarvis D, Kromhout H, d'Errico A, Payo F, Anto JM, Blanc PD. An international prospective general population-based study of respiratory work disability. Thorax. 2009;64(4):339–44.
8. Kaikkonen R, Harkanen T, Rahkonen O, Gould R, Koskinen S. Explaining educational differences in sickness absence: a population-based follow-up study. Scand J Work Environ Health. 2015;41(4):338–46.
9. Blanc PD, Burney P, Janson C, Toren K. The prevalence and predictors of respiratory-related work limitation and occupational disability in an international study. Chest. 2003;124(3):1153–9.
10. Kim JL, Blanc PD, Villani S, Olivieri M, Urrutia I, van Sprundel M, Storaas T, Le Moual N, Zock JP, Toren K. Predictors of respiratory sickness absence: an international population-based study. Am J Ind Med. 2013;56(5):541–9.
11. Saarinen K, Karjalainen A, Martikainen R, Uitti J, Tammilehto L, Klaukka T, Kurppa K. Prevalence of work-aggravated symptoms in clinically established asthma. Eur Respir J. 2003;22(2):305–9.
12. Lindstrom I, Pallasaho P, Luukkonen R, Suojalehto H, Karjalainen J, Lauerma A, Karjalainen A. Reduced work ability in middle-aged men with asthma from youth–a 20-year follow-up. Respir Med. 2011;105(6):950–5.
13. Gonzalez Barcala FJ, La Fuente-Cid RD, Alvarez-Gil R, Tafalla M, Nuevo J, Caamano-Isorna F. Factors associated with a higher prevalence of work disability among asthmatic patients. J Asthma. 2011;48(2):194–9.
14. Gonzalez-Barcala FJ, de la Fuente-Cid R, Tafalla M, Nuevo J, Caamano-Isorna F. Factors associated with health-related quality of life in adults with asthma. A cross-sectional study. Multidiscip Respir Med. 2012;7(1):32–6958. 7-32
15. White GE, Mazurek JM, Moorman JE. Work-related asthma and employment status–38 states and District of Columbia, 2006-2009. J Asthma. 2013;50(9):954–9.
16. Hakola R, Kauppi P, Leino T, Ojajarvi A, Pentti J, Oksanen T, Haahtela T, Kivimaki M, Vahtera J. Persistent asthma, comorbid conditions and the risk of work disability: a prospective cohort study. Allergy. 2011;66(12):1598–603.
17. Wenzel SE. Asthma phenotypes: the evolution from clinical to molecular approaches. Nat Med. 2012;18(5):716–25.
18. Boot CR, Vercoulen JH, van der Gulden JW, Orbon KH, Rooijackers JM, van Weel C, Folgering HT. Predictors of changes in sick leave in workers with asthma: a follow-up study. Int Arch Occup Environ Health. 2005;78(8):633–40.
19. Fell A, Abrahamsen R, Henneberger PK, Svendsen MV, Andersson E, Toren K, Kongerud J. Breath-taking jobs: a case-control study of respiratory work disability by occupation in Norway. Occup Environ Med. 2016;73(9):600–6.
20. WHO, Regional Office for Europe. WHO guidelines for indoor air quality: dampness and mould. Geneva: World Health Organization; 2009.
21. Henneberger PK, Liang X, Lillienberg L, Dahlman-Hoglund A, Toren K, Andersson E. Occupational exposures associated with severe exacerbation of asthma. Int J Tuberc Lung Dis. 2015;19(2):244–50.
22. Nyman H: Statistics from the Finnish Centre for Pensions: Statistical yearbook of pensioners in Finland 2015. 2016, 8/2016(http://www.etk.fi/wp-content/uploads/Statistical_yearbook_of_pensioners_in_Finland_2015.pdf):.
23. Kannisto J, Nyman H: Statistics from the Finnish Centre for Pensions: Earnings-related pension recipients in Finland 2015. 2016, http://www.etk.fi/wp-content/uploads/Earnings_related_pension_recipients_in_finland_2015.pdf:.
24. Polosa R, Thomson NC. Smoking and asthma: dangerous liaisons. Eur Respir J. 2013;41(3):716–26.
25. Le Moual N, Kauffmann F, Eisen EA, Kennedy SM. The healthy worker effect in asthma: work may cause asthma, but asthma may also influence work. Am J Respir Crit Care Med. 2008;177(1):4–10.
26. Haahtela T, Klaukka T, Koskela K, Erhola M, Laitinen LA. Working Group of the Asthma Programme in Finland 1994-2004: asthma programme in Finland: a community problem needs community solutions. Thorax. 2001;56(10):806–14.

3

Work-related diabetes distress among Finnish workers with type 1 diabetes: a national cross-sectional survey

Pirjo Hakkarainen[1*], Leena Moilanen[2], Vilma Hänninen[3], Jarmo Heikkinen[1] and Kimmo Räsänen[1]

Abstract

Background: Diabetes distress is common among people with type 1 diabetes, but knowledge is scarce regarding the perceived burden of reconciling work with this disease. This cross-sectional study investigated work-related diabetes distress among Finnish workers with type 1 diabetes.

Methods: A questionnaire was mailed to 2500 randomly sampled 18- to 65-year-old Finns with type 1 diabetes; 49.3 % responded. Work-related diabetes distress was measured by combining worry and exhaustion in reconciling work with diabetes. Self-perceived work-related diabetes distress was evaluated in the context of physical and psychosocial work conditions, job demands, work ability, general stress, diabetes acceptance, glycosylated hemoglobin (HbA1c) level, high blood glucose maintenance at work, and depressive symptoms. The data were analyzed with the use of cross-tabulation, chi-square tests, ANOVA analysis, Spearman correlation coefficients, and structural equation modeling.

Results: Of the respondents, 70 % experienced work-related diabetes distress. Problems with physical work conditions ($\beta = 0.27$), work ability ($\beta = -0.21$), difficulty in accepting diabetes ($\beta = 0.18$), and job demands ($\beta = 0.14$) were found to be associated with work-related diabetes distress. This distress was strongly associated with the maintenance of a high blood glucose level at work ($\beta = 0.34$). In turn, a high blood glucose level at work was associated with a high HbA1c level ($\beta = 0.29$). Work-related diabetes distress and depressive symptoms had a bi-directional association ($\beta = 0.06$ and $\beta = 0.14$). Difficulty accepting diabetes had three-dimensional associations: work-related diabetes distress ($\beta = 0.18$), depressive symptoms ($\beta = 0.13$), and high HbA1c level ($\beta = 0.12$). There was no notable association between work-related diabetes distress and general stress.

Conclusions: Work-related diabetes distress is common among workers with type 1 diabetes, and it may influence metabolic control. This stress could be prevented by adapting physical work conditions. People with type 1 diabetes should also be encouraged to pursue their full educational potential, and psychological support should be provided for those with difficulty accepting their diabetes.

Keywords: Type 1 diabetes, Work, Stress, Exhaustion, Blood glucose

Background

Diabetes distress is common among people with type 1 diabetes [1]. This psychological stress is related to living with diabetes and involves an emotional burden, physician-related and regimen-related stress, and diabetes-related interpersonal stress (i.e., lack of social support) [1–3]. Diabetes distress is strongly associated with poor diabetes self-management, and it is more common than depression among people with diabetes [3, 4].

Harmful work stress occurs when job demands exceed people's resources for handling their jobs [5, 6]. It is a significant predictor of anxiety and depression [7–10]. In addition, self-reported exhaustion has been found to be associated with anxiety, depression, burnout, and poor work ability [11].

* Correspondence: pirjoirene.hakkarainen@uef.fi
[1]School of Medicine, Institute of Public Health and Clinical Nutrition, University of Eastern Finland, Kuopio, Finland
Full list of author information is available at the end of the article

The number of persons with type 1 diabetes is increasing in the workforce, but little is known about the relationship between work and type 1 diabetes [12, 13]. Previous studies have primarily focused on work productivity [14–16] and work disability [15, 17] among people with diabetes, but knowledge about the perceived burden of reconciling work with type 1 diabetes is scarce [18].

The aim of this cross-sectional study was to examine work-related diabetes distress among Finnish workers with type 1 diabetes. Self-perceived work-related diabetes distress was evaluated in the context of work conditions, job demands, work ability, general stress, diabetes acceptance, glycemic control, and depressive symptoms.

Methods

This study was carried out as part of a project called "People with Type 1 Diabetes in Worklife", conducted by the University of Eastern Finland and the Kuopio University Hospital in 2010–2012. The Research Ethics Committee of the Northern Savo Hospital District reviewed and approved the research protocol (18//2010).

The study questionnaire was constructed on the basis of previously validated worklife scales and diabetes questionnaires [19–24]. The questionnaire was mailed to a random sample of 2500 Finns with type 1 diabetes between the ages of 18 and 65 years and drawn from The Medication Reimbursement Register of The Social Insurance Institution of Finland, which includes all Finns with type 1 diabetes. Non-responders were sent two reminders. There were slightly over 40 000 persons with diagnosed type 1 diabetes in Finland in 2011 [25]. Thus, this random sample covered 6 % of the Finnish population with type 1 diabetes.

Altogether 2464 persons received the questionnaire (4 deceased and 32 unreachable), and 1214 returned the form. Thus the response rate was 49.3 %. We received 126 forms from respondents who reported having been diagnosed with another type of diabetes, and they were rejected. In addition, 25 respondents had been diagnosed after retirement, 16 were incapable of responding on account of a disability or serious illness, 15 declared that they were not working (in the last 12 months), 6 were not able to fill out the form in Finnish, and 13 had other reasons for not responding. These 75 uncompleted forms were also excluded from the study. Therefore the final sample included 1013 persons with type 1 diabetes.

There was a small difference in the gender distribution between the original sample and the respondents (proportion of men being 65.3 % in the original and 57.5 % among the respondents). The distributions of the age groups and residential provinces were similar in both groups (dispersion about 1 %).

We studied Finnish workers with type 1 diabetes. Of the total sample of 1013, those who were retired, unemployed, students, homemakers, and others who did not participate in worklife during the past 12 months were excluded, leaving 767 respondents to be included in the analysis.

Measurements

Work-related diabetes distress

On a scale of 1–3 (never; sometimes; often), the respondents rated how often they worried about their ability to do their job due to their diabetes. Using the same scale, they also rated how often they became exhausted by the need to reconcile their work with their diabetes. These variables correlated strongly (Spearman's correlation coefficient 0.64, $P < 0.001$). Thus the sum index "work-related diabetes distress" was calculated on the basis of these variables. In previous studies diabetes distress has been found to predict poor diabetes self-management and poor glycemic control [1, 26]. Diabetes-specific stress can also increase the risk of depression [27]. In addition, it has been found that diabetes distress mediates the relationship between depression and glycemic control [28].

Sociodemographic variables

The sociodemographic variables included gender, age, marital status, duration of diabetes, educational level, type of employment, and type of work.

Work-related variables

Problems with physical work conditions The respondents were asked: "Do problems in the work environment or with the physical load of work hinder you managing or coping with your work?" [19]. The options (1–4) were not present/no harm; troubles a little; troubles a lot; cannot say. For our statistical analysis, those who reported option 4 = cannot say ($n = 13$) were combined with option 1 = not present/not harm. In a previous study, it was found that people who had a high physical load at work perceived diabetes self-management as a burden [29].

Problems with psychosocial work conditions The respondents were asked: "Do problems in the work community or the mental load of work hinder you managing or coping with your work?" [19]. The options (1–4) were not present/no harm; troubles a little; troubles a lot; cannot say. For our statistical analysis, those who reported option 4 = cannot say ($n = 15$) were combined with option 1 = not present/no harm. Problems with psychosocial work conditions have been found to predict mental distress and depression [30, 31].

Job demands Five questions of the Job Content Questionnaire [20] that have been widely used to assess job demands [32] and job strain [33] were included in the questionnaire. The questions were (a) "My job requires me to work very fast", (b) "My job requires me to work very hard", (c) "My job requires an inordinate amount of work", (d) "My job requires an intense pace", (e) "I have enough time to get my job done." For our further analyses, the scale of question e was reversed. The respondents rated these features of their jobs on a scale of 1–5 (fully agree to fully disagree). From these items, a sum index was calculated. Job demands have been found to form a risk factor for perceived stress and psychological distress [34–36].

Health-related variables

Depressive symptoms To assess current depressive symptoms or a high risk of depression, we asked the respondents to answer "yes" or "no" to the following two questions: "During the past month, have you often felt down, depressed, or hopeless?" and "During the past month, have you often felt little interest or pleasure in doing things?". A sum index was calculated. These two questions have been developed for screening purposes and have proven to be sensitive and specific for the screening of depression [21]. A bi-directional relation has been found between diabetes distress and depressive symptoms: diabetes distress predicting depressive symptoms and depressive symptoms amplifying diabetes distress [37]. Depression can also cause poor diabetes self-care [38].

Work ability Work ability was measured with the use of the Work Ability Score (WAS), which measures self-reported work ability by comparing a person's current work ability with the person's lifetime best on a scale of 0–10 (0 = completely unable to work to 10 = work ability as its best) [22, 39]. This single-item question is the first item of the widely used Work Ability Index, WAI [40]. Both, WAS and WAI have been found to predict stress, general and mental health, and sick leaves [22].

General stress General stress was asked by the question: "Do you feel stress these days?" [23]. The respondents rated their perceived stress on a scale of 0–4 (not at all – very much). In previous studies stress has generally been found to predict anxiety and depression [9].

Diabetes-related variables

Glycosylated hemoglobin level The respondents were asked to report their last glycosylated hemoglobin (HbA1c) level using the categories ≤60 mmol/mol (≤7.5 %), 61–70 mmol/mol (7.6–8.5 %), 71–80 mmol/mol (8.6–9.5 %), and ≥81 mmol/mol (≥9.6 %) [24].

High blood glucose level at work On a scale of 1–5 (never to always), the respondents rated how often they kept their blood glucose level higher at work than usual.

Difficulty in accepting diabetes On a scale of 0–2 (no; yes, a little; yes, a lot), the respondents were asked: "Do you have difficulty in accepting your diabetes?" Difficulty in accepting diabetes has been found to be associated with reduced self-care, a high HbA1c level, diabetes distress, and depressive symptoms [41].

Severe hypoglycemia events in the past 12 months On a scale of 0–3 (no; once; 2–3 times; more often), the respondents were asked: "Have you had hypoglycemic events in which help has been needed in the last 12 months?".

Statistical analysis

The number of missing values varied between 0 and 22 among the studied variables. Missing values were substituted by the mean (ratio scaled factors) or mode (nominal and ordinal scaled factors).

For further analysis, we dichotomized the nominal scaled variables gender, marital status, type of employment, and type of work. Educational level, physical work conditions, psychosocial work conditions, general stress, HbA1c level, high blood glucose level at work, difficulty in accepting diabetes, and severe hypoglycemic events were ordinal scaled, and they were treated as continuous variables. We computed age and duration of diabetes as original continuous scores and calculated the values for work-related diabetes distress, job demands, depressive symptoms, and self-rated work ability as additive sums.

The distributions of the relevant variables in the sample were analyzed in association with work-related diabetes distress by cross-tabulation, the chi-square test, and an ANOVA analysis (Table 1). Spearman's correlations were calculated between the background and independent and dependent variables (Table 2).

We used structural equation modeling (SEM) [42] for analyzing the correlational multivariate data simultaneously. Basically, SEM conjoins the methodology of multiple regression and path analysis, in which the hypothetical causal relations are defined on the basis of previous research and theory. We used this method to clarify the association between the independent variables (physical and psychosocial work conditions, job demands, self-rated work ability, difficulty in accepting diabetes, and general stress) and the dependent variables (work-related diabetes distress, HbA1c level, high blood glucose level at work, and depressive symptoms). These potential and theoretically relevant variables were placed in the model according to previous studies [1, 9, 22, 26–31, 34–38, 41]. Standardized (β) and non-standardized (B) regression coefficients were computed

Table 1 Characteristics of the respondents according to their work-related diabetes distress

	All N = 767	Never stressed n = 230 (30.0 %)	Sometimes stressed n = 379 (49.4 %)	Often stressed n = 158 (20.6 %)	P-value
Gender n (%)					<0.001[a]
Male	430 (56.1)	150 (34.9)	213 (49.5)	67 (15.6)	
Female	337 (43.9)	80 (23.7)	166 (49.3)	91 (27.0)	
Age, years (mean ± SD)	36.2 ± 12.4	34.4±12.9	36.3±11.8	38.7±12.6	0.004[b]
Marital status, n (%)					0.895[a]
Married or cohabiting	478 (62.3)	142 (29.7)	235 (49.2)	101 (21.1)	
Unmarried, divorced, widowed	289 (37.7)	88 (30.4)	144 (49.8)	57 (19.7)	
Duration of diabetes, years (mean ± SD)	8.5 ± 4.8	9.1±4.7	8.1±4.8	8.6±4.7	0.050[b]
Educational level, n (%)					0.003[a]
Basic education	182 (23.7)	60 (33.0)	78 (42.9)	44 (24.2)	
Vocational school	264 (34.4)	68 (25.8)	142 (53.8)	54 (20.5)	
Technical or vocational college	217 (28.3)	56 (25.8)	112 (51.6)	49 (22.6)	
University or university of applied science	104 (13.6)	46 (44.2)	47 (45.2)	11 (10.6)	
Employment, n (%)					0.318[a]
Entrepreneur	68 (8.9)	16 (23.5)	34 (50.0)	18 (26.5)	
Employee	699 (91.1)	214 (30.6)	345 (49.4)	140 (20.0)	
Type of work, n (%)					0.016[a]
Mental work	324 (42.2)	115 (35.5)	150 (46.3)	59 (18.2)	
Physical work	443 (57.8)	115 (26.0)	229 (51.7)	99 (22.3)	
Problems with physical work conditions, n (%)					<0.001[a]
Not present/no harm/cannot say	469 (61.1)	198 (42.2)	220 (46.9)	51 (10.9)	
Troubles a little	248 (32.3)	29 (11.7)	145 (58.5)	74 (29.8)	
Troubles a lot	50 (6.5)	3 (6.0)	14 (28.0)	33 (66.0)	
Problems with psychosocial work conditions, n (%)					<0.001[a]
Not present/no harm/cannot say	415 (54.1)	176 (42.4)	193 (46.5)	46 (11.1)	
Troubles a little	263 (34.3)	45 (17.1)	150 (57.0)	68 (25.9)	
Troubles a lot	89 (11.6)	9 (10.1)	36 (40.4)	44 (49.4)	
Job demands, points (mean ± SD)	15.5 ± 4.0	14.1±3.6	15.5±3.8	17.4±4.3	<0.001[b]
Depressive symptoms, points (mean ± SD)	2.6 ± 0.9	2.2±0.5	2.6±0.8	3.3±0.9	<0.001[b]
Work ability, points (mean ± SD)	8.1 ± 1.7	8.8±1.3	8.2±1.5	6.8±2.1	<0.001[b]
General stress, n (%)					<0.001[a]
No	61 (8.0)	38 (62.3)	20 (32.8)	3 (4.9)	
Little	221 (28.8)	76 (34.4)	121 (54.8)	24 (10.9)	
Somewhat	322 (42.0)	92 (28.6)	168 (52.2)	62 (19.3)	
Quite a lot	127 (16.6)	20 (15.7)	57 (44.9)	50 (39.4)	
Very much	36 (4.7)	4 (11.1)	13 (36.1)	19 (52.8)	
HbA1c level[c], n (%)					<0.001[a]
≤ 60 mmol/mol (≤7.5 %)	255 (33.2)	90 (35.3)	131 (51.4)	34 (13.3)	
61–70 mmol/mol (7.6 %–8.5 %)	271 (35.3)	85 (31.4)	135 (49.8)	51 (18.8)	
71–80 mmol/mol (8.6 %–9.5 %)	176 (22.9)	43 (24.4)	86 (48.9)	47 (26.7)	
≥ 81 mmol/mol (≥ 9.6 %)	65 (8.5)	12 (18.5)	27 (41.5)	26 (40.0)	

Table 1 Characteristics of the respondents according to their work-related diabetes distress *(Continued)*

High blood glucose level at work, n (%)					<0.001[a]
Never	148 (19.3)	94 (63.5)	42 (28.4)	12 (8.1)	
Quite seldom	208 (27.1)	68 (32.7)	120 (57.7)	20 (9.6)	
Sometimes	226 (29.5)	45 (19.9)	133 (58.8)	48 (21.2)	
Quite often	150 (19.6)	20 (13.3)	74 (49.3)	56 (37.3)	
Always	35 (4.6)	3 (1.3)	10 (28.6)	22 (62.9)	
Difficulty in accepting Type 1 diabetes, n (%)					<0.001[a]
No	568 (74.1)	211 (37.1)	271 (47.7)	86 (15.1)	
Yes, a little	160 (20.9)	16 (10.0)	96 (60.0)	48 (30.0)	
Yes, a lot	39 (5.1)	3 (7.7)	12 (30.8)	24 (61.5)	
Severe hypoglycemia events in 12 months prior to enrollment, n (%)					0.023[a]
No	593 (77.3)	183 (30.9)	300 (50.6)	110 (18.5)	
Once	89 (11.6)	26 (29.2)	41 (46.1)	22 (24.7)	
2–3 times	53 (6.9)	17 (32.1)	24 (45.3)	12 (22.6)	
More often	32 (4.2)	4 (12.5)	14 (43.8)	14 (43.8)	

[a]Chi-square test
[b]ANOVA analysis
[c]Self-reported

[see Additional file 1], and a path diagram was drawn (Fig. 1). Standardized regression coefficients (β) were interpreted as weak if <0.10, moderate if 0.10–0.30, and strong if >0.50 [42]. Model fit was estimated with the GFI (goodness of fit index) and the RMSEA (root mean square error of approximation). A GFI (0–1) of >0.90 indicated a good model, and >0.95 indicated an excellent model. The RMSEA should be <0.08, and a value of <0.05 was considered excellent [43].

All of the analyses were performed with SPSS for Windows, Rel. 19.0.0.2. 2010 (SPSS Inc., Chicago, IL, USA) and IBM SPSS®Amos 21.0.0.

Results

The descriptive statistics of the 767 participants are presented in Table 1. The mean age of the participants was 36 (SD 12.4, range 18–64) years, 56 % were men, and 62 % were married or cohabiting. The majority (91 %) worked as wage-earners, and over half worked in physical tasks (at least 50 % of their working time). The mean of the sum index for job demands was 16 (SD 4.0, range 5–25), that for depressive symptoms was 2.6 (SD 0.9, range 2–4), and the mean for self-rated work ability was 8.1 (SD 1.7, range 0–10). The mean duration of diabetes was 8.5 (SD 4.8, range 0–38) years, and 23 % declared that they had had one or more severe hypoglycemic events in the last 12 months.

Of the respondents, 30 % had never experienced work-related diabetes distress, 49 % reported having work-related diabetes distress sometimes, and 21 % reported such stress often (Table 1). The higher the HbA1c level, the more common work-related diabetes distress was. Of the respondents with good metabolic control, 13 % reported that they were often stressed. In contrast, among those with poor metabolic control, 40 % were often stressed. Of those who had experienced more than 3 severe hypoglycemia events in the past 12 months, 44 % reported often experiencing stress, whereas 19 % of those without such events had often been stressed. Altogether 63 % of those who always kept their blood glucose level higher at work than usual reported often having work-related diabetes distress.

Among the respondents with the highest education, work-related diabetes distress was reported markedly less often (Table 1). Those who perceived problems with physical or psychosocial work conditions experienced diabetes-related stress more often than the others. In addition, work-related diabetes distress was more common among those with much difficulty accepting their diabetes (62 %).

The correlations between the background, independent, and dependent variables are presented in Table 2. Work ability, problems with physical or psychosocial work conditions, difficulty in accepting diabetes, job demands, and general stress had the highest correlation with the dependent variables.

Figure 1 presents the path diagram of the structural equation modeling, which was adjusted for gender, age, educational level, and duration of diabetes. The regressions lower than 0.10 were removed from the final path diagram.

Problems with physical work conditions (β = 0.27), self-rated work ability (β = -0.21), difficulty in accepting diabetes (β = 0.18), and job demands (β = 0.14) were moderately associated with work-related diabetes

Table 2 Correlation table for variables used in the structural equation modeling

	2	3	4	5	6	7	8	9	10	11	12	13	14
1 Gender	,076*	-,019	-,085*	-,002	-,172**	-,052	-,142**	-,036	-,124**	-,155**	-,224**	-,132**	-,097**
2 Age		,178**	-,096**	-,260**	,101**	,151**	,029	,061	,055	,158**	-,139**	-,054	-,003
3 Educational level			,035	,073*	,093**	-,083*	-,008	,082*	,077*	-,064	-,136**	-,074*	-,027
4 Duration of diabetes				,067	,029	-,043	-,113**	-,023	-,002	-,038	,146**	-,023	,003
5 Work ability					-,365**	-,396**	-,189**	-,184**	-,393**	-,433**	-,107**	-,229**	-,432**
6 Problems with psychosocial work conditions						,417**	,219**	,314**	,402**	,387**	,101**	,222**	,394**
7 Problems with physical work conditions							,151**	,310**	,314**	,464**	,071*	,290**	,307**
8 Difficulty in accepting Type 1 diabetes								,132**	,202**	,328**	,182**	,219**	,278**
9 Job demands									,332**	,310**	,067	,191**	,199**
10 General stress										,342**	,124**	,228**	,465**
11 Work-related diabetes distress											,180**	,393**	,434**
12 HbA1c level												,333**	,202**
13 High blood glucose level at work													,274**
14 Depressive symptoms													

*P Correlation is significant at the level 0.05 (two-tailed). **P Correlation is significant at the level 0.01 (two-tailed)

distress. Work-related diabetes distress was moderately associated with the blood glucose level being maintained at a high level at work ($\beta = 0.34$). In turn, a high blood glucose level at work was associated with high HbA1c level ($\beta = 0.29$). In addition, physical work conditions were associated with keeping blood glucose high at work.

There was no notable association between general stress and work-related diabetes distress in the multivariate analysis. General stress ($\beta = 0.26$), self-rated work ability ($\beta = -0.25$), problems with psychosocial work conditions ($\beta = 0.16$), and difficulty in accepting diabetes ($\beta = 0.13$) were associated with depressive symptoms. Work-related diabetes distress and depressive symptoms

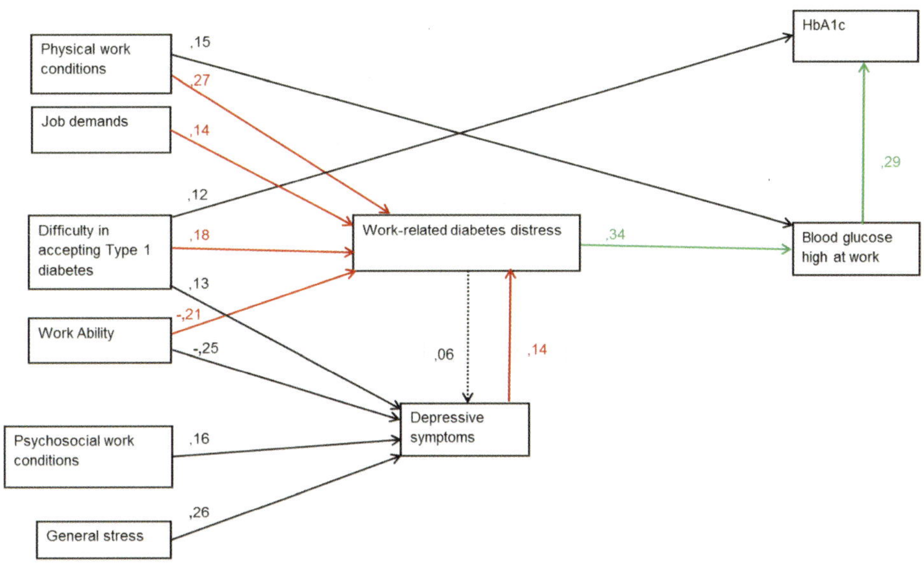

Fig. 1 Path diagram of work-related, diabetes-related, and health-related variables with work-related diabetes distress. All of the path coefficients were standardized (β). This model was adjusted for gender, age, education level, and duration of diabetes. Gender was associated with HbA1c level (-,16) and work-related diabetes distress (-,10). Age was associated with a high blood glucose level at work (-,13) and depressive symptoms (-,11). Level of education was associated with the HbA1c level (-,12). Duration of diabetes was also associated with the HbA1c level (,16). Red arrows show the predictors of work-related diabetes distress. Green arrows indicate how work-related diabetes distress mediates the effect of these predictors on metabolic control.

showed a bi-directional association: diabetes distress was associated with depressive symptoms ($\beta = 0.06$) and depressive symptoms were associated with diabetes distress ($\beta = 0.14$) (Fig. 1). Separately, the associations were 0.19 for both directions.

Of the independent variables, only difficulty in accepting type 1 diabetes was associated with the three dependent variables: work-related diabetes distress, depressive symptoms, and HbA1c level.

The structural equation model was an excellent fit for the data, the GFI being 0.982 and the RMSEA being 0.039.

Discussion

Working people with type 1 diabetes have work stress, just as their healthy colleagues do. They can also have diabetes distress, including diabetes self-management, and, in addition, work-related diabetes distress. We studied work-related diabetes distress in a representative national sample. The structural equation model enabled us to assess the theory-based associations of work-related, health-related, and diabetes-related factors with work-related diabetes distress.

In our study, work-related diabetes distress mediated the effect of independent variables on metabolic control. This finding is in a line with a previous study among people with diabetes [28].

We found an important association between problems with physical work conditions and work-related diabetes distress. The work environment and physical work load may be modifiable to better fit the needs of workers [44]; such an adjustment would probably decrease work-related diabetes distress. A high level of job demands, indicated by the pace and amount of work, was also associated with work-related diabetes distress. High job demands per se have previously been reported to be related to stress at work [9, 34]. It seems then that the same factors that increase stress in general also increase work-related diabetes distress. On the other hand, mental work and a high educational level seemed to protect workers from stress in our study. Therefore, persons with type 1 diabetes should be encouraged to use their full potential in pursuing their education.

Work ability showed a moderate association with work-related diabetes distress. We measured work ability using the Work Ability Score (WAS). This single-item score comes from the first question of the widely used Work Ability Index [40]. WAS has been found to be reliable and valid, and it is an easy method to assess work ability [22, 39]. Persons with type 1 diabetes and an excellent work ability probably have uncomplicated diabetes. Diabetes complications and other co-morbidities decrease work ability and induce work-related diabetes distress. In previous studies, work ability has been shown to correlate with productivity loss [45], as well as with mortality and disability [33]. A low WAS among workers with type 1 diabetes challenges occupational health personnel and employers to develop opportunities for part-time work and to modify jobs to match workers' resources or arrange other means of support.

Difficulty in accepting diabetes was the only independent variable associated with the three dependent variables: work-related diabetes distress, depressive symptoms, and HbA1c level. These associations have been found also in an earlier study [41]. Learning to live with diabetes is a lifelong process; thus the duration of diabetes is not the "point" in how well a person has been empowered and has accepted his or her diabetes after receiving the diagnosis [46]. People develop and sustain various behavior patterns over time [47]. Although workplace health promotion may be one way to promote a change in health behavior [48], individual health care and support in self-management activities is needed to meet the different and varying needs of people diagnosed with diabetes [46, 47].

In previous studies, high diabetes distress was found to be correlated with poor diabetes empowerment, low overall and mental quality of life, low income, unhealthy diet, physical inactivity, poor glycemic control, hypoglycemic reactions, and future complications [3, 4, 38]. In addition, individual (e.g., knowledge and motivation) and environment-related (e.g., social support) issues affect the self-management of diabetes. Too, depression may cause poor diabetes self-care. Self-management education, coping skills, and the ability to solve problems have been found to decrease diabetes-related distress [38]. As a result, counseling, training, and coping courses for persons with diabetes are needed to support the self-management of diabetes.

An interesting result of our study was a lack of a notable association between general stress and work-related diabetes distress in the multivariate analysis. The latter seems therefore to be an independent phenomenon of general stress in the worklife of people with type 1 diabetes.

In this study, work-related diabetes distress was associated to the greatest degree with the blood glucose level being kept at a high level at work. If the physical work load is unpredictable, the risk of hypoglycemia increases. Furthermore, an inability or reluctance to self-monitor blood glucose at work may lead to the blood glucose level being kept high at work. Therefore a tendency to keep the blood glucose level high at work as a coping strategy may partly be due to a realistic fear of hypoglycemia and partly due to personal challenges in reaching good metabolic control. As far as we know, there are no reports concerning the problem of keeping blood glucose levels too high at work. The complications of poor metabolic control are well known, but the frequency and reasons for voluntarily maintaining a high blood glucose level are not. Therefore further studies are needed on this phenomenon.

Work-related diabetes distress had a bi-directional association with depression. Similar associations have also been found in other studies [37]. When both directions were estimated in the same model the association from depressive symptoms to work-related diabetes distress was stronger than vice versa. Nevertheless, as these directions are cross-sectional associations, we cannot make any causal inferences. It is reasonable to conclude that diabetes-related stress can increase the risk of depression [27, 28], and, obviously, depression-prone people also tend to feel stress about their work ability [49]. Screening for the risk of depression among workers with type 1 diabetes may facilitate early intervention aimed at improving work ability.

One of the strengths of our study was the size of the randomized sample ($n = 2500$), which covered 8.3 % of the working-aged Finns with type 1 diabetes. Even though only half of the recipients returned the questionnaire, the respondents seemed to form a good representation of working-aged Finns with type 1 diabetes since the sample was not biased in terms of demographic distributions. In addition, the sample size was big enough to enable a comparison of workers who had never experienced work-related diabetes distress with those who often felt such stress. Our sample represented workers extensively from different organizations and types of occupations. Furthermore, the questionnaire was based on several validated scales that included questions related to health, work ability, and worklife.

Using SEM, we were able to assess the associations, and the paths were dictated on a theoretical basis. Due to the cross-sectional nature of the study, the causal relations between the variables could not be confirmed, however. As the study was based on self-reporting, biases especially in the recall of the HbA1c level and the assessment of other study factors could have affected the results. Nonetheless, self-reported measurements are widely used due to practical reasons in data collection of large study samples (11, 29, 48). All of the participants were Finnish which may limit the generalizability of our results. We think that the results would be applicable to other Western countries, which have same kind of labour legislation and where health care is available for the whole population.

Conclusions

In conclusion, work-related diabetes distress was found to be common among workers with type 1 diabetes. Problems with physical work conditions, work ability, difficulty in accepting diabetes, job demands, as well as depressive symptoms proved to be associated with work-related diabetes distress. Work-related diabetes distress seems to mediate the adverse effects of these factors on metabolic control through the maintenance of a high blood glucose level at work. Reconciling work with diabetes may be challenging. Some of the factors associated with work-related diabetes distress are modifiable, and some are not. Vocational guidance should encourage people with type 1 diabetes to use their full potential in pursuing their education. Occupational health personnel, employers, and superiors at work can facilitate and support the self-monitoring of blood glucose at work. They can also collaborate with people with diabetes to devise means for adapting work to fit their needs. We suggest that even minor work arrangements may be enough to diminish work-related diabetes distress.

Abbreviations

ANOVA: analysis of variance; GFI: goodness of fit index; HbA1c: glycosylated hemoglobin; RMSEA: root mean square error of estimation; SEM: structural equation modeling; WAI: Work Ability Index; WAS: Work Ability Score.

Competing interests

The authors declare that they have no competing interests.

Authors' contributions

PH participated in study design, researched the data, performed the statistical analyses, and wrote and edited the manuscript; LM participated in study design and helped research the data and edit the manuscript; VH participated in the study design and helped research the data and edit the manuscript; JH participated in the study design and helped edit the manuscript; KR participated in the study design, supervised the study, and helped write and edit the manuscript. KR is the guarantor of this work and, as such, had full access to all the data in the study and takes responsibility for the integrity of the data and the accuracy of the data analysis. All authors read and approved the final manuscript.

Acknowledgements

The authors acknowledge all those who participated in this study by filling out and returning the questionnaire. The authors also express their gratitude to Erja Huttunen, registered nurse (Kuopio University Hospital), Kimmo Ronkainen, a senior data manager (University of Eastern Finland), Marja-Leena Lamidi, a statistician (University of Eastern Finland), Merja Turunen, a data manager (University of Eastern Finland) and Georgianna Oja, ELS, for their valuable help during this study.

Grant support

Our study has been funded by The Finnish Work Environment Fund, The Social Insurance Institution of Finland, the Foundation of Kyllikki and Uolevi Lehikoinen, The Finnish Diabetes Association, and the Foundation of Occupational Health in Finland.

Author details

[1]School of Medicine, Institute of Public Health and Clinical Nutrition, University of Eastern Finland, Kuopio, Finland. [2]Department of Medicine, Kuopio University Hospital, Kuopio, Finland. [3]Department of Social Sciences, University of Eastern Finland, Kuopio, Finland.

References

1. Egede LE, Dismuke CE. Serious psychological distress and diabetes: a review of the literature. Curr Psychiatry Rep. 2012. doi:10.1007/s11920-011-0240-0.

2. Polonsky WH, Fisher L, Earles J, Dudl RJ, Lees J, Mullan J, et al. Assessing psychosocial distress in diabetes: development of the Diabetes Distress Scale. Diabetes Care. 2005;28:626–31.
3. Joensen LE, Tapager I, Willaing I. Diabetes distress in type 1 diabetes – a new measurement fit for purpose. Diabet Med. 2013. doi:10.1111/dme.12241.
4. Hermanns N, Kulzer B, Krichbaum M, Kubiak T, Haak T. How to screen for depression and emotional problems in patients with diabetes: comparison of screening characteristics of depression questionnaires, measurement of diabetes-specific emotional problems and standard clinical assessment. Diabetologia. 2006. doi:10.1007/s00125-005-0094-2.
5. Folkman S, Lazarus RS, Pimley S, Novacek J. Age differences in stress and coping processes. Psychol Aging. 1987. doi:10.1037/0882-7974.2.2.171.
6. Velasco Garrido M, Bittner C, Harth V, Preisser A. Health status and health-related quality of life of municipal waste collection workers – a cross-sectional survey. J Occup Med Toxicol. 2015. doi:10.1186/s12995-015-0065-6.
7. Clays E, De Bacquer D, Leynen F, Kornitzer M, Kittel F, De Backer G. Job stress and depression symptoms in middle-aged workers – prospective results from the Belstress study. Scand J Work Environ Health. 2007. doi:10.5271/sjweh.1140.
8. Lunau T, Wahrendorf M, Dragano N, Siegrist J. Work stress and depressive symptoms in older employees: impact of national labour and social policies. BMC Public Health. 2013. doi:10.1186/1471-2458-13-1086.
9. Melchior M, Caspi A, Milne BJ, Danese A, Poulton R, Moffitt TE. Work stress precipitates depression and anxiety in young, working women and men. Psychol Med. 2007. doi:10.1017/S0033291707000414.
10. Szeto ACH, Dobson KS. Mental disorders and their association with perceived work stress: an investigation of the 2010 Canadian Community Health Survey. J Occup Health Psych. 2013. doi:10.1037/a0031806.
11. Glise K, Hadzibajramovic E, Jonsdottir IH, Ahlborg Jr G. Self-reported exhaustion: a possible indicator of reduced work ability and increased risk of sickness absence among human service workers. Int Arch Occup Environ Health. 2010. doi:10.1007/s00420-009-0490-x.
12. Balfe M, Brugha R, Smith D, Sreenan S, Doyle F, Conroy R. Why do young adults with type 1 diabetes find it difficult to manage diabetes in the workplace? Health Place. 2014. doi:10.1016/j.healthplace.2013.12.016.
13. Young J, Waclawski E, Young JA, Spencer J. Control of type 1 diabetes mellitus and shift work. Occup Med (Lond). 2013. doi:10.1093/occmed/kqs176.
14. Brod M, Christensen T, Thomsen TL, Bushnell DM. The impact of non-severe hypoglycemic events on work productivity and diabetes management. Value in Health. 2011. doi:10.1016/j.jval.2011.02.001.
15. Franciosi M, Lucisano G, Amoretti R, Capani F, Bruttomesso D, Di Bartolo P, et al. Costs of treatment and complications of adult type 1 diabetes. Nutr Metab Cardiovasc Dis. 2012. doi:10.1016/j.numecd.2012.03.002.
16. Hex N, Bartlett C, Wright D, Taylor M, Varley D. Estimating the current and future costs of type 1 and type 2 diabetes in the UK, including direct health costs and indirect societal and productivity costs. Diabet Med. 2012. doi:10.1111/j.1464-5491.2012.03698.x.
17. Dray-Spira R, Herquelot E, Bonenfant S, Gueguen A, Melchior M. Impact of diabetes mellitus onset on sickness absence from work – a 15-year follow-up of the GAZEL occupational cohort study. Diabet Med. 2013. doi:10.1111/dme.12076.
18. Weijman I, Ros WJG, Rutten GEHM, Schaufeli WB, Schabracq MJ, Winnubst JAM. The role of work-related and personal factors in diabetes self-management. Patient Educ Couns. 2005. doi:10.1016/j.pec.2004.10.004.
19. Aromaa A, Koskinen S, editors. Health and functional capacity in Finland: baseline results of the Health 2000 Health Examination Survey. Helsinki: National Public Health Institute; 2004.
20. Karasek R, Brisson C, Kawakami N, Houtman I, Bongers P, Amick B. The job content questionnaire (JCQ): an instrument for internationally comparative assessments of psychosocial job characteristics. J Occup Health Psych. 1998;4:322–55.
21. Whooley MA, Avins AL, Miranda J, Browner WS. Case-finding instruments for depression: two questions are as good as many. J Gen Intern Med. 1997. doi:10.1046/j.1525-1497.1997.00076.x.
22. Ahlstrom L, Grimby-Ekman A, Hagberg M, Dellve L. The work ability index and single-item question: associations with sick leave, symptoms, and health – a prospective study of women on long-term sick leave. Scand J Work Environ Health. 2010;36(5):404–12.
23. Elo AL, Leppanen A, Jahkola A. Validity of a single-item measure of stress symptoms. Scand J Work Environ Health. 2003. doi:10.5271/sjweh.752.
24. DEHKO. Development Programme for the Prevention and Care of Diabetes in Finland 2000–2010. Tampere: Finnish Diabetes Association; 2001.
25. Diabetes in Finland (FinDM) database, 2011. The National Institute for Health and Welfare (THL).
26. Fisher L, Mullan JT, Arean P, Glasgow RE, Hessler D, Masharani U. Diabetes distress but not clinical depression or depressive symptoms is associated with glycemic control in both cross-sectional and longitudinal analyses. Diabetes Care. 2010. doi:10.2337/dc09-1238.
27. Rotella F, Mannucci E. Diabetes mellitus as a risk factor for depression: a meta-analysis of longitudinal studies. Diabetes Res Clin Pract. 2013. doi:10.1016/j.diabres.2012.11.022.
28. van Bastelaar KM, Pouwer F, Geelhoed-Duijvestijn PH, Tack CJ, Bazelmans E, Beekman AT, et al. Diabetes-specific emotional distress mediates the association between depressive symptoms and glycaemic control in type 1 and type 2 diabetes. Diabet Med. 2010. doi:10.1111/j.1464-5491.2010.03025.x.
29. Weijman I, Ros WJ, Rutten GE, Schaufeli WB, Schabracq MJ, Winnubst JA. Frequency and perceived burden of diabetes self-management activities in employees with insulin-treated diabetes: relationships with health outcomes. Diabetes Res Clin Pract. 2005. doi:10.1016/j.diabres.2004.08.004.
30. Rugulies R, Aust B, Madsen IEH, Bur H, Siegrist J, Bültman U. Adverse psychosocial working conditions and risk of severe depressive symptoms: do effects differ by occupational grade? Eur J Pub Health. 2012. doi:10.1093/eurpub/cks071.
31. Finne LB, Christensen JO, Knardahl S. Psychological and social work factors as predictors of mental distress: a prospective study. Plos One. 2014. doi:10.1371/journal.pone.0102514.
32. Canivet C, Choi B, Karasek R, Moghaddassi M, Staland-Nyman C, Ostergren PO. Can high psychological job demands, low decision latitude, and high job strain predict disability pensions? A 12-year follow-up of middle-aged Swedish workers. Int Arch Occup Environ Health. 2013. doi:10.1007/s00420-012-0766-4.
33. von Bonsdorff MB, Seitsamo J, von Bonsdorff ME, Ilmarinen J, Nygard CH, Rantanen T. Job strain among blue-collar and white-collar employees as a determinant of total mortality: a 28-year population-based follow-up. BMJ Open. 2012. doi:10.1136/bmjopen-2012-00086.
34. Adriaenssens J, De Gucht V, Maes S. Causes and consequences of occupational stress in emergency nurses, a longitudinal study. J Nurs Manag. 2013. doi:10.1111/jonm.12138.
35. Elovainio M, Heponiemi T, Kuusio H, Jokela M, Aalto A-M, Pekkarinen L, et al. Job demands and job strain as risk factors for employee wellbeing in elderly care: an instrumental-variables analysis. Eur J Pub Health. 2014. doi:10.1093/eurpub/cku115.
36. Seidler A, Thinschmidt M, Deckert S, Then F, Hegewald J, Nieuwenhuijsen K, et al. The role of psychosocial working conditions on burnout and its core component emotional exhaustion – a systematic review. J Occup Med Toxicol. 2014. doi:10.1186/1745-6673-9-10.
37. Ehrmann D, Kulzer B, Haak T, Hermanns N. Longitudinal relationship of diabetes-related distress and depressive symptoms: analysing incidence and persistence. Diabet Med. 2015. Accepted manuscript online: 22 Jul 2015. doi: 10.1111/dme.12861.
38. Ahola AJ, Groop PH. Barriers to self-management of diabetes. Diabet Med. 2013. doi:10.1111/dme.12105.
39. El Fassi M, Bocquet V, Majery N, Lair ML, Couffignal S, Mairiaux P. Work ability assessment in a worker population: comparison and determinants of Work Ability Index and Work Ability score. BMC Pub Health. 2013. doi:10.1186/1471-2458-13-305.
40. Tuomi K, Ilmarinen J, Jahkola A, Katajarinne L, Tulkki A. Work ability index (2nd rev ed). Finnish Institute of Occupational Health: Helsinki; 1998.
41. Schmitt A, Reimer B, Kulzer T, Haak A, Gahr A, Hermanns N. Assessment of diabetes acceptance can help identify patients with ineffective diabetes self-care and poor diabetes control. Diabet Med. 2014. doi:10.1111/dme.12553.
42. Kline RB. Principles and practice of structural equation modelling. 3rd ed. New York: The Guilford Press; 2011.
43. Hu L, Bentler PM. Cutoff criteria for fit indexes in covariance structure analysis: conventional criteria versus new alternatives. Struct Equa Modeling. 1999. doi:10.1080/10705519909540118.
44. Varekamp I, van Dijk FJ. Workplace problems and solutions for employees with chronic diseases. Occup Med (Lond). 2010. doi:10.1093/occmed/kqq076.
45. Ilmarinen J. Work ability – a comprehensive concept for occupational health research and prevention. Scand J Work Environ Health. 2009;1:1–5.
46. Kneck Å, Fagerberg I, Eriksson LE, Lundman B. Living with diabetes—Development of learning patterns over a 3-year period. Int J Qual Stud Health Well-being. 2014. doi:10.3402/qhw.v9.24375.
47. Audulv Å. The over time development of chronic illness self-management patterns: a longitudinal qualitative study. BMC Public Health. 2013;13:452. doi:10.1186/1471-2458-13-452.

48. Mache S, Jensen S, Linnig S, Jahn R, Steudtner M, Ochsmann E, Preuss G. Do overweight workers profit by workplace health promotion, more than their normal-weight peers? Evaluation of a worksite intervention. J Occup Med Toxicol. 2015. doi:10.1186/s12995-015-0068-3.
49. Shiri R, Kaila-Kangas L, Ahola K, Kivekas T, Viikari-Juntura E, Heliovaara M, et al. The relation of co-occurring musculoskeletal pain and depressive symptoms with work ability. J Occup Environ Med. 2013. doi:10.1097/JOM.0b013e3182a4ffc4.

4

Malignant mesothelioma incidence by nation-wide cancer registry

Kristinn Tomasson[1], Gunnar Gudmundsson[2,3], Haraldur Briem[4] and Vilhjalmur Rafnsson[5*]

Abstract

Background: Malignant mesothelioma caused by asbestos exposure has a long latency period. A ban on asbestos use may not be apparent in decreased incidence in the population until after several decades. The aim was to evaluate changes in the incidence of malignant mesothelioma, and the possible impact of the asbestos ban implemented in Iceland in 1983.

Methods: This is a population study on aggregate level; the source of data was the Icelandic Cancer Registry, the National Cause-of-Death Registry, and the National Register. Volume of asbestos import was obtained from Customs Tariff. The import figures reflect fairly accurately the amount used, as there are no mines in the country.

Results: Asbestos import peaked in 1980 at 15.0 kg/capita/year, diminishing to 0.3 kg/capita/year ten years after the ban in 1983, and to zero in the most recent years. Seventy-nine per cent of the cases of malignant mesothelioma were men, and 72 % were of pleural origin. Mesothelioma incidence increased steadily from 1965 to 2014, when it reached 21.4 per million among men, and 5.6 among women. Mortality in 2014 was 22.2 per million among men, and 4.8 among women.

Conclusion: Malignant mesothelioma incidence and mortality increased in the population during the period, despite the ban on asbestos use from 1983. This is in agreement with the long latency time for malignant mesothelioma. In line with the previously high per capita volume of asbestos import, many buildings, equipment, and structures contain asbestos, so there is an on-going risk of asbestos exposure during maintenance, renovations and replacements. It is thus difficult to predict when the incidence of malignant mesothelioma will decrease in the future. During the last ten-year period, the incidence in Iceland was higher than the recently reported incidence in neighbouring countries.

Keywords: Malignant mesothelioma, Cancer registry, Incidence rates, Death registry, Mortality, Asbestos import, Relative risk, Trend, Population

Background

Malignant mesothelioma is a cancer of mesothelial serosa; its primary location is pleura, peritoneum, pericardium, and tunica vaginalis. Since the association between malignant mesothelioma and asbestos exposure was first described by Wagner and co-workers in 1960 [1], it has been established and recognized that asbestos is the dominant cause of malignant mesothelioma, according to studies from several national mesothelioma registries [2–5]. Today, all types of asbestos, chrysotile, crocidolite, amosite, anthophyllite, tremolite, and actinolite are considered causes of human malignant mesothelioma according to the International Agency for Research on Cancer (IARC) report [6] where epidemiological, experimental, and mechanistic studies have been evaluated. Chrysotile asbestos was the last type to be definitively included as a cause of malignant mesothelioma [7–9]. The time from first exposure to asbestos until diagnosis of malignant mesothelioma is called the induction/latency time. This period can be from 20 to 50 years [10–12], with a shorter latency in the heavily exposed population and longer latency among groups with low-level exposure.

* Correspondence: vilraf@hi.is
[5]Department of Preventive Medicine, University of Iceland, Stapi/ Hringbraut, Reykjavik, Iceland
Full list of author information is available at the end of the article

In the case of crocidolite exposed cohort the risk of malignant mesothelioma increases from 10–15 years following first exposure and persists for as long as the exposed persons survive, however stops increasing after 30–40 years [13]. The long latency period poses difficulties in occupational studies; however the risk of malignant mesothelioma caused by asbestos is dose-dependent [4, 14, 15], and malignant mesothelioma occurs at very low-level exposure, indeed lower than the eight-hour occupational threshold limit value generally established at 0.1 fibre/ml air, and no safe dose has been found, below which there is no risk of malignant mesothelioma [16].

In addition to asbestos exposure, other casual associations with malignant mesothelioma include radiation treatment for Hodgkin lymphoma and non-Hodgkin lymphoma [17, 18]. Malignant mesothelioma has also been found as a second cancer among testis and prostate cancer patients treated with radiotherapy [19, 20]. At one time, the Simian Virus 40 was thought to play a role in the aetiology of malignant mesothelioma; however, according to IARC, there is inadequate evidence to consider Simian Virus 40 a carcinogen to humans [21]. Erionite is a fibrous mineral belonging to a group of minerals called zeolite and fluoro-edenite another type of fibrous mineral have been associated with malignant mesothelioma in specific areas in Turkey, Mexico and Sicily [22–25]. Erionite is classified as a human carcinogen according to IARC [6], and is widely prevalent in the US [26] and in Iceland [27].

Mortality information on mesothelioma is compiled internationally in the WHO database [28]. Information on the incidence of malignant mesothelioma is commonly obtained from special national malignant mesothelioma registers [2–5], or the cancer registry, Surveillance, Epidemiology, and End Results (SEER) [29]. Where cancer registries and special occupational disease registries can be compared on the national level, the cancer registries show numerical superiority compared with the occupational disease registries, as reported in studies from some Scandinavian countries [30–33]. The setting in Iceland, where the cancer registry was established in 1955 [34], and where there is access to comprehensive population registries as well as general use of a personal identifier, provides an opportunity to study malignant mesothelioma incidence.

The aim of the study was to describe the long-term changes in incidence of malignant mesothelioma up to 2014, and to evaluate the possible impact of the asbestos ban implemented in 1983.

Methods

This is a population-based observational study and the source of data was the Icelandic Cancer Registry. The registry is nation-wide and includes all cases of cancer since 1955 [34]. The registry has virtually complete coverage, and over 95 % of diagnoses are histologically confirmed [34, 35]. We asked for information from the registry on all cases of cancer with ICD-10 code C45 mesothelioma (the accurate location was read from the decimal figure, pleura, peritoneum, and other and unspecified sites), and ICD-O codes 9050, 9051, 9052, and 9053, mesothelioma, with the behaviour code /3, malignant, primary site. Different versions of the ICD were in use during the operation of the registry, and they were standardized by the registry to ICD-10. Besides the information on the location and morphology of the cases, we obtained information on encrypted personal identification number, gender, age, year and age at diagnosis. The registry does not routinely collect information on occupational or environmental exposure, or survival of the reported cancer cases.

Statistics Iceland maintains the National Cause-of-Death Registry [36]. The registry is nation-wide and includes causes of death according to death certificates. The ICD-10 code C45 was available for 1996–2014.

Three broad categories of exposure to asbestos have been described. The first is for miners and millers of raw asbestos and people employed by manufacturers of asbestos products, such as asbestos cement factories, often associated with heavy exposure. The second category is for workers such as carpenters, plumbers, shipbuilders, machine engineers, and insulators who use asbestos products, and other less-exposed occupations such as seamen, fishermen, and various factory workers. The third category is for groups and individuals with short-term or low-level exposure to asbestos, often non-occupational, including family members of asbestos workers, people living near an asbestos industry, and those dwelling or working in buildings containing asbestos. Asbestos production or mining activities have never occurred in Iceland, so the asbestos exposure in question would be of the second category, involving, for example, the building industry, fishing, and geothermal industry, and of the third category.

Information on the volume of annual import of asbestos and goods containing asbestos was obtained from Statistics Iceland [36], according to Customs Tariff, the Directorate of Customs [37], codes under 2524, 6811, 6812, 6813, and 8708 with mention of asbestos, and corresponding codes from older versions of the Customs Tariffs. The amount of asbestos in the Customs Tariff was declared in metric tons and types of asbestos were not indicated.

To estimate the incidence rates for malignant mesothelioma, the numerator used was the number of cases during ten-year periods 1965–1974, 1975–1984, 1985–1994, 1995–2004, and 2005–2014, with the corresponding population figures of those 15 years of age or older [38] obtained from Statistics Iceland [36]. The ten-year rates were compared with the rate in the first period

1965–1974, calculating relative risk (RR), and 95 % confidence intervals (CI). Similarly, the mortality rates were estimated in eight- and ten-year periods 1996–2004, and 2005–2014.

The incidence rates, 95 % CI of the rates, and statistical analyses were performed using the software packet Epi-Info, and Microsoft Excel 7.

The National Bioethics Committee (VSNb2010150400 06/03.03) approved the study, and the Data Protection Commission was notified of the study and did not make remarks on the way it was conducted.

Results

Information on the annual import of asbestos was available for the period 1976 to 2014, and is shown in Fig. 1. Import volume peaked in the year 1980 at 3500 tons, corresponding to 1500 tons per 100,000 inhabitants, or 15.0 kg/capita/year of asbestos. This huge import coincided with extensive construction of district heating systems, where the main feeding pipes consisted of asbestos cement pipes, and geothermal hot water was piped 20 to 50 km into houses of communities with greater than 10,000 inhabitants. The ban against asbestos use with certain exceptions was implemented in 1983, and that year, import volume decreased considerably, to increase again over a five-year period, and peaking again in 1992 with 800 tons, corresponding to 299 tons per 100,000, or 0.3 kg/capita/year of asbestos. We do not have an explanation for this temporary increase in asbestos import; however, it is clear that this volume involves asbestos cement used in building materials and pipes, or similar articles, as friction material in brake linings and clutches, and fabricated asbestos fibres seldom exceeded 20–30 tons per year in the early period, and did not ever reach an annual volume of one ton during the last ten years of the period.

In table 1, the number of cases of malignant mesothelioma, ten-year annual incidence rates and 95 % confidence intervals, are shown for men and women. Among men, the rates increase steadily through this 50 -year period; however, the changes over the period are not straightforward for women, where the rates are low, and no cases occur in the period 1975–1984.

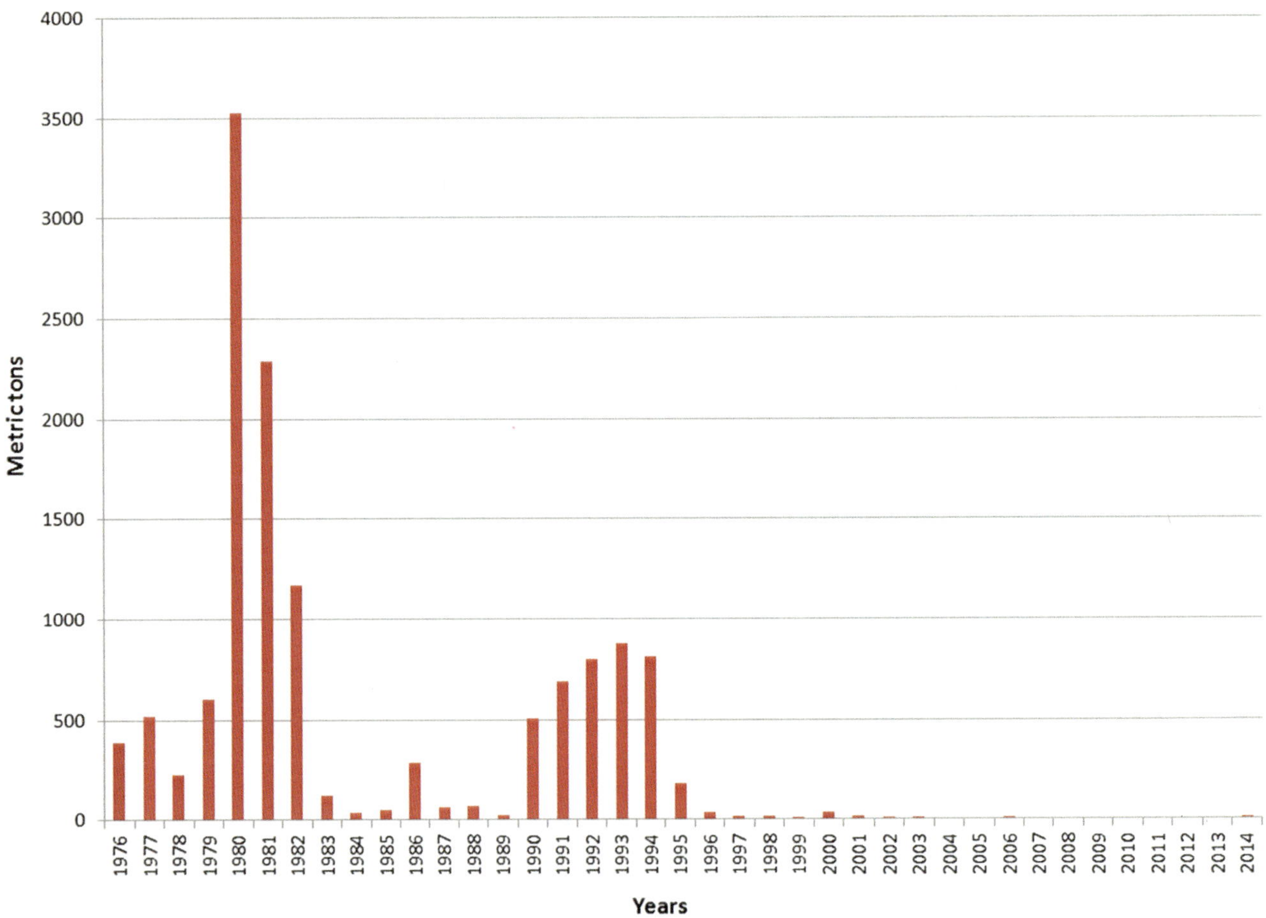

Fig. 1 Annual weight of import in metric tons by tariff numbers with mention of asbestos

Table 1 Number of malignant mesothelioma cases in ten years periods by gender, annual incidence per million, and 95 % confidence interval (CI)

		1965–1974	1975–1984	1985–1994	1995–2004	2005–2014
Male	Number of cases	1	4	9	19	27
	Incidence per 10^6	1.4	4.8	9.4	17.6	21.4
	95 % CI	0.1–7.1	1.5–11.6	4.6–17.2	10.9–26.9	14.4–30.7
Female	Number of cases	2	0	3	4	7
	Incidence per 10^6	2.9	-	3.1	3.7	5.6
	95 % CI	0.5–9.6	-	0.8–8.5	1.2–8.8	2.4–11.0

Table 2 shows age distribution of malignant mesothelioma cases by gender, with the highest number in the age group 70 to 79. In table 3, location and histological diagnosis are shown by gender. In ninety-seven per cent of cases among men, the mesothelioma is located in the pleura, but among women, 56 % is pleura and 44 % is located in peritoneum. Malignant mesothelioma NOS (M-9050/3) is the dominant histological type for both genders.

In table 4, the number of deaths due to malignant mesothelioma according to death certificates, and annual mortality rates is shown by gender. The period available for mortality was 18 years, and no obvious increase over this short observational period and limited volume of data is noted. However, the rates and the RR were high.

Table 5 shows again the number of cases per ten-year periods through 1965 to 2014, and the relative risk, where the first ten-year period, 1965–1974 is the reference. Among men, the relative risk increases over the years, and the trend is statistically significant. The pattern is not so clear among women; however the relative risks increase over the years, but the trend is not statistically significant.

Discussion

There is still a rising incidence of malignant mesothelioma in Iceland, particularly among men. The increase may be real; however, it may also be partly a reflection of improvement in the diagnoses, and greater watchfulness for the cancer. The ban on asbestos use in 1983 may not have been as influential in Iceland as in neighbouring countries [39]. No case of malignant mesothelioma has ever been reported as an occupational disease in Iceland, so such registration of cases is even less effective than in the other Scandinavian countries [30–33]. The observed incidence of malignant mesothelioma in the last ten-year period is high and consistent with the high incidence rate reported by countries in the global overview. Only Australia, Great Britain, Belgium and the Netherlands had higher rates [12]. This is noteworthy, as there are no asbestos mines and there never has been any asbestos production industry in Iceland. However, the import figures are astonishingly high in relation to the population. In a report on disease burden due to asbestos in European countries, the age-adjusted mortality rate of malignant mesothelioma was highest in Iceland, 25 per million people [40]. That figure is not much higher than the rate 22.2 found in the present study, in spite of some differences in methodologies used to calculate the rates.

Table 2 Number of malignant mesothelioma cases and deaths by age categories, and gender

		<50	50–59	60–69	70–79	>80	Total
Male	Number of cases	3	8	16	20	13	60
Female	Number of cases	2	1	4	5	4	16
Male	Number deceased	1	5	7	18	11	42
Female	Number deceased	0	0	4	4	2	10

In the past the volume of the asbestos import was among the highest per capita in a European study [40], and this was confirmed in the present study. The description of the import of asbestos in the present study shows the same pattern as has been observed in previous studies on asbestos use, where a ban has been established; the national consumption of asbestos has diminished from high per capita use to an almost immeasurably small amount in the past few years [39, 40]. In these recent years, it is the friction material in brake linings and clutches that is still important [41]. However, other sources of asbestos exposure are related to home maintenance and renovation [42], and the maintenance of the asbestos-containing structure of the extensive hot water supply systems in Iceland. During the last 20 years, labour inspection, the Administration for Occupational Safety and Health [43], has been enforcing safe handling of asbestos in maintenance work. According to information from the cancer registry, no cluster of malignant mesothelioma has been identified at time of diagnosis in the areas with known erionite occurrence in the country.

Malignant mesothelioma is not the only cancer attributed to asbestos exposure. There is sufficient evidence that asbestos exposure causes lung, larynx and ovarian cancer, and limited evidence that it causes colorectal, pharynx and stomach cancers [6]. Lung cancer is the most important and is generally more frequent than malignant mesothelioma in asbestos-exposed cohort studies. However, lung cancer caused by asbestos is under-recognized and

Table 3 Number of malignant mesothelioma by sites, gender, and morphology

		M-9050/3 NOS n (%)	M-9051/3 Fibrous n (%)	M-9052/3 Epithelioid n (%)	M-9053/3 Biphasic n (%)	Total
Male	Pleura	40 (69.0)	1 (1.7)	14 (24.1)	3 (5.2)	58
	Peritoneum	-	-	1 (100)	-	1
	Other and unspecified sites	1 (100)	-	-	-	1
Female	Pleura	8 (88.9)	-	1 (11.1)	-	9
	Peritoneum	6 (85.7)	-	1 (14.3)	-	7

often confounded by cigarette smoking [44]. Because of the firm association between asbestos exposure and malignant mesothelioma, its incidence or mortality has been taken as an indicator of asbestos exposure in the population. In a recent study of McCormack and co-workers, malignant mesothelioma mortality was used to estimate asbestos-related lung cancer in different populations [45], and smoking habits were taken into account. In the two models used in that study to estimate asbestos-related lung cancer mortality, the proportion of lung cancers that are a consequence of asbestos exposure ranged between 6.6 to 9.3 % in Iceland [45].

The use of the National Register for the source of denominator strengthens the study. Personal identification numbers, which we had access to in encrypted form, are used in the comprehensive population registers in Iceland, and they ensure that we did not double count cases or dead persons. The National Cause-of-Death Registry, the source of information of number of deaths from malignant mesothelioma, has been reported as good in the global evaluation, and was categorized as high quality overall and ranked in the same category as data from 23 developed countries, including the US and the UK [46]. The autopsy rate is about 14 % of all deaths during the study period [36].

The figures from the two sources of information concerning number of incident cases, and number of deaths due to malignant mesothelioma per calendar year or age categories are not in agreement in the present study. This is partly because there is a natural lag between the diagnosis and the death, further more an autopsy study has revealed that about 45 % of male cases of mesothelioma may remain undiagnosed [47], while still another Italian study has shown that the overall concordance between histo-pathological diagnosis and death certification was about 75 % [48].

To the strength of the study we count the use of the Icelandic Cancer Registry for the source of malignant mesothelioma incidence, in which more than 95 % of the diagnoses in the registry are histologically verified [34, 35], and in the present study all cases were with morphological diagnosis.

The relatively high proportion of peritoneal mesotheliomas among females may raise concern of diagnostic error, and as the cases were not histologically reviewed by an expert pathologist for the purpose of this study, we count this as a limitation of the study.

The study material originates from the comprehensive population registries in Iceland, which are considered to

Table 4 Number of malignant mesothelioma deaths in eight and ten years periods, annual mortality per million per ≥ 15 years (yr), with 95 % confidence interval (CI), and relative risk (RR) and 95 % confidence intervals (CI) during 1996 to 2014, among men and women, first period is the reference

		1996–2004	2005–2014	RR	95 % CI
Male	Number of deaths	14	28		
	Mortality per 10^6	14.4	22.2	1.54	0.82–3.00
	95 % CI	8.2–23.6	15.0–31.7		
Female	Number of deaths	4	6		
	Mortality per 10^6	4.1	4.8	1.17	0.32–4.69
	95 % CI	1.3–9.8	1.9–9.9		

Table 5 Number of incident cases of malignant mesothelioma in ten years periods, and relative risk (RR) and 95 % confidence intervals (CI) during 1965 to 2014 among men and women, first period is the reference

		Number of cases	RR	95 % CI
Male	1965–1974	1	Ref.	
	1975–1984	4	3.34	0.37–29.84
	1985–1994	9	6.53	0.83–51.57
	1995–2004	19	12.24	1.64–91.39
	2005–2014	27	14.90	2.03–109.7
	Trend, *p*-value <0.000			
Female	1965–1974	2	Ref.	
	1975–1984	0	-	
	1985-1994	3	1.07	0.18–6.43
	1995–2004	4	1.26	0.23–6.89
	2005–2014	7	1.92	0.40–9.22
	Trend, *p*-value 0.11			

be of high quality; however these are from one country only, which may limit the generalizability of the results. The characteristics of the background population are known and the population is homogenous, being 99 % white Caucasian, with uniform financing of the health care system, also of high quality. The country belongs to the developed countries [45]; however, it differs from other European countries in that heavy industry has expanded during the study period, with aluminium and ferrosilicon plants having been set up to harvest abundant electric power resources.

Conclusion

The incidence rates of malignant mesothelioma seem to be increasing in Iceland, which indicates that there is no reduction yet of the influence of previous asbestos exposure on the population, despite the ban, first implemented in 1983, in an attempt to diminish the use of asbestos. The previous per capita asbestos import rate was among the highest in Europe. The findings of the high incidence and mortality of malignant mesothelioma is in agreement with the long latency for malignant mesothelioma. The incidence during the last ten-year period in the present study is higher than the recently reported incidence in neighbouring Scandinavian countries.

Abbreviations

CI, confidence intervals; IARC, International Agency for Research on Cancer; ICD-10, International Classification of Diseases, 10th version; ICD-O, International Classification of Diseases for Oncology, Third Edition; RR, relative risk; SEER, Surveillance Epidemiology and End Results; UK, United Kingdom; US, United States

Acknowledgements

We thank the Icelandic Cancer Registry for providing data on the cases of malignant mesothelioma and histology.

Funding

This study has no external funding.

Authors' contributions

KT, GG, HB, and VR actively participated in design the study, and planning of analyses. VR obtained the data, performed the statistical analyses and drafted the manuscript. All authors had full access to all of the data in the study, critically reviewed the manuscript for important intellectual content; approved the final version of the submitted manuscript. VR is the guarantor. The manuscript's guarantor affirms that the manuscript is an honest, accurate, and transparent account of the study being reported; that no important aspects of the study have been omitted.

Competing interests

The authors declare that they have no competing interests.

Author details

[1]Department of Occupational Medicine, Administration of Occupational Safety and Health, Reykjavik, Iceland. [2]Faculty of Medicine, University of Iceland, Reykjavik, Iceland. [3]Department of Respiratory Medicine and Sleep, Landspitali University Hospital, Fossvogur, 108 Reykjavik, Iceland. [4]Centre for Health Security and Communicable Disease Control, Directorate of Health, Reykjavik, Iceland. [5]Department of Preventive Medicine, University of Iceland, Stapi/ Hringbraut, Reykjavik, Iceland.

References

1. Wagner JC, Sleggs CA, Marchand P. Diffuse pleural mesothelioma and asbestos exposure in the North Western Cape Province. Br J Ind Med. 1960; 17:260–71.
2. Leigh J, Driscoll T. Malignant mesothelioma in Australia, 1945–2002. Int J Occup Environ Health. 2003;9:206–17.
3. Marinaccio A, Binazzi A, Di Marzio D, et al. Incidence of extrapleural malignant mesothelioma and asbestos exposure, from the Italian national register. Occup Environ Med. 2010;67:760–5.
4. Lacourt A, Gramond C, Audignon S, et al. Pleural mesothelioma and occupational exposure to asbestos, miniral wool, and silica. Am J Respir Crit Care Med. 2013;187:977–82.
5. Rake C, Gilham C, Hatch J, Darnton A, Hodgson J, Peto J. Occupational, domestic and environmental mesothelioma risk in the British population: a case–control study. Br J Cancer. 2009;100:1175–83.
6. International Agency for Research on Cancer. IARC Monographs on Evaluation of Carcinogenic Risk to Humans: Volume 100c: Arsenic, Metals, Fibres, and Dust. WHO Press, 2012.
7. Nicholson WJ. The carcinogenicity of chrysotile asbestos – a review. Ind Health. 2001;39:57–64.
8. Lemen RA. Chrysotile asbestos as a case of mesothelioma: application of the Hilll causation model. Int J Occup Environ Health. 2004;10:233–9.
9. Kanarek MS. Mesothelioma from chrysotile asbestos: update. Ann Epidemiol. 2011;21:688–97.
10. Marinaccio A, Binazzi A, Cauzillo G, et al. Analysis of latency time and its determinants in asbestos related malignant mesothelioma cases of the Italian register. Eur J Cancer. 2007;43:2722–8.
11. Hilliard AK, Lovett JK, Mc Gavin CR. The rise and fall in incidence of malignant mesothelioma from a British Naval Dockyard, 1979–199. Occup Med (Lond). 2003;53:209–12.
12. Bianchi C, Bianchi T. Malignant mesothelioma: global incidence and relationship with asbestos. Ind Health. 2007;45:379–87.
13. Berry G, de Klerk NH, Reid A, Ambrosini GL, Fritschi L, Olsen NJ, Merler E, Musk AW. Malignant pleural and peritoneal mesotheliomas in former millers and miners of crocidolite at Wittenoom. Western Australia Occup Envrion Med. 2004;61:e14.
14. Iwatsubo Y, Pairon JC, Boutin C, et al. Pleural mesothelioma: dose response relation at low levels of asbestos exposure in a French population-based case–control study. Am J Epidemiol. 1998;148:133–42.
15. Rödelsperger K, Jöckel KH, Pohlabeln H, Römer W, Woitowitz HJ. Asbestos and man-made vitreous fibers as risk factors for diffuse malignant mesothelioma: results from a German hospital-based case–control study. Am J Ind Med. 2001;39:262–75.
16. Occupational Safety and Health Administration. https://www.osha.gov/SLTC/asbestos/. Accessed December 15, 2015
17. De Bruin ML, Burgers JA, Baas P, et al. Malignant mesothelioma after radiation treatment for Hodgkin lymphoma. Blood. 2009;113:3679–81.
18. Chirieac LR, Barletta JA, Yeap BY, et al. Clinicopathologic characteristics of malignant mesothelioma arising in patients with a history of radiation for Hodgkin and non-Hodgkin lymphoma. J Clin Oncol. 2013;31:4544–9.
19. Travis LB, Fossa SD, Schonfeld SJ, et al. Second cancers among 40 576 testis cancer patients: focus on long-term survivors. J Natl Cancer Inst. 2005;97:1354–65.
20. Farioli A, Violante FS, Mattioli S, Curti S, Kriebel D. Risk of mesothelioma following external beam radiotherapy for prostate cancer: a cohort analysis of SEER database. Cancer Causes Control. 2013;24:1535–45.
21. International Agency for Research on Cancer. IARC Monographs on the Evaluation of Carcinogenic Risk to Humans: Malaria and Some Polymaviruses (SV40, BK, JC, and Merkel Cell Viruses). 104: World Health Organization Press; 2013 (Monograph).

22. Lilis R. Fibrous zeolites and endemic mesothelioma in Cappadocia. Turkey J Occup Med. 1981;23:548–50.
23. Baris I, Simonato L, Artvinli M, et al. Epidemiological and environmental evidence of the health effects of exposure to erionite fibres: a four-year study in the Cappadocia region of Turkey. Int J Cancer. 1987;39:10–7.
24. Ortega-Guerrero MA, Carrasco-Nunez G, Barragan-Campos H, Ortega MR. High incidence of lung cancer and malignant mesothelioma linked to erionite fibre exposure in a rural community in Central Mexico. Occup Environ Med. 2015;72:216–8.
25. Paoletti L, Batisti D, Bruno C, et al. Unusually high incidence of malignant mesothelioma in a town of eastern Sicily: an epidemiological and environmental study. Arch Environ Health. 2000;55:392–8.
26. Van Gosen BS, Blitz TA, Plumlee GS, Meeker GP, Pierson MP. Geologic occurrences of erionite in the United States: an emerging national public health concern for respiratory disease. Environ Geochem Health. 2013;35:419–30.
27. Eroinite from Svignaskard, Norðurardalur, Myrasysla, Western Region, Iceland. http://www.mindat.org/locentry-438519.html. Accessed January 15, 2016.
28. Delgermaa V, Takahashi K, Park EK, Le GV, Hara T, Sorahan T. Global mesothelioma death reported to World Health Organization between 1994 and 2008. Bull World Health Organ. 2011;89:716–724C.
29. Price B, Ware A. Mesothelioma trend in the United States: an update based on Surveillance, Epidemiology, and End Results program data for 1973 through 2003. Am J Epidemiol. 2003;159:107–12.
30. Andersson E, Toren K. Pleural mesotheliomas are underreported as occupational cancer in Sweden. Am J Ind Med. 1995;27:577–80.
31. Dano H, Skov T, Lynge E. Underreporting of occupational cancers in Denmark. Scand J Work Environ Health. 1996;22:55–7.
32. Karjalainen A, Pukkala E, Mattson K, Tammilehto L, Vainio H. Trends in mesothelioma incidence and occupational mesotheliomas in Finland in 1960–1995. Scand J Work Environ Health. 1997;23:266–70.
33. Mowe G, Andersen A, Osvoll P. Trends in mesothelioma incidence in Norway 1960–1988. Tox Ind Health. 1991;7:47–52.
34. Jonasson JG, Tryggvadottir L. Krabbamein á Íslandi. Upplýsingar úr Krabbameinsskránni fyrir tímabilið 1955–2010. (Cancer in Iceland. Information from the Cancer Registry for the period 1955–2010); 2012. http://www.krabbameinsskra.is/?id=krabbamein_a_islandi. Accessed 15 November 2015.
35. Sigurdardottir GL, Jonasson JG, Stefansdottir S, Jonsdottir A, Olafsdottir GH, Olafsdottir EJ, Tryggvadottir L. Data quality at the Icelandic Cancer registry: comparability, validity, timeliness and completeness. Acta Oncol. 2012;51:880–9.
36. Statistic Iceland. http://www.hagstofa.is/. Accessed December 15, 2015
37. Directorate of Customs. https://www.tollur.is/english/businesses/customs/import-duties/customs-tariff/. Accessed December 15, 2015.
38. Mc Donald AD, McDonald JC. Malignant mesothelioma in North America. Cancer. 1980;46:1650–6.
39. Jarvholm B, Burdorf A. Emerging evidence that the ban on asbestos use in reducing the occurrence of pleural mesothelioma in Sweden. Scand J Public Health. 2015;43:875–81.
40. Kameda T, Takahashi K, Kim R, Jiang Y, Movahed M, Park EK, Rantanen J. Asbestos: use, bans and disease burden in Europe. Bull World Health Organ. 2014;92:790–7.
41. Salazar N, Cely-Garcia MF, Breysse PN, Ramos-Bonilla JP. Asbestos exposure among transmission mechanics in automotive repair shop. Ann Occup Hyg. 2015;59:292–306.
42. Olsen NJ, Franklin PJ, Reid A, et al. Increasing incidence of malignant mesothelioma after exposure to asbestos during home maintenance and renovation. Med J Aust. 2011;195:271–4.
43. Administration of Occupational Safety and Health. http://www.vinnueftirlit.is/english. Accessed January 15, 2016.
44. Henderson DW, Rödelsperger K, Woitowitz HJ, Leigh J. After Helsinki: a multidisciplinary review of the relationship between asbestos exposure and lung cancer, with emphasis on studies published during 1997–2004. Pathology. 2004;36:517–50.
45. McCormack V, Peto J, Byrnes G, Straif K, Boffetta P. Estimating the asbestos-related lung cancer burden from mesothelioma mortality. Br J Cancer. 2012; 106:575–84.
46. Mathers CD, Fat DM, Rao C, Lopez AD. Counting the dead and what they died from: an assessment of the global status of cause of death data. Bull World Health Org. 2005;83(3):171–7.
47. Delendi M, Riboli E, Peruzzo P, Stanta G, Cocchi A, Gardiman D, Sasco AJ, Giarelli L. Comparison of diagnoses of cancers of the respiratory system on death certificates and at autopsy. IARC Sci Publ. 1991;112:55–62.
48. Bruno C, Comba P, Maiozzi P, Vetrugno T. Accuracy of death certification of pleural mesothelioma in Italy. Eur J Epidemiol. 1996;12:421–3.

5

Selected toxic and essential heavy metals in impacted teeth and the surrounding mandibular bones of people exposed to heavy metals in the environment

Piotr Malara[1*], Agnieszka Fischer[2] and Beata Malara[3]

Abstract

Background: The elemental composition of bones and teeth can allow exposure to heavy metals in the environment to be estimated. The aim of this study was to determine whether impacted mandibular teeth and the surrounding bones can be used as biomonitoring media to assess exposure to heavy metals.

Methods: The research materials were 67 impacted lower third molars and samples of the cortical bone removed when the wisdom teeth were surgically extracted. The samples were from people living in two areas with different environmental concentrations of heavy metals. The cadmium, chromium, copper, iron, lead, manganese, and zinc concentrations in the samples were determined by atomic absorption spectrometry with flame atomization.

Results: The cadmium and lead concentrations in the impacted third molars and the bones surrounding the teeth were significantly higher for people living in the relatively polluted Ruda Slaska region than for people living in Bielsko-Biala region. Significantly higher chromium, copper, manganese, and zinc concentrations were found in the bones surrounding the impacted teeth from people living in Ruda Slaska than in the bones surrounding the impacted teeth from people living in Bielsko-Biala. The cadmium concentrations in impacted teeth and the surrounding bones were significantly positively correlated.

Conclusion: The results indicated that impacted mandibular teeth and the surrounding mandibular bones may reflect the exposure of people to cadmium and lead in the environment. This conclusion, however, must be verified in future research projects designed to exclude the possibility of additional dietary, occupational, and other types of exposure to heavy metals.

Keywords: Tooth chemistry, Bone, Heavy metals, Cadmium, Lead, Atomic absorption spectrometry, Biomonitoring, Environmental exposure

Background

The elemental compositions of the bones and teeth of a person can provide information on the diet and health of that person and the exposure of the person to chemicals in the environment [1–3]. In the field of forensic medicine, research has been performed on the use of the elemental compositions of bones and teeth to identify murder victims and ancient human remains [4]. Links between the concentrations of certain metallic elements in children's teeth and behavioural deficits have been described [5].

Bones and teeth are calcified tissues, and hydroxyapatite is the main component of both. Bones and teeth are chemically stable, although it is believed that certain trace elements may accumulate in them by replacing calcium in the hydroxyapatite structure [6].

Deciduous teeth are mainly used in environmental studies because they are easily obtained after being naturally shed. Information on exposure to metals in the environment during childhood can be provided by

* Correspondence: malara@dentaris.pl
[1]Institute of Engineering Materials and Biomaterials, Silesian University of Technology, 18a Konarskiego str, 44-100 Gliwice, Poland
Full list of author information is available at the end of the article

deciduous teeth [7, 8]. Deciduous teeth start to develop *in utero*, and the last deciduous teeth are replaced with permanent teeth when a child is 12–13 years of age [9]. Deciduous and permanent teeth are morphologically and histologically similar, so environmental exposure to metals may also be assessed by analysing permanent teeth [10]. However, the availability of permanent teeth for analysis is a problem because it is unacceptable to extract permanent teeth for biomonitoring purposes. It should be noted that tooth enamel is constantly in direct contact with the environment of the oral cavity. This means that many physiological and pathological factors that affect the oral cavity (such as the carious process, the consumption of food, and the use of drugs) can affect the elemental compositions of the surface layers of teeth [11].

Although hydroxyapatite is the main component of teeth and bones, the structures of teeth and bones have different histological remodelling dynamics [12]. At the structural level, there are two types of bone, cortical and cancellous bone. Cancellous bone can provide information on recent exposure to metals, whereas cortical bone can accumulate trace elements over much longer periods [13]. Determining the elemental composition of cortical bone is preferred to determining the elemental composition of cancellous bone because cortical bone has a compact structure and is less sensitive to contamination during sampling and sample preparation [14]. Generally speaking, concentrations of trace elements are usually higher in cancellous bone than in cortical bone. Similarly, concentrations of trace elements are usually higher in the metaphyseal areas than in the shafts of long bones [15].

No indications have been reported of elements in the mineralogical structures of a tooth being released once the tooth has been formed [12]. In contrast, elements can be released from bone into the blood in a range of physiological and pathological situations [13].

Knowledge gaps

An impacted tooth is a fully developed tooth that has, for any of a number of reasons, not erupted and has remained entirely covered in bone tissue in the jaw [16]. Impacted teeth could be valuable for use in biomonitoring studies. An impacted tooth is isolated from the oral cavity, and blood is the only source of elements to the structure of such a tooth. The third molars in the mandible are the most commonly impacted teeth. The third molars in the mandible become completely developed when a person reaches an age of between 17 and 21 years, when all of the other teeth are present in the dental arch and bone growth is complete [9]. It is very often necessary to surgically remove impacted teeth for orthodontic or surgical reasons [17]. Removed impacted teeth are waste materials that can be used in research studies. The elemental compositions of impacted teeth are of particular interest for the reasons given above. A certain amount of overlying bone has to be removed to allow an impacted tooth to be extracted [18]. It is possible, with skilful surgery, to acquire both impacted teeth and overlying bone samples suitable for analysis. This allows calcified tissues from the same anatomical area but with different histological and physiological characteristics to be analysed. An impacted tooth and the overlying bone structure will in fact have been in direct contact with each other over the lifetime of the individual to whom they belong.

The mandibular bone has an unusual anatomy, with a relatively thick layer of cortical bone and very little cancellous bone. An impacted tooth will be covered almost exclusively with cortical bone [16, 17]. The overlying bone may be collected when an impacted tooth is removed, and the elemental compositions of the bone and tooth can be determined [18].

No information is currently available on whether heavy metal concentrations in an impacted tooth and the surrounding mandibular bone reflect heavy metal concentrations in the environment. It is difficult to acquire such information because heavy metals in tooth and bone structures can come from a range of different types of exposure that can occur simultaneously.

Potential interactions between elements within the structures of calcified tissues mean that it is necessary to determine both toxic and essential elements when biomonitoring studies are performed to investigate the effects of environmental or occupational exposure on the accumulation of elements in tissues [19].

Aim of the study

The aim of the study was to determine whether impacted mandibular teeth and the surrounding bones reflect environmental exposure to heavy metals and can be used as biomonitoring materials. To achieve this, cadmium, chromium, copper, iron, lead, manganese, and zinc were determined in samples of impacted teeth and the surrounding bone from people who will have been exposed to different ranges and concentrations of heavy metals where they live.

Methods

Patients and samples

The material used in the study consisted of 67 impacted lower third molars and 67 samples of the mandibular cortical bones surrounding the impacted teeth. The samples came from people from 18 to 40 years of age. Each person supplied one tooth and one bone sample. The samples were collected from 23 women and 11 men living in Ruda Slaska and 23 women and 10 men living in

Bielsko-Biala. Ruda Slaska and Bielsko-Biala are cities in southern Poland, 52 km apart, and polluted with heavy metals to different degrees (see Table 1) [20, 21]. A map showing the locations of Ruda Slaska and Bielsko-Biala is shown in Fig. 1.

Ruda Slaska has a population of more than 140,000, and it is in the "Upper Silesian industrial district" in which high heavy metals concentration have repeatedly been found in the air for many years [20]. The air quality is considered to be one of the best factors representing the overall environmental burden and having the most important impact on human health [22]. The economy of Ruda Slaska has been profoundly restructured, but heavy industry is still a crucial part of the economy. Bielsko-Biala has a population of more than 170,000, and is the capital of Podbeskidzie. Bielsko-Biala has a strong tourism industry and a relatively clean environment. Pollutants in Bielsko-Biala mainly come from local "low emission" sources and emissions in Slovakia and the Czech Republic transported in the atmosphere. Although, the region of Bielsko-Biala is known to have raising environmental issues concerning mainly the air quality, the data shown in Table 1 indicate that lead and cadmium in PM10 levels in the air of Bielsko-Biala are lower than concentrations of these heavy metals in the air of Ruda Slaska (0,024 ± 0,021 vs. 0,040 ± 0,015 for Pb and 0,58 ± 0,41 vs. 0,84 ± 0,45 for Cd in PM10 in year 2015; and 0,027 ± 0,021 vs. 0,044 ± 0,022 for Pb and 0,65 ± 0,53 vs. 1,40 ± 1,21 for Cd in PM10 in year 2014). It must be remembered that human teeth represent a long term accumulation of heavy metals. As the mean age of the population under the study (25,7 ± 7,2 y) and the periods of time when the wisdom teeth are formed and the rate of mineralization is the highest (between 12 and 17 years of age), Table 1 contains the historical data showing the lead levels in the air of Bielsko-Biala and Ruda Slaska in years 2002–2006. In those years the lead levels in the air of Upper Silesia Region were higher than the lead levels in the air of Bielsko-Biala. Taking into account the data shown in Table 1, we decided to use Bielsko-Biala as a reference area. As we intended to limit to the lowest possible level the influence of industry and motor traffic, only samples from people who lived from 6 to 14 km from the city centre were analysed. It must be emphasised that the area was not free from long-range emission, but free of industry with typical occupational setting in agriculture and paperwork. The participants from Bielsko-Biala were grouped into those who lived 6–10 km from the city centre (21 people) and those who lived 10–14 km from the city centre (12 people).

Each participant in the study declared that he or she had lived in either Ruda Slaska or Bielsko-Biala since birth and had never left that area for more than 2 months. All of the participants declared that they were non-smokers and had not been exposed to cigarette smoke at home (i.e., they were not passive smokers). None of the participants regularly took medication or dietary supplements. None of the participants had ever worked in an industry known to increase exposure to heavy metals. All of the participants confirmed that they were not on special diets, that they bought their food from shops, and that they did not use any food grown on their own land. The medical histories of the participants were taken into consideration, but no additional medical examinations were performed. The participants were asked about their education levels, and the participants were divided into four groups: those who had only primary education, those who had vocational education, those who had secondary education, and those who had higher education. The research project was approved by the Silesian Medical University ethics committee.

The biological samples were collected when the participants had their impacted lower third molars surgically removed at an oral surgery clinic. Each procedure was carried out under local anaesthetic by a specialist oral and maxillofacial surgeon. The mandibular bone covering an impacted tooth was cut out using a piezo-surgical unit, then the tooth was extracted using elevators and forceps. Immediately after removal, the tooth and bone samples were washed with double-distilled water, then

Table 1 The average annual PM 10, Cd in PM 10 and Pb concentrations in the air in Bielsko-Biala and Ruda Slaska [20]

	Year	2015[a]	2014[a]	2006	2005	2004	2003	2002
Pb [μg/m^3]	Bielsko-Biala	0,024 ± 0,021	0,027 ± 0,021	0,04	0,02	0,04	0,05	0,04
	Ruda Slaska	0,040 ± 0,015[b]	0,044 ± 0,022[b]	0,07	0,06	0,05	0,08	0,07
Cd in PM10 [ng/m^3]	Bielsko-Biala	0,58 ± 0,41	0,65 ± 0,53	N/A	N/A	N/A	N/A	N/A
	Ruda Slaska	0,84 ± 0,45[b]	1,40 ± 1,21[b]	N/A	N/A	N/A	N/A	N/A
PM10 [μg/m^3]	Bielsko-Biala	36,80 ± 14,54	37,92 ± 14,61	0-36	0-43	40-58	35-43	30-42
	Ruda Slaska	39,17 ± 14,30[b]	43,33 ± 15,36[b]	40-60	46-56	31-57	41-72	41-63

[a]data obtained from the database of Regional Inspectorate for Environmental Protection in Katowice (Wojewodzki Inspektorat Ochrony Srodowiska in Katowice) http://powietrze.katowice.wios.gov.pl

[b]data from the air quality monitoring station in Katowice

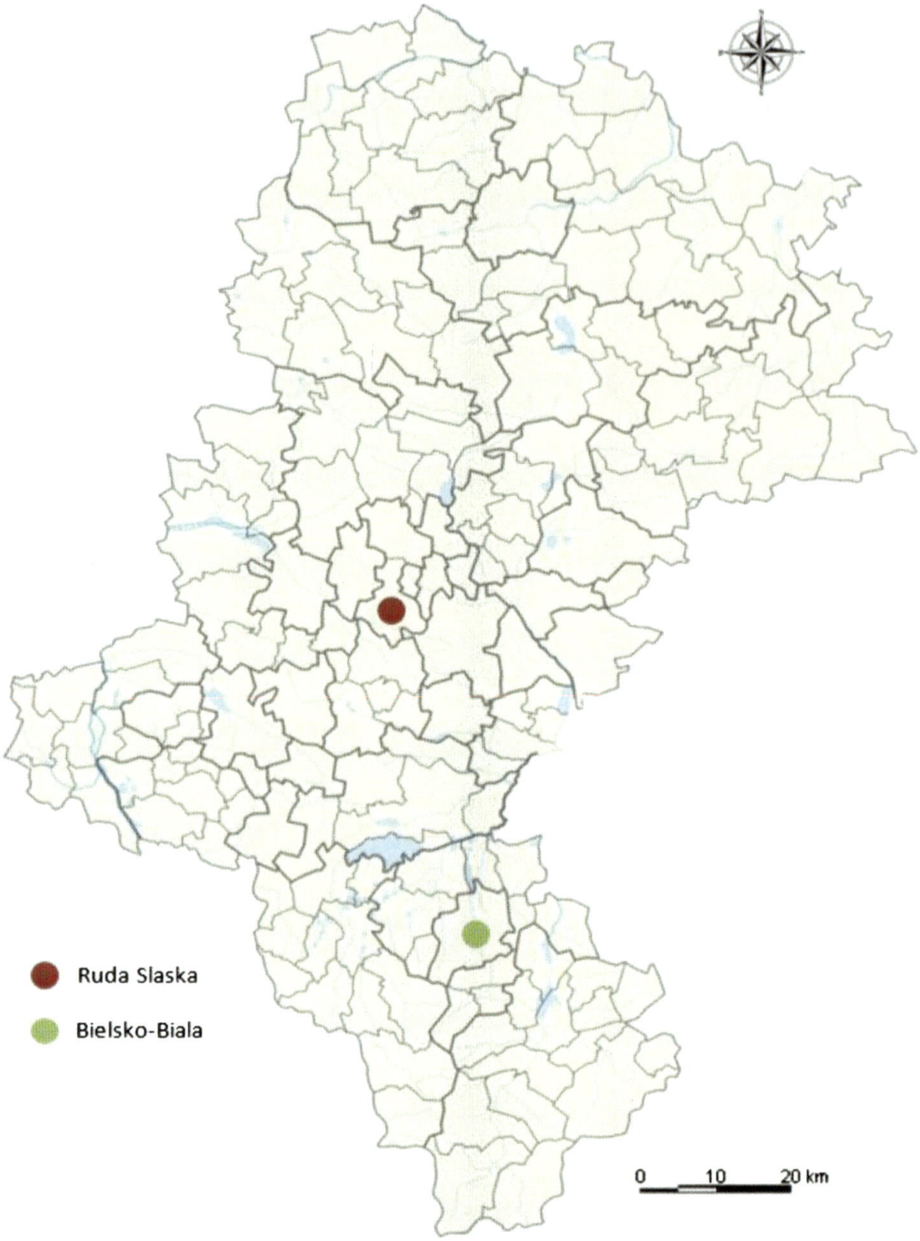

Fig. 1 A section of a map of Poland showing the location of Ruda Slaska and Bielsko-Biala

each sample was placed in a tightly sealed Teflon vessel and stored until it was prepared for analysis.

The samples were prepared following a chromium analysis procedure that has been described previously [23]. Each sample was dried at 105 °C until a constant weight was reached. Each sample was then pulverized, and the powder produced was stored in a desiccator. Each powdered sample was dried again at 105 °C for 4 h before being dissolved.

An aliquot of between 0.500 and 1.000 g of a dried and pulverized bone or tooth sample was dissolved in 3 mL of ultrapure concentrated nitric acid (Supra-Merck 65%; Merck, Darmstadt, Germany) in a Teflon vessel for 3 h at 120 °C. The clear solution produced was diluted to 10 mL with double-distilled water. All of the chemicals that were used were of the highest purity available.

Heavy metal analysis

The cadmium, chromium, copper, iron, lead, manganese, and zinc concentrations in the sample solutions were determined by flame atomization atomic absorption spectrometry using a Philips PYE Unicam SP-9 instrument (Philips, Amsterdam, The Netherlands). An air–acetylene mixture was used, and the absorption lines used for cadmium, chromium, copper, iron, lead, manganese, and zinc were 228.8, 357.9, 324.8, 248.3, 283.3, 279.5, and 231.9 nm, respectively.

Teeth and bones are histologically similar, so a certified bone meal reference material (SRM 1486; US National Institute of Standards and Technology, Gaithersburg, MD, USA) was analysed for cadmium, copper, iron, lead, manganese, and zinc and a certified bone ash reference material (SRM 1400; US National Institute of Standards and Technology) was analysed for chromium. The analyte concentrations we found and the certified concentrations are shown in Table 2. The precision of the method was close to 8%, and the accuracies for the different elements were between 3.01% and 6.99%.

Statistical analysis

The data for the teeth and bone samples were grouped by the area the donors of the samples lived in before statistical analyses were performed. The Kolmogorov–Smirnov goodness-of-fit test and plots of the results showed that concentrations of all the metals were not normally distributed. Subjecting the data to a natural logarithmic transformation caused the distributions to become normal. This allowed parametric tests to be used. The test procedures that were used have been described previously [24]. Student's t-test was performed to identify significant differences between the mean metal concentrations in the samples provided by people living in Bielsko-Biala and Ruda Slaska. Data have been treated in the same way in previous studies [8, 25, 26]. The ratios between the metal concentrations in impacted teeth and the surrounding bones ($Me_{(tooth)}/Me_{(bone)}$) were calculated, and Student's t-test was performed to identify significant differences between the ratios for the samples provided by people living in Bielsko-Biala and Ruda Slaska. Pearson's product–moment test was used to identify correlations between each element in the tooth and bone samples. Different numbers of samples were provided by men and women, so the non-parametric Mann–Whitney U test was used to determine the significances of the differences between the metal concentrations in the samples provided by men and women. Relatively few samples were analysed, so non-parametric tests were also used to determine the significances of the differences between the metal concentration in the samples provided by people with different educational backgrounds (for which the Kruskall–Wallis test was used) and between the metal concentrations in the samples provided by people living different distances from the Bielsko-Biala city centre (for which the Mann–Whitney U test was used). The statistical analyses were performed using Statistica 10.0 software (Statsoft, Tulsa, OK, USA). The statistical tests were performed using the 95% level to indicate a significant result.

Table 2 Certified and found heavy metal concentrations (µg/g) in the reference materials

Element	Certified value	Experimental value
Pb	1.335 ± 0.014	1.483 ± 0.024
Cd	0.011[a]	0.013 ± 0.010
Fe	99 ± 8	112 ± 14
Mn	1.16[a]	1.32 ± 0.36
Cr	0.03[b]	0.03 ± 0.010
Cu	0.8[a]	0.91 ± 0.07
Zn	147 ± 16	141 ± 12

SRM 1486 bone meal (Cd, Cu, Fe, Mn, Pb, and Zn concentrations) and SRM 1400 bone ash (Cr concentrations); both reference materials were supplied by the US National Institute of Standards and Technology (Gaithersburg, MD, USA)
[a]non-certified value
[b]SRM 1400 bone ash; non-certified value

Results

The 67 participants were between 18 and 40 years old. The mean ages (± the standard deviation) of the participants from Ruda Slaska and Bielsko-Biala were 24.9 ± 5.9 y (25.3 ± 5.7 years for women and 24.7 ± 6.2 years for men) and 26.1 ± 8.7 y (26.8 ± 7.9 years for women and 25.4 ± 8.5 years for men), respectively.

The mean concentrations of the seven metals that were analysed in the teeth and the bone surrounding the teeth provided by the people from the two different study areas are shown in Table 3. The Student's t-test results (the p-levels are shown in Tables 3) indicated that the cadmium and lead concentrations were significantly higher in the tooth and bone samples provided by people living in Ruda Slaska than in the samples provided by people living in Bielsko-Biala. The chromium, copper, manganese, and zinc concentrations were also significantly higher in the bone samples provided by the Ruda Slaska citizens than in the bone samples provided by the Bielsko-Biala citizens. The chromium and manganese concentrations in the bone samples from men from Ruda Slaska were significantly different from the chromium and manganese concentrations provided by women from Ruda Slaska (Table 4). There were no statistically significant differences between the metal concentrations in the impacted teeth from men and women living in Ruda Slaska (Table 4) and between the metal concentrations in bone and tooth samples from men and women living in Bielsko-Biala (Table 5). However, the reason(s) for these differences could not be identified because of the small numbers of samples provided.

No statistically significant differences were found in the metal concentrations in the teeth or bones from people living different distances from the Bielsko-Biala city centre (Table 6). No significant differences were found between the metal concentrations in samples from

Table 3 Descriptive statistics for the heavy metal concentrations (μg/g) in impacted wisdom teeth and in the bone surrounding the impacted teeth

		Samples from people living in Bielsko-Biala ($n = 33$)			Samples from people living in Ruda Slaska ($n = 34$)			p - level*
	Sample	Mean ± standard deviation	Min - Max	95% conf. limits of mean	Mean ± standard deviation	Min - Max	95% conf. limits of mean	
Pb	Teeth	10.29 ± 1.90	6.24 - 14.26	9.09 - 12.49	13.23 ± 1.93	6.26 - 18.10	11.21-15.25	0.038[a]
	Bone	3.53 ± 2.02	1.04 - 8.44	2.85 - 4.28	7.95 ± 2.66	2.06 - 13.30	7.02 - 8.88	<0.001[a]
Cd	Teeth	0.10 ± 0.02	0.07 - 0.14	0.09 - 0.12	0.12 ± 0.02	0.08 - 0.15	0.12 - 0.13	0.006[a]
	Bone	0.68 ± 0.36	0.05 - 1.38	0.55 - 0.81	0.97 ± 0.42	0.10 - 1.84	0.82 - 1.11	0.004[a]
Fe	Teeth	10.31 ± 1.99	7.14 - 14.87	9.60 - 11.01	10.48 ± 1.85	7.80 - 14.24	9.83 - 11.12	0.677
	Bone	19.08 ± 12.69	4.24 - 48.16	14.58 - 23. 58	17.61 ± 9.23	3.74 - 45.57	14.39 - 20.83	0.588
Mn	Teeth	3.58 ± 0.45	2.99 - 4.52	3.42 - 3.74	3.76 ± 0.45	2.94 - 4.69	3.60 - 3.92	0.960
	Bone	1.64 ± 1.10	0.12 - 4.03	1.25 - 2.03	4.05 ± 2.36	0.29 - 7.17	3.23 - 4.87	<0.001[a]
Cr	Teeth	5.73 ± 1.65	3.06 - 8.36	5.14 - 6.32	5.54 ± 1.57	3.63 - 8.67	4.99 - 6.09	0.767
	Bone	1.76 ± 1.70	0.19 - 13.74	0.96 - 2.56	3.79 ± 4.20	0.15 - 14.72	2.33- 5.26	0.016[a]
Cu	Teeth	8.83 ± 1.30	6.02 - 11.58	8.37 - 9.29	9.13 ± 1.11	6.02 -11.30	8.75 - 9.52	0.359
	Bone	6.86 ± 3.87	1.49 - 15.60	5.49 - 8.23	13.77 ± 7.73	4.39 - 27.74	11.07 - 16.47	<0.001[a]
Zn	Teeth	297.31 ± 44.73	201.36 - 382.02	281.44 - 313.17	314.87 ± 59.37	208.54 - 439.30	294.16 - 335.59	0.113
	Bone	155.76 ± 38.38	72.99 - 237.02	142.15 - 169.36	229.10 ± 107.96	85.78 - 443.74	191.43 - 266.77	<0.001[a]

n number of samples

* p-levels, determined using Student's t-tests, used to identify statistically significant differences between the mean heavy metal concentrations in the samples provided by people living in Bielsko-Biala and Ruda Slaska

[a] indicates the heavy metal concentrations in the samples provided by people living in Bielsko-Biala and Ruda Slaska were significantly different

people with different educational levels in either Ruda Slaska or Bielsko-Biala (Tables 7 and 8).

Descriptive statistics for the $Me_{(tooth)}/Me_{(bone)}$ ratios are shown in Table 9. Student's t-tests indicated that the differences between the ratios for the samples provided by people living in Ruda Slaska and Bielsko-Biala were not significantly different. Pearson's correlation coefficients for the relationships between the metal concentrations in the tooth and bone samples are shown in Table 10. Only the cadmium concentrations in the tooth and bone samples positively correlated, and this relationship was only found for the samples provided by people living in Ruda Slaska.

Discussion

The exposure of an organism to heavy metals can be assessed by analysing a range of tissues. Most tissues, however, mainly provide information on recent exposure, and the metal concentrations can vary considerably depending on the time between exposure and sample collection. For environmental biomonitoring, it is important to analyse tissues that reflect chronic exposure. Heavy metal concentrations in bones and teeth (the main mineral component of which is hydroxyapatite) reflect chronic exposure. Mineral turnover will be much faster in bones than in teeth because of the morphological and physiological

Table 4 Heavy metal concentrations (μg/g) in the samples provided by women and men living in Ruda Slaska

	Impacted teeth ($n = 34$)				Bone surrounding the impacted teeth ($n = 34$)			
Element	Women ($n = 23$) Median	Men ($n = 11$) Median	U-value	p - level*	Women ($n = 23$) Median	Men ($n = 11$) Median	U-value	p - level*
Pb	9.30	8.83	118	0.768	8.05	6.63	91	0.197
Cd	0.12	0.13	99	0.320	0.86	0.87	111	0.580
Fe	9.99	9.99	120	0.839	15.32	20.84	92	0.210
Mn	3.85	3.84	125	0.970	5.29	1.70	66	0.027[a]
Cr	4.72	5.79	83	0.113	4.47	1.31	51	0.006[a]
Cu	9.02	9.10	114	0.658	15.30	8.08	68	0.052
Zn	318.15	284.26	107	0.484	221.19	160.61	67	0.059

n number of samples

* p-levels, estimated using the Mann–Whitney U test, used to identify statistically significant differences between the metal concentrations in the samples provided by women and men

[a] indicates the mean concentrations in the samples provided by women and men were significantly different

Table 5 Heavy metal concentrations (μg/g) in the samples provided by women and men living in Bielsko-Biala

	Impacted teeth ($n = 33$)				Bone surrounding the impacted teeth ($n = 33$)			
Element	Women ($n = 23$) Median	Men ($n = 10$) Median	U-value	p - level*	Women ($n = 23$) Median	Men ($n = 10$) Median	U-value	p - level*
Pb	10.03	11.54	95.50	0.456	4.04	1.78	95.00	0.444
Cd	0.11	0.12	87.50	0.290	0.71	0.50	85.00	0.247
Fe	10.52	8.87	67.50	0.065	14.18	18.92	102.00	0.624
Mn	3.65	3.26	96.50	0.480	1.57	0.99	92.00	0.378
Cr	4.72	6.84	59.50	0.061	1.45	0.99	86.00	0.264
Cu	8.86	8.72	106.50	0.753	7.36	3.98	88.00	0.299
Zn	282.67	306.77	86.50	0.272	162.60	160.36	104.00	0.680

n the number of samples

* *p*-levels, estimated using the Mann–Whitney U test, used to identify statistically significant differences between the metal concentrations in the samples provided by women and men

characteristics of the tissues, so bones will reflect more recent exposure to heavy metals than will teeth. It is hardly possible for metals to be released from the structures of teeth.

Comparison with previous research

Teeth have been used to indicate environmental exposure to metals in many studies [27–29]. Deciduous teeth have mainly been used in such studies [7, 8]. Deciduous teeth meet the criterion that a good biomonitoring material should be easily accessible. In the study described here, we were able to use impacted permanent teeth and the surrounding mandibular bones as biomonitoring tissues.

We found differences in the cadmium and lead concentrations in the tooth samples provided by people living in the different study areas. The cadmium and lead concentrations in teeth provided by people living in Bielsko-Biala were 0.10 ± 0.02 and 10.29 ± 1.90 μg/g, respectively, and the cadmium and lead concentrations in teeth provided by people living in Ruda Slaska were 0.12 ± 0.02 and 13.23 ± 1.93 μg/g, respectively (Table 3). One reason for this could have been different environmental burdens of cadmium and lead in Bielsko-Biala and Ruda Slaska. Similar results have previously been found for deciduous teeth [7, 25] and permanent teeth [30–32]. In those studies, the cadmium and lead concentrations in teeth were found to reflect the cadmium and lead concentrations in different environmental compartments. The heavy metal concentrations in the samples of mandibular bone we analysed were within the concentration ranges found in other studies in which human bones have been analysed [4]. The mandibular bone samples we analysed reflected the cadmium, chromium, copper, lead, manganese, and zinc concentrations in environmental media in the areas in which the people who provided the samples lived.

A number of factors related to the sex of a person may affect heavy metal concentrations in the person's teeth. These factors include hormone concentrations [33, 34] and tooth formation and eruption times [9]. However, no differences have been found in the concentrations of a number of elements in deciduous and permanent teeth in males and females in a number of studies [35–37]. We found no differences in the heavy metal

Table 6 Heavy metal concentrations (μg/g) in the samples from people living different distances from the centre of Bielsko-Biala

	Impacted teeth ($n = 33$)				Bone surrounding the impacted teeth ($n = 33$)			
Element	6-10 km ($n = 21$) Median	10-14 km ($n = 12$) Median	U-value	p - level*	6-10 km ($n = 21$) Median	10-14 km ($n = 12$) Median	U-value	p - level*
Pb	10.79	10.03	125.50	0.125	3.74	4.36	88	0.160
Cd	0.10	0.11	87.00	0.149	0.62	0.77	85	0.129
Fe	11.32	8.98	81.50	0.099	14.52	13.53	101	0.359
Mn	3.45	3.42	104.00	0.421	1.14	1.69	98	0.312
Cr	4.68	5.39	100.50	0.349	1.29	1.49	104	0.421
Cu	8.79	8.86	113.50	0.653	7.09	5.91	125	0.985
Zn	293.94	294.23	98.50	0.312	170.71	156.67	125	0.985

n number of samples

* *p*-levels, estimated using the Mann–Whitney U test, used to identify statistically significant differences between the metal concentrations in the samples provided by people living different distances from the centre of Bielsko-Biala

Table 7 Heavy metal concentrations (μg/g) in the samples from people with different levels of education living in Ruda Slaska

	Impacted teeth ($n = 34$)						Bone surrounding the impacted teeth ($n = 34$)					
	Educational level						Educational level					
Element	Primary ($n = 6$) Median	Vocational ($n = 8$) Median	Secondary ($n = 11$) Median	Higher ($n = 9$) Median	H-value	p - level*	Primary ($n = 6$) Median	Vocational ($n = 8$) Median	Secondary ($n = 11$) Median	Higher ($n = 9$) Median	H-value	p - level*
Pb	14.63	12.41	11.89	11.83	9.88	0.196	7.69	7.22	7.80	8.04	1.171	0.982
Cd	0.12	0.12	0.14	0.11	7.90	0.481	0.64	0.86	1.20	0.91	4.112	0.249
Fe	9.14	9.74	9.94	11.92	7.47	0.098	25.45	18.69	15.32	13.37	7.772	0.873
Mn	3.84	3.84	3.85	3.94	1.58	0.901	3.82	3.42	4.23	3.91	1.653	0.884
Cr	5.09	5.79	4.66	5.79	4.32	0.229	1.34	1.99	4.47	1.45	4.121	0.249
Cu	8.60	9.05	9.84	8.77	1.58	0.664	10.40	10.56	15.08	8.45	1.980	0.577
Zn	356.55	274.80	288.92	321.86	4.65	0.207	136.11	187.74	212.39	210.62	2.691	0.442

n number of samples

* p-levels, estimated using the ANOVA Kruskal–Wallis test, used to identify statistically significant differences between the metal concentrations in the samples provided by people with different levels of education living in Ruda Slaska

concentrations in the impacted teeth from men and women from either Ruda Slaska or Bielsko-Biala (Tables 4 and 5, respectively). We found significant differences in the chromium and manganese concentrations in the mandibular bone samples from men and women living in Ruda Slaska (the more polluted study area). These differences could have been caused by men and women having different bone mineralization patterns, dietary habits, hormone concentrations, and occupational exposures. Unfortunately, these factors were not able to be analysed in this study.

We calculated of the $Me_{(tooth)}/Me_{(bone)}$ ratios for our samples. The ratios were higher for the samples from the residents of Bielsko-Biala than for the samples from the residents of Ruda Slaska, but the differences were not statistically significant (Table 9). However, the greatest differences between the ratios were obtained for lead (3,32 times higher ratio for the citizens of Bielsko-Biala), manganese (2,06 times higher ratio for the citizens of Bielsko-Biala) and copper (2,15 times higher ratio for the citizens of Bielsko-Biala). As these are the elements which easily substitute calcium in hydroxyapatite [19]. As bone reveals faster turnover of numerous elements, the lower levels of lead, manganese and copper are characteristic of the bones from the citizens of cleaner areas and influence significantly the $Me_{(tooth)}/Me_{(bone)}$ ratios. It would be valuable to compare the ratios obtained from our study to the results from other researchers, but to our best knowledge this is the first research work analysing occurrence of heavy metals in impacted wisdom teeth and the bone surrounding the teeth derived from the same individuals. The correlation analysis was performed to allow relationships between the metal concentrations in the samples to be assessed and interrelationships to be identified (Table 10). A significant positive correlation was only found between the cadmium concentrations in the tooth and bone samples from the inhabitants of Ruda Slaska (the Pearson's correlation coefficient was 0.36). This indicated that the cadmium concentration in the tooth structure increased as the

Table 8 Heavy metal concentrations (μg/g) in the samples from people with different levels of education living in Bielsko-Biala

	Impacted teeth ($n = 33$)						Bone surrounding the impacted teeth ($n = 33$)					
	Educational level						Educational level					
Element	Primary ($n = 7$) Median	Vocational ($n = 11$) Median	Secondary ($n = 9$) Median	Higher ($n = 6$) Median	H-value	p - level*	Primary ($n = 7$) Median	Vocational ($n = 11$) Median	Secondary ($n = 9$) Median	Higher ($n = 6$) Median	H-value	p - level*
Pb	14.08	13.20	12.02	11.70	5.126	0.162	3.44	3.81	4.54	4.11	3.460	0.326
Cd	0.12	0.11	0.12	0.10	2.109	0.549	0.34	0.65	0.84	0.67	13.959	0.096
Fe	8.72	9.92	8.79	11.94	7.660	0.536	13.44	13.16	12.05	16.70	8.352	0.046
Mn	3.26	3.89	3.19	3.73	6.063	0.109	0.86	1.22	1.59	1.52	2.054	0.561
Cr	5.95	5.39	4.72	4.54	2.956	0.398	0.86	1.45	1.96	1.12	4.016	0.259
Cu	8.25	8.86	8.86	9.16	2.208	0.530	6.93	7.09	8.52	4.76	2.025	0.567
Zn	328.10	263.94	282.67	293.94	6.303	0.097	101.80	172.83	162.60	165.19	11.124	0.091

n number of samples

* p-levels, estimated using the ANOVA Kruskal–Wallis test, used to identify statistically significant differences between the metal concentrations in the samples provided by people with different levels of education living in Bielsko-Biala

Table 9 Descriptive statistics for the $Me_{(tooth)}/Me_{(bone)}$ ratios (unitless) for the samples provided by people living in Bielsko-Biala and Ruda Slaska

	Coefficients $Me_{(tooth)}/Me_{(bone)}$ for the biological material from people living in Bielsko-Biala ($n = 33$)			Coefficients $Me_{(tooth)}/Me_{(bone)}$ for the biological material from people living in Ruda Slaska ($n = 34$)			p - level*
	Mean ± standard deviation	Min - Max	95% conf. limits of mean	Mean ± standard deviation	Min - Max	95% conf. limits of mean	
Pb	4.89 ± 4.14	0.97 - 17.49	3.42 - 6.35	1.47 ± 0.78	0.65 - 4.29	1.19 - 1.74	0.254
Cd	0.32 ± 0.22	0.08 - 2.43	0.15 - 0.48	0.19 ± 0.11	0.07 - 1.43	0.10 - 0.27	0.081
Fe	0.82 ± 0.59	0.18 - 2.80	0.61 - 1.02	0.78 ± 0.52	0.20 - 2.95	0.60 - 0.97	0.438
Mn	3.93 ± 2.53	0.88 - 26.36	2.32 - 5.55	1.91 ± 1.40	0.44 - 11.80	1.07 - 2.75	0.078
Cr	6.04 ± 3.61	0.59 - 31.28	3.69 - 8.38	4.47 ± 3.14	0.31 - 33.52	2.32 - 6.62	0.295
Cu	1.98 ± 1.59	0.50 -7.01	1.41 - 2.54	0.92 ± 0.56	0.30 - 2.57	0.73 - 1.12	0.059
Zn	2.08 ± 0.81	1.12 - 4.50	1.80 - 2.37	1.68 ± 0.89	0.67 - 4.47	1.37 - 1.99	0.086

n number of samples

* *p*-levels, estimated using Student's *t*-test, used to identify statistically significant differences between the $Me_{(tooth)}/Me_{(bone)}$ ratios for the samples provided by people living in Bielsko-Biala and Ruda Slaska

cadmium concentration in the surrounding bone increased. There could be closer relationships between heavy metal concentrations in teeth and mandibular bones in areas that are heavily polluted with heavy metals, although discrimination mechanisms tend to break down when an organism is exposed to high concentrations of heavy metals, and this decreases the number of correlations that are observed in tissues within the organism [19].

Strengths and limitations

The original aspect of the study was the analysis of heavy metals in impacted wisdom teeth and the mandibular bones surrounding the impacted teeth. To the best of our knowledge, no previous studies of heavy metals in these tissues in relation to the concentrations in the environment have been performed. However, there are numerous research works on occurrence of heavy metals in tooth hard tissues only, but they do not contain any information about metal concentration in bone surrounding the teeth [38–40]. Only a small number of samples could be analysed because of the generally limited indications for the surgical removal of wisdom teeth. We only analysed samples from people who declared that they had never worked in industries involving increased exposure to heavy metals, had never smoked cigarettes, did not regularly take medication or dietary supplements, and ate only food from shops (i.e., not grown on their own land). The participants all declared that they had not been regularly exposed to second-hand cigarette smoke recently, but most could not be sure that they had not been regularly exposed to second-hand smoke in childhood. These data were collected from the participants' medical histories, and no additional medical examinations were performed. These are undoubtedly important limitations of the study. It seems that impacted teeth and the surrounding alveolar bone can be used to assess environmental exposure to heavy metals in an area in which a person lives. This conclusion, however, must be verified in future research projects designed to exclude the possibility of additional dietary, occupational, and other types of exposure to heavy metals.

Table 10 Pearson's correlation coefficients describing relationships between metal concentrations in teeth and the bone surrounding the teeth

	Pb	Cd	Fe	Mn	Cr	Cu	Zn
Ruda Slaska	0.02	0.36*	-0.22	0.03	-0.04	-0.10	0.17
Bielsko-Biala	-0.14	-0.23	0.09	0.29	0.23	-0.05	-0.31

* indicates the correlation was significant at $p < 0.05$

Conclusions

The results of this study indicated that impacted mandibular teeth and the surrounding mandibular bone may reflect the environmental exposure of a person to cadmium and lead. An impacted tooth is isolated from the oral environment, so the elemental composition of the tooth will represent only elements delivered in blood while the tooth was forming. It is possible to obtain bone from around an impacted tooth when the tooth is surgically removed. The physiological and histological characteristics of bones and teeth mean that elements will be turned over more quickly in bone than in teeth. In this study, we found significant differences between the cadmium, chromium, copper, lead, manganese, and zinc concentrations in mandibular bones from people living in two areas in southern Poland with different environmental burdens of the heavy metals. The metal concentrations in the impacted teeth and surrounding bones did not correlate except for the cadmium concentrations in the samples provided by people living in the more polluted area (Ruda Slaska). More research is required to prove that impacted mandibular teeth and the surrounding bones can be used to assess environmental exposure to heavy metals. Future studies must exclude sources other than the blood of heavy metals to impacted teeth and the surrounding bones.

Acknowledgements
The authors would like to acknowledge help collecting the biological material used in the study provided by the staff of the Clinic of Oral and Maxillofacial Surgery in Ruda Slaska. The authors thank PhD student Jakub Galaszek for his involvement in the clinical part of the project.

Funding
This work was funded by the Medical University of Silesia in Katowice (contract no. KNW-1-124/K/4/0).

Authors' contributions
PM, AF, and BM conceived and designed the experiments. PM carried out the surgical procedures and prepared the biological material for the laboratory analyses. AF performed the sample treatments in the laboratory and determined the concentrations of the elements in the prepared samples. PM and BM analysed the data and wrote this paper. All authors read and approved the final manuscript.

Competing interests
The authors declare that they have no competing interest.

Author details
[1]Institute of Engineering Materials and Biomaterials, Silesian University of Technology, 18a Konarskiego str, 44-100 Gliwice, Poland. [2]Department of Toxicology, Medical University of Silesia, 4 Jagiellonska str, 41-200 Sosnowiec, Poland. [3]Institute of Medicine, Katowice School of Economics, 3 Harcerzy Wrzesnia str, 40-659 Katowice, Poland.

References
1. Nriagu JO, Pacyna JM. Quantitative assessment of worldwide contamination of air, water and soils by trace metals. Nature. 1988;333:134–9.
2. Larsen EH, Andersen NL, Moller A, Petersen A, Mortensen GK, Petersen J. Monitoring the content and intake of trace elements from food in Denmark. Food Addit Contam. 2002;1:33–46.
3. Purves D. Trace-element Contamination of the Environment. New York, NY, United States: Elsevier Science Pub. Co., Inc; 1985.
4. Castro W, Hoogewerff J, Latkoczy C, Almirall JR. Application of laser ablation (LA-ICP-SF-MS) for the elemental analysis of bone and teeth samples for discrimination purposes. Forensic Sci Int. 2010;195:17–27.
5. Chan TJH, Gutierrez C, Ogunseitan OA. Metallic Burden of Deciduous Teeth and Childhood Behavioral Deficits. Int J Environ Res Public Health. 2015;12: 6771–87.
6. Leventouri T, Antonakos A, Kyriacou A, Venturelli R, Liarokapis E, Perdikatsis V. Crystal structure studies of human dental apatite as a function of age. Int J Biol Materials. 2009;2009:1–17.
7. Bayo J, Moreno-Grau S, Martinez MJ, Moreno J, Angosto JM, Guillen-Perez JJ, Garcia-Marcos L, Moreno-Clavel J. Electroanalytical determination of cadmium and lead in deciduous teeth after microwave oven digestion procedure. J AOAC Int. 2001;84:111–6.
8. Hernandez-Guerrero JC, Jimenez-Farfan MD, Belmont R, Ledesma-Montes C, Baez A. Lead levels in primary teeth of children living in Mexico City. Int J Paediatr Dent. 2004;14:175–81.
9. Magnusson BO, Persliden B. Development and its aberrations. In: Magnusson BO, editor. Pedodontics: a systematic approach. Kopenhagen: Munksgaard; 1981. p. 42–54.
10. Bearer CF. How are children different from adults? Environ Health Perspect. 1995;103:7–12.
11. Tvinnereim HM, Eide R, Riise T. Heavy metals in human primary teeth: some factors influencing the metal concentrations. Sci Total Environ. 2000;255:21–7.
12. Hill PA. Bone remodelling. Br J Orthod. 1998;25:101–7.
13. Pye K. Isotope and trace element analysis of human teeth and bones for forensic purposes. In: Pye K, Croft DJ, editors. Forensic Geoscience—Principles, Techniques and Applications. London: Geological Society Publishing House; 2004.
14. Teitelbaum SL. Bone resorption by osteoblasts. Science. 2000;289:1504–8.
15. Dahl SG, Allain P, Marie PJ, Mauras Y, Boivin G, Ammann P, Tsouderos Y, Delmas PD, Christiansen C. Incorporation and distribution of strontium in bone. Bone. 2001;28:446–53.
16. Rafetto LK. Managing Impacted Third Molars. Atlas Oral Maxillofac Surg Clin North Am. 2015;27:363–71.
17. de Carvalho RW F, de Araújo Filho RC A, Vasconcelos BC. Assessment of factors associated with surgical difficulty during removal of impacted maxillary third molars. J Oral Maxillofac Surg. 2013;71:839–45.
18. Mantovani E, Arduino PG, Schierano G, Ferrero G, Gallesio G, Mozzati M, Russo A, Scully C, Carossa S. A split-mouth randomized clinical trial to evaluate the performance of piezosurgery compared with traditional technique in lower wisdom tooth removal. J Oral Maxillofac Surg. 2014;72: 1890–7.
19. Kwapulinski J, Brodziak B, Bogunia M. Relative change of elements in human osseous tissue. Bull Environ Contam Toxicol. 2003;70:1089–96.
20. Szczygiel A, Pillich A, Straszak K, editors. Estimation of the air quality in Silesian voivodiship in years 2002-2006 (in Polish: Ocena jakości powietrza w województwie śląskim w latach 2002-2006). Katowice: Wojewódzki Inspektorat Ochrony Środowiska w Katowicach; 2007.
21. http://powietrze.katowice.wios.gov.pl. Accessed 20 Nov 2016.
22. Bajor R, Sosnowska M, Tyczyński A. Atmospheric pollution in Silesian Voivodiship in years 2000-2001 [in Polish]. Katowice: Epidemiological Department in Katowice; 2002.
23. Malara P, Kwapuliński J. Determination of chromium in human premolar teeth by flame atomic absorption spectrometry. Chem Anal. 2005;50:481–6.
24. Miller JC, Miller JN. Statistics for analytical chemists. 3rd ed. London: Ellis Horwood Pub; 1993.
25. Gil F, Facio A, Villanneva E, Perez ML, Tojo R, Gil A. The association of tooth lead content with dental health factors. Sci Total Environ. 1996;192:183–91.
26. Malara P, Kwapuliński J, Malara B. The influence of lead on occurrence of some essential elements in teeth. Acta Toxicol. 2004;12:47–53.
27. Brown CJ, Chenery SR, Smith B, Mason C, Tomkins A, Roberts GJ, Sserunjogi L, Tiberindwa JV. Environmental influences on the trace element content of teeth - implications for disease and nutritional status. Arch Oral Biol. 2004;49: 705–17.
28. Oprea C, Szalanski PJ, Gustova MV, Oprea IA, Buzguta V. Multivariate comparison of elemental concentrations in human teeth. Appl Radiat Isotopes. 2009;67:2142–5.
29. Mora AM, Arora M, Harley KG, Kogut K, Parra K, Hernández-Bonilla D, Gunier RB, Bradman A, Smith DR, Eskenazi B. Prenatal and postnatal manganese teeth levels and neurodevelopment at 7, 9, and 10.5 years in the CHAMACOS cohort. Environ Int. 2015;84:39–54.
30. Alomary A, Al-Momani IF, Massadeh AM. Lead and cadmium in human teeth from Jordan by atomic absorption spectrometry: Some factors influencing their concentrations. Sci Total Environ. 2006;369:69–75.
31. Arruda-Neto JDT, Geraldo LP, Prado GR, Garcia F, Bittencourt-Oliveira MC, Sarkis JES, Martinez-Lusardo F, Lima-Cazorla L, Rosa-Medero D, Rodrigues TE, Genofre GC. Study of metals transfer from environment using teeth as biomonitor. Environ Int. 2010;36:243–6.
32. Malara P, Kwapulinski J, Malara B. Do the levels of selected metals differ significantly between the roots of carious and non-carious teeth? Sci Total Environ. 2006;369:59–68.
33. Rahnama M, Błoniarz J. Changes of the calcium metabolism in mineralized tissues of rats during experimental postmenopausal osteoporosis. Bull Vet Instytut Pulawy. 2004;48:467–70.
34. Rahnama M, Marciniak A. Influence of estrogen deficiency on the level of magnesium in rat mandible and teeth. Bull Vet Instytut Pulawy. 2002;46:267–71.
35. Halling A, Lofman O, Nosratabadi AR, Tagesson C, Oster B. Aluminum concentration in deciduous teeth is dependent on tooth type and dental status. Acta Odontol Scand. 2001;59:356–60.

36. Bayo J, Moreno-Grau S, Martinez MJ, Moreno J, Angosto JM, Guillen-Perez JJ, Garcia-Marcos L, Moreno-Clavel J. Environmental and physiological factors affecting lead and cadmium levels in deciduous teeth. Arch Environ Contam Toxicol. 2001;41:247–54.
37. Nowak B, Chmielnicka J. Relationship of lead and cadmium to essential elements in hair, teeth and nails of environmentally exposed people. Ecotoxicol Environ Saf. 2000;46:265–74.
38. Arora M. The spatial distribution of lead in teeth as a biomarker of prenatal and neonatal lead exposure. PhD thesis; University of Sydney, Faculty of Dentistry; 2005.
39. Gulson BL. Tooth analyses of sources and intensity of lead exposure in children. Environ Health Perspect. 1996;104:306–12.
40. Shepherd TJ, Dirks W, Manmee C, Hodgson S, Banks DA, Averley P, Pless-Mulloli T. Reconstructing the life-time lead exposure in children using dentine in deciduous teeth. Sci Total Environ. 2012;15:214–22.

6

Health status of male steel workers at an electric arc furnace (EAF)

Roberto Cappelletti[1*], Marcello Ceppi[2], Justina Claudatus[1] and Valerio Gennaro[1,2]

Abstract

Background: The aim of this retrospective cohort study was to determine if the workers of an Electric Arc Furnace (EAF), which recycles scrap, had higher mortality and morbidity due to possible exposure to pollutants at work. EAFs do not run on coke ovens. In EAFs 40 % of the particulate matter (PM) is made up of PM $_{2.5}$. The foundry dust contained iron, aluminum, zinc, manganese, lead, chromium, nickel, cadmium, mercury, arsenic, polycyclic aromatic hydrocarbons (PAHs), polychlorinated biphenyls and dioxins.

Methods: *Mortality study*: a cohort of 331 exposed workers (6731 person-years) was studied from 19/03/1979 to 31/12/2009 (mean follow up 20.7 years). The group of exposed workers was compared to the general population and to a small control group of 32 workers from the same company.
Morbidity study: rates of exemption from health fee for the seven major diseases of 235 exposed workers were compared to the rates of exemption in the Province of Trento.

Results: *Mortality study*: an excess mortality was found in the exposed workers as compared to the *general population* (SMR 1.13; 95 % CI: 0.76–1.62; 29 deaths) and to the *internal group* (RR 2.34; 95 % CI: 0.39–95.7). The mortality rate was increased for *all tumours* (SMR 1.36; 95 % CI: 0.75–2.29; 14 cases), for lung cancer (SMR 3.35; 95 % CI 1.45–6.60; 8 cases), for *ischemic heart disease* (SMR 1.27; 95 % CI: 0.35–3.26; 4 cases), for *chronic liver disease* (SMR 1.16; 95 % CI: 0.14–4.20; 2 cases) and for *injury and poisoning* (SMR 1.32; 95 % CI: 0.48–2.88; 6 cases).
Morbidity study: there was a statistically significant increase of diabetes, rheumatoid arthritis, hypertension and cardiovascular diseases in exposed workers.

Conclusions: With the limitations of this relatively small cohort, we found a statistically significant increase of diabetes, cardiovascular diseases and deaths due to lung cancer in exposed workers. These findings cannot be explained by PAH exposure alone; metal particulates are the most important pollutants in the working area of EAFs. A reliable method for measuring metal PM in tissues is urgently needed for exposure assessment. This study underlines the necessity to maximize the standards of security toward *foundry dusts/diffuse emission*. Further studies on EAF's are needed to confirm our findings and to increase statistical power.

Keywords: Steel workers, Electric arc furnace (EAF), Diffuse emission, Injury, Diabetes, Hypertension, Cardiovascular disease, Foundry dust, Lung cancer, Rheumatoid arthritis

Background

The correlation between increased rate of mortality for some tumours (mainly for lung cancer) and working in a steel foundry is well-known [1–13]. In 1987 the International Agency for Research on Cancer (IARC) classified iron and steel founding as being carcinogenic to humans (Group 1) [13]. There is still no agreement on which of the following agents (alone or in combination with) are responsible for the adverse effects on health in steel workers, i.e. polycyclic aromatic hydrocarbons (PAHs) and silica [2, 6, 11, 12], chromium and nickel [3, 9, 11, 12], iron dust and mixture of dusts [2], oil mist [2, 10], welding fumes [2, 11], particulate matter (PM) containing nickel and arsenic [14]. The Electric Arc Furnaces (EAFs) play an increasingly important role in modern steel production. Today the percentage of electric arc furnace

* Correspondence: cappellettiroberto@valsugana.com
[1]International Society of Doctors for the Environment (ISDE Italy), via della Fioraia 17/19, 52100 Arezzo, Italy
Full list of author information is available at the end of the article

steel of the overall steel production in the EU-27 is 41.8 % [15]. In Italy with 61 % and in Spain with 77 %, the production of EAF steel is significantly higher than steel production via the blast furnace/basic oxygen furnace route [15]. In Italy there are 35 EAFs which employ 40,000 adepts. EAFs do not run on coke ovens. A coke oven produces, benzo-[a]-pyrene, benzene, coke dust and other PAHs, which may cause lung tumours [16–18]. These facts may generate the misleading idea that EAFs, not been equipped with a coke oven, are less hazardous to health. In iron foundries the proportion of ultrafine particle is considerably higher as compared to outdoor ambient air [19]. In EAFs, 40 % of the particulate matter (PM) is made up of $PM_{2.5}$ [20]. Ample data has been published on the damage caused by $PM_{2.5}$ and ultrafine PM (PM $_{<0.1}$) in humans [21]. $PM_{2.5}$ has been recently classified by IARC as being carcinogenic for humans (Group 1) [22]. Metal particulate matter poses additional risks [23–25]: it can persist over a long period of time both in the environment and in the body tissues [26, 27]. Metal content enhances oxidative stress and promotes the release of pro-inflammatory mediators [24]. Evidence of increased DNA damage and lipid peroxidation through oxidative stress has been found in foundry workers [28]. Long term exposure of steel workers to air particles containing nickel or arsenic can induce histone modification as an epigenetic mechanism leading to cancer [14]. In EAFs there is also an exposure to polychlorinated-biphenyls (PCBs) and polychlorinated dibenzo-p-dioxin/dibenzofurans (PCDD/Fs) [29, 30]. As of yet no epidemiological occupational studies have been carried out in EAFs. This type of steel foundry could represent an ideal model for studying the effect on health of the metal particulate matter. In the present study we report the data of mortality and morbidity of an EAF located in an alpine valley in the municipality of Borgo Valsugana (Italy). We tested the hypothesis that the various substances in Table 1, released as fine and ultrafine PM through *diffuse emissions*, could have produced adverse health effects in the workers. By definition *diffuse emissions* occur during regular operations, as opposed to *fugitive emissions* that happen during irregular operations [15].

EAF characteristics

The EAF of Borgo Valsugana, in the Province of Trento (Trentino), Italy, produces roughly 550,000 tons/year (110 tons/h) of semi-finished products (steel billets) from scrap recycling. At the beginning of the activity in 1979, when working only on a 4^{Th} hole extraction, up to 80 Kg of dust per hour were estimated to be released into the environment as *diffuse emissions*. There have been several technical interventions throughout the years and a doghouse and canopy hoods were installed. In 2011 total quantities of *diffuse emissions* were evaluated to be 2–5 kg/h of dust, as compared to 0.2–0.6 kg/h present in the channelled emissions [31]. Emissions from this steel foundry were found to be present in a perimeter of 2 km around the foundry, containing PCDD/F and PCB [32]. *Diffuse emissions* in EAFs arise mainly from the charging of the oven and can be minimized by isolating the oven area and by

Table 1 Composition of foundry dust[a] and corresponding toxicological data

Elements	mg/kg of dusts	% of total	IARC Classification[b]	non-cancer health effects
Iron (Fe)	197000	78		Intestine, liver, heart
Aluminium (Al)	18970	7.64		Central Nervous System (CNS), bone
Zinc (Zn)	14340	5.68		Intestine, genitourinary, CNS [67, 73]
Manganese (Mn)	12500	4.95		CNS [74]
Total hydrocarbons	2960	1.17	(see P.A.H.)	(see P.A.H.)
Lead (Pb)	2860	1.13	2A (inorganic compounds) and 2B	CNS, liver, kidney [75]
Chromium (Cr) (total)	2230	0.88	1	Skin, bone, kidney [75]
Copper (Cu)	810	0.32		Liver, kidney, skin, bone, teeth
Nickel (Ni)	510	0.20	1 (compounds) and 2B	Skin, bone, teeth, diabetes [25, 56]
Cadmium (Cd)	30	0.0118	1	Liver, kidney, eye, bone, diabetes [57]
P.A.H.	3.66–44.67	0.009	1 (benzo[a]pyrene), 2A, 2B and 3	Heart (attack), teratogenic [16]
Mercury (Hg)	9	0.0035	2B (methyl mercury) and 3	CNS, liver, kidney, diabetes [56]
Arsenic (As)	4	0.0015	1	CNS, diabetes [56]
Polychlorinated biphenyls (PCB)	0.092–0.693	0.0001	1	Endocrine disruptor, teratogenic
Dioxins (PCDD/F)	107.8 ng/TEQ	/	1	Endocrine disruptor, teratogenic [44]

[a]from Agenzia Provinciale per la Protezione dell'Ambiente (APPA) of Trento, 12th December 2006 (dioxins excluded)
[b]International Agency for Research on Cancer (IARC) classification: group 1: carcinogenic for humans; group 2A: probable carcinogenic for humans; group 2B: possible carcinogenic for humans; Group 3: unclassified as to carcinogenic for humans

capturing them and transferring them into ducted emissions for further treatment.

Methods

The company record books, which had been confiscated by the General Prosecutor of Trento during an inquiry about pollution, were utilized to study the workers. 20 % of the workers were hired via temp agency, and therefore it was impossible to study this group of workers. Dimension of the cohort, mean duration of employment, person-years, average time of follow-up, age at entry, and drop outs are summarized in Table 2. Seventeen workers, registered as "technical employee", were excluded. The status of life (alive or dead) was certified by the respective municipality where each worker resided, and partially by directly verifying medical records. Causes of death were obtained, when possible, from the death certificate of the National Institute of Statistics (ISTAT). Otherwise, the Nominal Registry for the causes of death (2005–2009) at the Provincial Health Agency (APSS) in Trento and the medical records found at the Hospital of Borgo Valsugana were utilized. In the absence of medical records, three cases of death were not included in the specific causes of death, although there were testimonies which we judged trustworthy (one death possibly due to myocardial infarction, one to a car accident and one to carbon monoxide poisoning). Steel production in Borgo Valsugana began on 19/03/1979, when this study was started. Subjects were enrolled to the study on the day they were employed. The follow-up began on the date of employment (not before 19th march 1979) and terminated either with the death or on 31st of December 2009. Status of life was verified. A worker was classified as "being exposed" after having worked at the foundry for at least one year.

Analysis of mortality

331 male "workers" were enrolled to the study. 32 male subjects, whose life status was known, were chosen as controls (clerks, managers and a watchman). Women were excluded from the study. The high percentage of drop outs in the control group (30.4 %) could be explained by the high mobility of these subjects, making it difficult to trace them. The person-years were calculated by age groups for periods of five years from 1979 to 2009 (6 groups). *Expected deaths* for *all causes* and for each specific disease were evaluated by utilizing the rate of mortality in the Region Trentino-Alto Adige [33]. Every five years the specific rate of mortality was applied to each age group, using an arithmetic average of the yearly rates. Be it that the years 2004 and 2005 were lacking, the average depends on the years available. Standardized Mortality Ratios (SMR), 95 % Confidence Interval (95 % CI) and p values (p) were calculated for the main pathologies and causes of death. STATA software (Statacorp 2009) was utilized for the calculations [34]. Other factors, beside the occupational risk factors, were analysed, when present in the medical records, like smoking and alcohol consumption.

Analysis of morbidity

Exemption from health fees in the group of workers employed for more than one year was adopted as a surrogate for the prevalence of disease and compared to the rate observed in the Province of Trento. The analysis was limited to seven exemptions, that accounted for more than 2/3 of the total exemptions in the province of Trento, i.e. patients suffering from malignant tumours (code 048); hypertension with organ damage ("complicated" hypertension is used in this study as synonym: code 0031); hypertension (without any organ damage: code 0A31); diabetes mellitus (code 013); cardiopulmonary vascular diseases (cardiovascular disease is used as synonym: code 0A02); rheumatoid arthritis (code 006) and asthma (code 007). The status of exemption from health fees for the given pathology for 299 residents in the Province of Trento up to the 28th of January 2011 was obtained from the APSS of Trento. 235/299 male

Table 2 Principal characteristics of the foundry worker cohort

Cohort foundry workers			
	Workers ≥ 1 year (exposed)	Control group (office work)	Workers < 1 year
Workers studied	331	32	111
Mean duration of employment (median)	8.6 (5.5) years	5.6 (3.1) years	<1 year
Lost to the follow-up	22 (6 %)	15 (31 %)	16 (12 %)
Person-years	6731.0	491.3	2387.1
Average duration of the follow-up (range)	20.5 (1.2–30.8) years	15.5 (0.2–30.8) years	21.0 (2.2–30.8) years
Mean age at entry	31.1 years	35.5 years	29.2 years
Observed deaths (n.)	29	1	7
Not included	17 (exposition not certain) + 3 females	12 females	
TOTAL	373	59	127

subjects (workers and clerks), having one or more than one year of employment at the steel foundry, were studied. The workers studied for health fee exemptions were less than those studied for mortality, because workers not residing in the Province of Trento were excluded, and residents in some municipalities were accidentally excluded in the formulation of the request of data to APSS. The census of the provincial population was taken in January 2011. The rates of exemption registered in the Province of Trento were calculated by dividing the total number of exemption for a certain disease by the number of males over 20 years of age reported for on the 1st of January 2011. We utilized the Mantel-Haenszel method to adjust the result for age; three age groups were utilized: 20–64, 65–74, 75 and over. 17 out of 64 non-exposed workers, exempt from health fees, were inserted into an additional cohort for an internal comparison. The remaining 47 were excluded since they did not fulfil the criteria of this study: 4 women, 34 workers employed under one year; and 9 technical employees.

Results

Analysis of mortality

Table 3 shows the observed and expected number of deaths of the foundry workers for *all causes* and for the main groups of diseases (cause-specific mortality). The SMR for all causes was 1.13 (95 % CI:0.76–1.62), when the general male population was used as the reference. Average age at death was 54 years. There was an increase of *all cancers* (SMR 1.36; 95 % CI: 0.75–2.29; 14 cases), that was statistically significant for lung cancer (SMR 3.35; 95 % CI: 1.45–6.6; 8 cases). With the exception of the 8 cases of lung cancer, the other deaths due to malignant tumours were localized in 6 different sites (oesophagus, stomach, colon-rectum, pancreas, testicle and multiple myeloma). There was also a non-statistically significant increase for *ischemic cardiac diseases* (SMR 1.27; 95 % CI: 0.35–3.26; 4 cases) *chronic liver diseases* (SMR 1.16; 95 % CI: 0.14–4.2; 2 cases), *injuries and poisoning* (SMR 1.32; 95 % CI: 0.48–2.88; 6 cases). When computing the overall mortality SMR (all causes) for different time lengths of employment (1–4; 5–9; ≥10) there was an inverse relationship (Table 4), indicating a strong *healthy survivor effect* [35]. This cohort is characterised by a high turn-over of the personnel: 25 % of the total cohort of blue-collar workers was employed less than 1 year, 55 % less than 5 years. There were no lung cancers before 3 years of exposure. In workers who died from lung cancer, the mean age at death was 63.7 years, while the mean age at death from lung cancer in the Province of Trento was 72.1 years (2003–2006). Seven out of eight deaths from lung cancer occurred between 2005 and 2009. SMRs by exposure duration and by time since first exposure for all tumours and lung cancer are synthetized in Tables 4 and 5. In 91 workers employed at present, the habit of smoking was reported only for 17 workers (18.7 %). As compared to the smoking habit of the general population in the Province of Trento (29 % smokers; 29.2 % ex-smokers) [36], there was a 12 % excess of smokers in this small sample of workers. Regarding alcohol consumption, 2 workers declared that they consumed a moderate quantity of wine daily, whereas 11 denied alcohol intake. In 8 workers, who died from lung cancer, only in 6 did we obtain information on their smoking habit: 1 was not a smoker, 2 were ex-smokers and 3 had been smokers (20 cigarettes/per day). Six exposed workers died because of *injuries or poisoning*: 4 being fortuitous non work-related traumata, one death due to work-related trauma and one due to suicide. Three of these deaths occurred while still being employed, whereas three occurred successively. Mean length of employment time was 10.6 years (range 2–17 years). 331 exposed workers were confronted with 32 white collar workers of the same company. In this *internal* confrontation the Relative Risk ratio (RR) was 2.34 (95 % CI: 0.39–95.72). We calculated the avoidable deaths to be 16.6 (95 % CI: 0–28.7). Finally, we studied the workers with less than one year of employment separately. The SMR for all causes was 0.97 (95 % CI 0.39–2.0). Seven workers, employed under one year, died as follows: four cases of *injury and poisoning* (SMR: 2,56; 95 % CI: 0.8–6.1; 3 suicides, 1 car accident), 1 case of gastrointestinal

Table 3 Mortality of workers exposed ≥ 1 year (reference: general population)

ICD 9[a]	ICD 10	Cause of death	Observed	Expected	SMR	95 % CI	*P*
001 - 999	A00–T98	**All causes**	29[b]	25.69	1.13	0.76–1.62	0.527
140 - 239	C00–D48	**All tumours**	14	10.27	1.36	0.75–2.29	0.283
162	C33–C34	**Malignant tumors of the larynx, trachea, bronchi, lungs**	8	2.39	**3.35**	**1.45–6.60**	**0.010**
410 - 414	I20–I25	**Ischemic heart disease**	4	3.14	1.27	0.35–3.26	0.768
571	K70; K73–K74	**Chronic liver disease**	2	1.72	1.16	0.14–4.20	0.837
800 - 999	S00–T99	**Injury and poisoning**	6	4.53	1.32	0.48–2.88	0.604

[a]Till 2002. [b]In the absence of medical records, 3 cases were not included in the specific causes of deaths. CI = Confidence Interval
In bold, statistically significant value

Table 4 SMRs by years of exposure (employment) for selected causes of death

ICD 9	Cause of death	Years of exposure											
		0 - < 1 year			1–<5 years			5–<10 years			10 + years		
		Obs	SMR	95 % CI	Obs	SMR	95 % CI	Obs	SMR	95 % CI	Obs	SMR	95 % CI
001–999	All causes	7	0.97	0.39–2.00	11	1.29	0.64–2.31	9	1.21	0.55–2.30	9	0.94	0.43–1.79
140–239	All tumours	2	0.75	0.09–2.71	5	1.68	0.54–3.92	4	1.32	0.36–3.38	5	1.17	0.38–2.73
162	Malignant tumors of the larynx, trachea, bronchi, lungs	1	1.66	0.04–9.25	3	4.35	0.90–12.71	3	4.11	0.85–12.01	2	2.06	0.25–7.45

Obs observed death, *Exp* expected death, *CI* confidence interval

haemorrhage (liver cirrhosis for alcohol abuse), 2 cases due to cancer (SMR 0.75; 95 % CI: 0.09–2.71; 1 cancer of the larynx, 1 pancreatic cancer) (see also Table 4).

Analysis of morbidity

88 out of 235 workers had 118 health fee exemptions (50.2 %). The rate of exemption for all diseases in the Province of Trento is about 28 % for the male sex. Table 6 summarizes the rates of health fee exemption of exposed workers as compared to the rate exemption found in the Province of Trento. The rate of exemption in exposed workers was statistically significant for diabetes (RR = 2.24; $p = 0.0002$), hypertension (RR = 2.01; $p = 0.0018$), and rheumatoid arthritis (RR = 6.18; $p = 0.013$). After adjustment for age (Mantel Haenszel method), the increased rate of cardiovascular diseases also became statistically significant. As foreseen, by *internally comparing* the workers, less fee exemptions were requested among the non-exposed group: in fact, there were only two cases (048 and 0A31) versus the expected 8.5. The exemption 048 (malignant tumour) was referred to a night watchman.

Discussion

Limitations

EAFs are small plants as compared to integrated foundries which include all the production phases starting from the initial processing of the iron ore. EAFs use scrap as raw material and in the case of Borgo Valsugana only semi-finished products are obtained. Therefore, this cohort is relatively smaller as compared to other studies on foundries and may have a limited statistical power. We did not have access to a similar *external* comparison *group* of workers to minimize the *healthy worker effect* (HWE) [35, 37–42]. Instead, we compared mortality and morbidity of 331 exposed workers (≥1 year) with the *general population* of the Region Trentino Alto Adige (Table 3) and also with a small group of clerks working at the same foundry (Table 7). Although this internal comparison was numerically limited, the relative risk ratio between exposed workers/non-exposed clerks in our study was well above the unity (RR 2.34), in line with a previous study [2]. We could not differentiate among the different type of work tasks, because no data were available in the Registration Book. In this factory the working environment was constituted by a single non-divided shed, so that all workers were exposed to the same pollutant/s. Some tasks (e.g. continuous casting, furnace workers) could have had a higher level of exposure than others (e.g. maintainers, operators), but in this small plant it was not infrequent to go from a type of task to another. Besides age, other confounders, like diet and the socio-economical level were not considered in this study. On the other hand, having studied both mortality and morbidity has the advantage of a more comprehensive evaluation of the problem, bearing in mind the pyramid phenomenon of effects on health.

Healthy worker effect

The lower SMR of workers as compared to the general population is due to the so-called *healthy worker effect* (HWE), arising largely from employment selection factors [35, 37–42]. In the absence of workplace hazards, all cause SMRs for Caucasian men is 0.70–0.85 [9]. In this study we found a SMR of 1.13 (95 % CI: 0.76–1.62), which is similar to what has been found

Table 5 SMRs by time since first exposure for selected causes of death (workers exposed ≥ 1 year)

ICD 9	Cause of death	Years since first exposure											
		1–<10 years				10–<20 years				20 + years			
		Obs	Exp	SMR	95 % CI	Obs	Exp	SMR	95 % CI	Obs	Exp	SMR	95 % CI
001–999	All causes	8	6.18	1.29	0.56–2.55	7	8.03	0.87	0.35–1.80	14	11.48	1.22	0.67–2.05
140–239	All tumours	2	1.59	1.26	0.15–4.54	4	3.11	1.29	0.35–3.29	8	5.56	1.44	0.62–2.84
162	Malignant tumors of the larynx, trachea, bronchi, lungs	1	0.36	2.78	0.07–15.48	1	0.75	1.33	0.03–7.43	6	1.27	4.72	1.73–10.28

Table 6 Health fees exemptions of 235 workers[a] compared to the exemptions of the provincial population

	Workers ($n = 235$)	Province of Trento (PT) (n. of male population ≥ 20 years = 203332)			PT, Adjusted for age (Mantel Haenszel)	
Diseases	n. of cases	n. of cases	RR	P	RR	95 % CI
Tumours	12	9655	1.08	0.7580	1.19	0.69–2.04
Cardiovascular Diseases	5	8676	1.50	0.1067	**1.74**	1.07–2.82
Diabetes	25	9630	**2.24**	**0.0002**	**2.39**	1.67–3.41
Rheumatoid Arthritis	3	420	**6.18**	**0.0133**	**6.17**	2.00–19.02
Asthma	2	1968	0.88	1.0000	1.08	0.27–4.31
Non-complicated Hypertension	30	11655	**2.23**	**0.0001**	**2.44**	1.75–3.40
Complicated Hypertension	14	6033	**2.01**	**0.0181**	**2.22**	1.35–3.65

[a]male sex, exposed ≥ 1 year
In bold statistically significant values. "Cases" refer to health fees exemptions

by others [5, 7, 8]. We attributed the inverse dose–response relationship for *all causes* (Table 4) to a *healthy survivor effect*, a component of the *healthy worker effect* [35]. The *healthy survivor effect* is attributed to a strong selection throughout the years due to an early dropping out from work by those workers who are feeble [35, 37–42].

Mortality for lung cancer

Our data confirm what has been already reported in literature: there is a high statistically significant increase ($p = 0.01$) of deaths due to lung cancer (8 cases observed versus the expected 2.39). In this study there are limited data regarding the habit of smoking and alcohol consumption amongst the workers. However, it does not seem that differences in life style could justify the high rate of mortality for lung cancer. The precocious median age at death for lung cancer in the exposed workers (minus 8.4 years) as compared to the Province of Trento suggests the presence of carcinogenic factors other than cigarette smoking. The relationship between environmental pollution due to particulate matter and lung cancer is well-known [43].

Gradient effect

In this study no dose–response relationship was found for tumours when considering the duration of employment. On the other hand, when considering the time since the first exposure, there was an increase of SMRs for all tumours and lung cancer after 20 years (Table 5). While an increasing risk with employment duration supports causal inference, the absence of an increasing risk with employment duration is not a strong evidence against it [9, 37]. In mortality studies of steel workers the absence of a gradient effect for cancer deaths is rather frequent: among 7 studies, that reported dose–response assessment [1, 3–7, 9], 3 studies found no dose–response relationship [1, 6, 9], while 4 studies found a certain dose–response relationship [3–5, 7]. There can be several explanations for this. First, the *healthy survivor effect* should be taken into consideration. Secondly, there is a *competition between diseases* so that those who die, e.g. from cardiovascular disease or injuries, have no time to develop cancer. Thirdly, the length of employment does not always correlate with the level of exposure. In the case of steel workers, urine or serum analysis of metals do not always correlate with metal PM content in tissue, so a reliable method for measuring fine and ultrafine metal PM in tissue is urgently needed [26]. Finally, the difficulty of evidencing a dose–response relationship imply that the substances in question have their characteristic way of reacting. A given substance may accumulate in the tissues over time and induce a cancer slowly throughout life [44].

Injuries

Though not statistically significant, we found an excess (+32 %) of injuries. Increase of mortality for injuries is frequently reported in steel worker studies [2, 5, 9, 45].

Table 7 Internal comparison between workers exposed ≥ 1 year and the non-exposed workers (white collars)

Groups (N. of subjects)	Observed	Expected	SMR	95 % CI	Person Years
Exposed Workers ≥ 1 year (n.331)	29	25.69	1.13	0.76–1.62	6731.0
Non-exposed (controls) (n.32)	1	2.09	0.47	0.01–2.67	491.3
Comparison exposed/non exposed workers			RR: 2.34	0.39–95.72	
Avoidable deaths			16.6	0–28.7	

Barreto et al. observed in Brazil an increase of mortality due to car accidents [45] and suggested that work-related factors could be rotating shift work, high levels of noise and mental illness, which is "a major health problem in steel workers" [45]. The Chinese study found that increased mortality for injuries paralleled increased mortality for all causes when certain types of exposures are concerned (iron, welding fumes, coal, asbestos, heat, PAHs and benzene), but not for other types of exposures (silica, wood and CO) [2]. Neurobehavioral function alterations have been documented in steel workers [46, 47]. Recent animal studies on neurological toxicity of metal particulates on a nanometric scale have shown that these particles have a high tropism for the brain [48]: they can cause an alteration of the sensorial and cognitive functions, damage to the blood–brain barrier, the neural cells, the glial cells and myelin. Finally, it is recognized that subjects exposed to nanoparticulates may have an altered function of their mental health [48–50]. Therefore, we consider it possible that high levels of metal particulates and neurotoxic substances (Table 1) could cause subtle effects on the capability of reaction and attention and could explain the increased number of accidents in steel workers. Further studies are needed.

Morbidity

Our study shows a statistical significant increase of diabetes, rheumatoid arthritis, hypertension and cardiovascular diseases in exposed workers as compared to the population of the province (Table 4). We used the exemption of health fees as a surrogate for the prevalence of diseases. As is known, the analysis of the exemption from health fees may give results, which underestimate the real prevalence of diseases. We assumed that, when internal comparisons are made, the rate of exemption from health fees is a good indicator of health status of a given population in the absence of other data. The validity of this assumption, is confirmed by the results obtained from the internal analysis of the health fee exempted cohort, comparing exposed workers to *non-exposed* workers: there were only two applications for exemption from health fees in the small group of controls. Age was shown not to be a confounding element. At present in the Italian Health System, who suffers from a chronic disease may request the exemption from health fees, independently from his/her socio-economic status. The seven diseases considered in this study account for more than 2/3 of the total number of exemptions for diseases in the Province of Trento, so we consider them relevant in assessing a health status. There is no evidence that this cohort of steel workers had better access to health care than the general population. We confirm what Martinez et al. [51] found in Brazil, i.e. a high prevalence of diabetes and hypertension in foundry workers: the prevalence of diabetes in Brazil was 11.5 %, and we observed a prevalence of 10.6 % in the foundry workers of Borgo Valsugana. Martinez et al. also reported more cases of diabetes in the exposed workers as compared to clerks. Diabetes is the most frequent chronic disease in industrialized countries and it is now increasingly evident that it is also associated with environmental toxic agents like heavy metals and PCDD/Fs [52–57]. Moreover, the relationship between hypertension/cardiovascular diseases and air pollutants is well known [58–67].

Diffuse emissions/foundry dust

This study shows a notable deterioration of the health status of the exposed workers, as compared to the referral groups. This negative finding could be due to the working conditions. We do not have detailed information on PM concentration and metal content of the air within the foundry, although we assume that it has a similar composition and proportion of the elements found in the dust which had deposited (Table 1). The level of PNOC (particulates not otherwise classified) might have been quite high, sometimes exceeding the limits of 10 mg/Nm^3 established by the ACGIH. In 2007, the local Environment Protection Agency (APPA) reported that the quantity of diffuse emissions during charging of the electric arc furnace of Borgo Valsugana was *"some grams per normal cubic meter and could be perceived by the naked eye"*. The working conditions in this EAF have improved after the instalment of new canopy hoods and with the automation of several working processes. The danger of foundry dusts inhaled through diffuse emission is inherent to the deposition of metal PM in body tissue and to the release of toxic and carcinogenic metals. Common steel can release nickel and chromium in body tissues by corrosion. Regarding fine and ultrafine metal PM there is a tremendous lack of knowledge concerning tissue distribution, clearance (half-life) and toxic health effects. Data on PM level and composition in the air of steel foundries, as well as the health risk assessment on metal exposure, are available from other studies [14, 28, 68, 69]. In fact, Angelo Borroni (Polytechnic University of Milan) studied over 400 samples of air taken within the working areas of 10 Italian EAFs from 1985–2005; in the *oven working area* the levels of PNOC, manganese, lead, silica and calcium oxide were not infrequently (roughly 1/8) above the limits determined by the ACGIH (silica is no longer utilized as a refractory material since 1990) (unpublished data). Furthermore, Liu et al. reported that the health risk assessment on metal exposure in foundries showed that the cancer risk for cadmium, chromium and nickel were all above 1×10 (−6) [28]. To avoid underestimation of health risk assessment we suggest to consider steel *"foundry dusts" in toto*, as the sum of the individual risks can neglect the synergistic effect of its single pollutants. Foundry dust should be considered a *"high hazard"* pollutant. PAH exposure alone cannot explain the excess of diabetes in our study, that may better correlate with heavy metals and PCDD/F. Exposure to PAH in EAFs has been reported to be in the median range as compared to other types of industries [70]. Therefore, PAH exposure does not seem to be so relevant in EAFs as compared to other substances present in the foundry dust, i.e. fine and ultrafine metal PM deriving from high temperature fusion processes. To limit the diffuse emissions of the EAFs, which contain dangerous micropollutants like PCCD/F, the European Commission has underlined the necessity of total enclosure buildings [15]. On the other hand, nowadays the EU regulation allows for over 98 % cut down of the total dust produced by the oven. This means that up to 27 kg/h of dust could be released into the environment, when roughly 1360 kg of dust per hour is produced as is the case in Borgo Valsugana. Unfortunately, as of yet, in Europe there are still EAFs plants which work only with a fourth hole extraction [15].

Conclusions

With the limitations of this relatively small cohort (331 exposed workers, 6731 person-years) and the lack of a consistent comparison group of workers, this study shows a significant increased risk of lung tumours, diabetes, rheumatoid arthritis, hypertension and cardiovascular diseases as compared to the general population. This outcome may be attributed to working conditions in the EAF, where the numerous toxic and carcinogenic substances contained in the *foundry dust/diffuse emissions* represent the most important risk factors for quantity and biological plausibility. PAHs alone cannot explain the increased prevalence of diabetes. A reliable method for measuring metal PM in tissue is urgently needed for a better exposure assessment in future studies. Our data underline the importance to maximize the standards of security for *foundry dust/diffuse emissions* in EAF, so as to protect *in primis* the workers and then the population living around this foundries [71, 72]. Further studies on EAF's are needed to confirm our findings and to increase statistical power with pooled analyses.

Competing interests

The authors declare that they have no competing interests.

Authors' contributions

VG and RC have made substantial contributions to the conception and design of the study, MC has performed the statistical analysis, JC the linguistic supervision, RC the acquisition of the data and the preliminary draft of the manuscript. All authors have been involved in drafting and revising the manuscript. All authors have read and approved the final manuscript.

Acknowledgement

We thank the Procura della Repubblica (Crown Prosecution Service) of Trento for kindly having permitted to access the data. We thank Professor Angelo Borroni for having kindly provided important data and Dr. Silvano Piffer for his valuable advice.

Author details

[1]International Society of Doctors for the Environment (ISDE Italy), via della Fioraia 17/19, 52100 Arezzo, Italy. [2]Istituto di Ricovero e Cura a Carattere Scientifico (IRCCS) Azienda Ospedaliera Universitaria "San Martino" Istituto Nazionale per la Ricerca sul Cancro (IST), largo R. Benzi 10, 16132 Genoa, Italy.

References

1. Andjelkovich DA, Mathew RM, Richardson RB, Levine RJ. Mortality of iron foundry workers: I. Overall findings. J Occup Med. 1990;32(6):529–40.
2. Hoshuyama T, Pan G, Tanaka C, Feng Y, Yu L, Liu T, et al. Mortality of iron-steel workers in Anshan, China: a retrospective cohort study. Int J Occup Environ Health. 2006;12(3):193–202.
3. Finkelstein MM, Wilk N. Investigation of a lung cancer cluster in the melt shop of an Ontario steel producer. Am J Ind Med. 1990;17(4):483–91.
4. Fletcher AC, Ades A. Lung cancer mortality in a cohort of English foundry workers. Scand J Work Environ Health. 1984;10:7–16.
5. Koskela RS, Hernberg S, Karava R, Jarvinen E, Nurminen M. A mortality study of foundry workers. Scand J Work Environ Health. 1976;2 Suppl 1:73–89.
6. Moulin JJ, Portefaix P, Wild P, Mur JM, Smagghe G, Mantout B. Mortality study of workers producing ferroalloys and stainless steel in France. Br J Ind Med. 1990;47:537–43.
7. Sorahan T, Faux AM, Cooke MA. Mortality among a cohort of United Kingdom steel foundry workers with special reference to cancers of the stomach and lung, 1946–90. Occup Environ Med. 1994;51(5):316–22.
8. Lloyd JW, Lundin Jr FE, Redmond CK, Geiser PB. Long-term mortality study of steelworkers. IV. Mortality by work area. J Occup Med. 1970;12(5):51–157.
9. Park RM, Ahn YS, Stayner LT, Kang SK, Jang JK. Mortality of Iron and steel Workers in Korea. Am J Ind Med. 2005;48:194–204.
10. Bourgkard E, Wild P, Courcot B, Diss M, Ettlinger J, Goutet P, et al. Lung cancer mortality and iron oxide exposure in a French steel-producing factory. Occup Environ Med. 2009;66:175–81.
11. Rodriguez V, Tardon A, Kogevinas M, Prieto CS, Cueto A, Garcia M, et al. Lung Cancer Risk in Iron and Steel Foundry Workers: A Nested Case Control Study in Asturias, Spain. Am J Ind Med. 2000;38:644–50.
12. Tossavanien A. Estimated risk of lung cancer attributable to occupational exposures in iron and steel foundries. IARC Sci Publ. 1990;104:363–7.
13. IARC Monographs on the Evaluation of Carcinogenic Risks to Humans. Overall Evaluations of Carcinogenicity: An Updating of IARC Monographs. 1987 - Volumes 1 to 42 Supplement 7, p. 224–25.
14. Cantone L, Nordio F, Hou L, Apostoli P, Bonzini M, Tarantini M, et al. Inhalable Metal-Rich Air Particles And Histone H3K4 Dimethylation And H3K9 Acetylation In A Cross-Sectional Study Of Steel Workers. Environ Health Perspect. 2011;119:964–9.
15. European Commission. Best Available Techniques (BAT) Reference Document for: Production of Iron and steel. Integrated Pollution Prevention and Control (IPPC). 2013; 8.2:419–479. http://eippcb.jrc.ec.europa.eu/reference/BREF/IS_Adopted_03_2012.pdf
16. IARC. Coke production. IARC Monogr Eval Carcinog Risk Chem Hum. 1984; 34:101–31.
17. Giua R, Spartera M, Viviano G, Ziemacki G, Carbotti G. [Cancer risk for coke oven workers in the steel plant of Taranto]. [Article in Italian]. Epidemiol Prev. 2005;29(5–6):42–4.
18. Lloyd JW. Long-term mortality study of steelworkers. V. Respiratory cancer in coke plant workers. J Occup Med. 1971;13(2):53–68.
19. Cheng YH, Chao YC, Wu CH, Tsai CJ, Uang SN, Shih TS. Measurements of ultrafine particle concentrations and size distribution in an iron foundry. J Hazard Mater. 2008;158(1):124–30.

20. International Institute for Applied Systems Analysis (IIASA). Modelling Particulate emissions in Europe. A Framework to Estimate Reduction Potential and Control Costs. 2002. Interim Report IR-02-076.
21. Nemmar A, Holme JA, Rosas I, Schwarze PE, Alfaro Moreno E. Recent Advances in Particulate Matter and Nanoparticle Toxicology: A Review of the in Vivo and in Vitro Studies. Biomed Res Int. 2013; doi:10.1155/2013/279371.
22. International Agency for Research on Cancer – World Health Organization – Press release n. 221/17-10-2013.
23. Schwarze PE, Ovrevik J, Lag M, Refsnes M, Nafstad P, Hetland RB, et al. Particulate Matter Properties And Health Effects: Consistency of Epidemiological and Toxicological Studies. Hum Exp Toxicol. 2006;25:559–79.
24. Ghio AJ. Biological Effects Of Utah Valley Ambient Air – Particles In Humans: A Review. J Aerosol Med. 2004;17(2):157–64.
25. Fletcher GG, Rossetto FE, Turnbull JD, Nieboer E. Toxicity, Uptake and Mutagenicity of Particulate and Soluble Nickel Compounds. Environ Health Perspect. 1994;102 Suppl 3:69–79.
26. Lee JA, Kim MK, Paek HJ, Kim MK, Lee JK, Jeong J, et al. Tissue distribution and excretion kinetics of oral administered silica nanoparticles in rats. Int J Nanomedicine. 2014;9 Suppl 2:251–60.
27. Shaw BJ, Handy R. Physiological Effects Of Nanoparticles On Fish: A Comparison Of Nanometals Versus Metal Ions. Environ Int. 2011;37(6):1083–97.
28. Liu HH, Lin MH, Liu PC, Chan CI, Chen HL. Health risk assessment by measuring plasma malondialdehyde (MDA), urinary 8-hydroxydeoxyguanosine (8-OH-dG) and DNA strand breakage following metal exposure in foundry workers. J Hazard Mater. 2009;170:699–704.
29. Chen HL, Shih TS, Huang PC, Hsieh CY, Lee CC. Exposure of arc-furnace plant workers to polychlorinated dibenzo-p-dioxins and dibenzofurans (PCDD/F). Chemosphere. 2006;64:666–71.
30. Cottica D, Grignani E, Ghitti R, Festa D, Apostoli P. [Measurement of chemical agents in metallurgy field: electric steel plant]. [Article in Italian]. G Ital Med Lav Ergon. 2012;34(3):236–41.
31. Borroni A. Relazione del consulente tecnico del GUP (Expert report for the General Prosecutor). [In Italian]. Tribunale Ordinario di Trento, Ufficio del Giudice per le Udienze Preliminari N. 6346/08 R.G. Notizie Di Reato, N.1841/09 GIP. P.35. https://docs.google.com/open?id=0B9jXgSdelYflRUw0c1ZybU9RRENRTmxMRy1nN0Vjdw. Accessed 26 Sept 2011.
32. Rada EC, Ragazzi M, Schiavon M. Assessment of the local role of a steel making plant by POPs deposition measurements. Chemosphere. 2014;110:53–61.
33. Istituto Superiore di Sanità. [Cause-Specific Mortality In Italy: 1980–2003 and 2006–2008]. [Italian]. http://www.iss.it/site/mortalita/Scripts/SelCause.asp
34. StataCorp. Stata: Release 11. Statistical Sofware. College Station: StataCorp LP; 2009.
35. Baillargeon J. Characteristics of the Healthy Worker effect. Occup Med. 2001; 16:359–66.
36. Studio PASSI. [Smoking habitus in Trentino, Italy 2008–2011]. [Article in Italian]. http://www.trentinosalute.net/content/download/1775/11715/version/1/file/Fumo+TN_28.5.pdf
37. Li CY, Sung FC. A review of the healthy worker effect in occupational epidemiology. Occup Med. 1999;49:225–9.
38. Gennaro V, Ceppi M, Montanaro F. Reanalysis of mortality in a petrochemical plant producing vinyl chloride and polyvinyl chloride]. [Article in Italian]. Epidemiol Prev. 2003;27(4):221–5.
39. Gennaro V, Ceppi M, Crosignani P, Montanaro F. Reanalysis of updated mortality among vinyl and polyvinyl chloride workers: Confirmation of historical evidence and new findings. BMC Public Health. 2008;8:21.
40. Gennaro V, Ricci P, Lewis AG, Crosignani P. [Epidemiology's and epidemiologists vices and virtues]. [Article in Italian]. Epidemiol Prev. 2009; 33(4-5 Suppl 2):49–56.
41. Gennaro V, Tomatis L, Business Bias. How Epidemiologic Studies May Underestimate or Fail to Detect Increased Risks of Cancer and Other Diseases. Int J Occup Environ Health. 2005;11:356–9.
42. Boffetta P, Sali D, Kolstad H, Coggon D, Olsen J, Andersen A, et al. Mortality of short term workers in two International cohorts. J Occup Environ Med. 1998;40(12):1120–6.
43. Raaschou-Nielsen O, Andersen ZJ, Beelen R, Samoli E, Stafoggia M, Weinmyr G, et al. Air pollution and lung cancer incidence in 17 European cohorts: prospective analyses from the European Study of Cohorts for Air Pollution Effects (ESCAPE). Lancet oncol. 2013;14(9):813–22.
44. Kogevinas M. Epidemiological approaches in the investigation of environmental causes of cancer: the case of dioxin and water disinfection by-products. Environ Health. 2011;10 Suppl 1:53.
45. Barreto SM, Swerdlow AJ, Smith PG, Higgins CD, Andrade A. Mortality from injuries and other causes in a cohort of 21800 Brazilian steel worker. Occup Environ Med. 1996;53:343–50.
46. Blond M, Netterstrom B, Laursen P. Cognitive function in a cohort of Danish steel workers. Neurotoxicology. 2007;28(2):328–35.
47. Blond M, Netterstrom B. Neuromotor function in a cohort of Danish steel workers. Neurotoxicology. 2007;28(2):336–44.
48. Sharma HS, Sharma A. Neurotoxity of Engineered Nanoparticles from Metals. CNS Neurol Disord Drug Targets. 2012;11:65–80.
49. Hubbs AF, Mercer RR, Stanley A, Benkovic SA, Harkema J, Sriram K, et al. Nanotoxicology – A Pathologist perspective. Toxicol Pathol. 2011;39:301–24.
50. Lafuente JV, Sharma A, Patnaik R, et al. Diabetes exacerbates Nanoparticles Induced Brain Pathology. CNS Neurol Disord Drug Targets. 2012;11:26–36.
51. Martinez MC, Latorre MR. Risk Factors for Hypertension and Diabetes Mellitus in Metallurgic and Siderurgic Company's Workers. Arq Bras Cardiol. 2006;87:424–32.
52. Thayer KA, Heindel JJ, Bucher JR, Gallo MA. Role of environmental chemicals in diabetes and obesity: a National Toxicology Program workshop review. Environ Health Perspect. 2012;120(6):779–89.
53. Rignell-Hydbom A, Rylander L, Hagmar L. Exposure to persistent organochlorine pollutants and type 2 diabetes mellitus. Hum Exp Toxicol. 2007;26(5):447–52.
54. Lee DH. Persistent organic pollutants and obesity-related metabolic dysfunction: focusing on type 2 Diabetes. Epidemiol Health. 2012; doi:10.4178/epih/e2012002.
55. Fujiyoshi PT, Michalek JE, Matsumura F. Molecular epidemiologic evidence for diabetogenic effects of dioxin exposure in U.S. Air force veterans of the Vietnam war. Environ Health Perspect. 2006;114(11):1677–83.
56. Chen YW, Yang CY, Huang CF, Hung DZ, Leung YM, Liu SH. Heavy metals, islet function and diabetes development. Review. Islets. 2009;1(3):169–76.
57. Soisungwan S, Moore MR. Emerging Roles of Cadmium and Heme Oxygenase in Type-2 Diabetes and Cancer Susceptibility. Tohoku J Exp Med. 2012;228:267–88.
58. Brook RD, Brook JR, Urch B, Vincent R, Rajagopalan S, Silverman F. Inhalation of fine particulate air pollution and ozone causes acute arterial vasoconstriction in healthy adults. Circulation. 2002;105:1534–6.
59. Urch B, Silverman F, Corey P, Brook JR, Luzic KZ, Rajopagalan S, et al. Acute blood pressure responses in healthy adults during controlled air pollution exposure. Environ Health Perspect. 2005;113:1052–5.
60. Guo Y, Tong S, Zhang Y, Barnett AG, Jia Y, Pan X. The relationship between particulate air pollution and emergency hospital visits for hypertension in Beijing, China. Sci Total Environ. 2010;408:4446–50.
61. Chiarelli PS, Pereira LAA, Saldiva PHN, Ferreira-Filho C, Garcia MLB, Braga ALF, et al. The association between air pollution and blood pressure in traffic controllers in Santo André, São Paulo, Brazil. Environ Res. 2011;111:650–5.
62. Bartoli CR, Wellenius GA, Diaz EA, Lawrence J, Coull BA, Akiyama I, et al. Mechanisms of inhaled fine particulate air pollution-induced arterial blood pressure changes. Environ Health Perspect. 2009;117:361–6.
63. Nascimento LFC, Francisco JB. Particulate matter and hospital admission due to arterial hypertension in a medium-sized Brazilian city. Cad Saúde Pública. 2013;29(8):1565–71.
64. Nemmar A, Al-Maskari S, Ali BH, Al-Amri IS. Cardiovascular and lung inflammatory effects induced by systemically administered diesel exhaust particles in rats. Am J Physiol. 2007;292(3):664–70.
65. Nemmar A, Dhanasekaran S, Yasin J, Ba-Omar H, Fahim MA, Kazzam EE, et al. Evaluation of the direct systemic and cardiopulmonary effects of diesel particles in spontaneously hypertensive rats. Toxicolog. 2009;262(1):50–6.
66. Cavallari JM, Eisen EA, Fang SC, Schwartz J, Hauser R, Herrick RF, et al. $PM_{2.5}$ metal exposures and nocturnal heart rate variability: A panel study of boilermaker construction workers. Environ Health. 2008;7:36.
67. Kodavanti UP, Schladweiler MC, Gilmour PS, Wallenborn JG, Mandavilli BS, Ledbetter AD, et al. The role of particulate matter-associated zinc in cardiac injury in rats. Environ Health Perspect. 2008;116:13–20.
68. Borroni A. [Risk's profiles and solutions. Report from research activity with the Istituto Superiore per la Prevenzione e la Sicurezza sul Lavoro (ISPESL): "Research of good practices in employment sectors in small and medium iron and steel foundry. Electric steel foundry]. [Article in Italian]. Milan, May 2005. http://www.safetyworkingareas.org/Download/aziende-a-rischio-atex/Metallurgie.pdf

69. Cottica D, Grignani E, Ghitti R, Festa D, Apostoli P. [Measurment of chemical agents in metallurgy field: electric steel plant]. [Article in Italian]. G Ital Med Lav Ergon. 2012;4(3):236–41.
70. Bergamaschi E, Catalani S, Folesani G, Venco P, Bodini E, Guidetti F, et al. Environmental and biological monitoring of exposure to Polycyclic Aromatic Hydrocarbons in workers of an electric steel foundry]. [Article in Italian]. Med Lav. 2005;96(5):390–402.
71. Casella C, Garrone E, Gennaro V, Orengo MA, Puppo A, Stagnaro E, et al. Health conditions of the general population living near a steel plant]. [Article in Italian]. Epidemiol Prev. 2005;29(5–6):77–85.
72. Comba P, Pirastu R, Conti S, De Santis M, Iavarone I, Marsili G, et al. Environment and health in Taranto, southern Italy: epidemiological studies and public health recommendation]. [Article in Italian]. Epidemiol Prev. 2012;36(6):305–20.
73. Xiong D, Fang T, Yu L, Sima X, Zhu W. Effects of nano-scale TiO_2, ZnO and their bulk counterparts on zebrafish: Acute toxicity, oxidative stress and oxidative damage. Sci Total Environ. 2011;409:1444–52.
74. Karki P, Lee E, Aschner M. Manganese Neurotoxicity: a Focus on Glutamate Transporters. Review Ann Occup Environ Med. 2013;25:4.
75. Tchounwou PB, Yedjou CG, Patlolla AK, Sutton DJ. Heavy Metals Toxicity in the Environment. EXS. 2012;101:133–64.

7

Prevalence, habits and personal attitudes towards smoking among health care professionals

Brankica Juranić[1*], Željko Rakošec[2], Jelena Jakab[1], Štefica Mikšić[1], Suzana Vuletić[3], Marul Ivandić[4] and Ivka Blažević[1]

Abstract

Background: Tobacco use is the second major cause of morbidity and the 4th most common health risk factor in the world. Medical professionals have a critical role in the process of smoking cessation both as advisers and behavioural models for the citizens. The aim of this study was to investigate the prevalence of smoking among health care professionals, their smoking habits and personal attitudes toward smoking, role and the responsibility of health care professionals in the prevention of smoking.

Results: Out of the total number of examinees, 175 (35,1%) are active smokers, 29 (5,8%) are former smokers, and 295 (59,1%) are non-smokers. Nurses with secondary education disagree the most with the claim that passive smoking is more harmful to health ($\chi 2$ test, p = .008), also with the claim that the introduced Smoking Act is fair to smokers ($\chi 2$ test, p = .021). More nurses with secondary education disagree completely or partially that one should pay attention to smoking in the presence of non-smokers ($\chi 2$ test, p = .012).

Conclusion: Training programs for health care workers are needed to improve their ability in smoking cessation techniques to provide active support to their patients.

Keywords: Attitude, Habits, Prevalence, Smoking

Background

Worldwide, tobacco use is the second major cause of morbidity and the 4th most common health risk factor in the world. It causes diseases such as lung cancer, chronic obstructive pulmonary disease and coronary heart disease [1, 2].

All modern states are responsible for the preservation and improvement of their citizen's health and are therefore obliged to undertake systematic legal action to fight tobacco smoking. A comprehensive approach to reduction of this global pandemic is a priority, which can be seen in EU anti-smoking strategy [3]. This strategy offers extensive smoking prevention and cessation activities, including education measures and restrictions on tobacco marketing [4–7].

According to "The Survey on Tobacco use in the adult population of Croatia" conducted in 2014/2015., 31% of Croatians are smokers. As an EU member country, Croatia implements a stricter enforcement of new laws against smoking which was first brought in 1999. The Act on the Restriction of the Use of Tobacco Products imposes a total smoking ban in all workplaces, all public areas where people work or stay, open areas such as school yards, hospital areas, sports stadiums, arenas, open-air theatres, tram and bus stations. Smoking is also banned in all enclosed public areas including bars, restaurants and cafes [8].

It is of major importance to assess habits and attitudes toward smoking of medical professionals, given their critical role in the process of smoking cessation both as advisers and behavioural models for the citizens [9]. Especially important is the way they see themselves in a role of helping smokers who wish to quit [10]. This mostly applies to nurses, given the fact that they

* Correspondence: juranicbrankica@gmail.com
[1]Faculty of Medicine, Josip Juraj Strossmayer University of Osijek, Cara Hadrijana 10/E, HR-31000 Osijek, Croatia
Full list of author information is available at the end of the article

represent the biggest working group among healthcare professionals, thus having a major impact on their colleagues and patients regarding smoking habits.

Two important findings emerged from a number of studies are that health professionals have more success in convincing patients to stop smoking if they are not smokers [11]; and smokers who rely on a support and advice of their healthcare provider have more chances to quit than those who try it on their own [12–14]. Despite all this, and despite the well-known damages of smoking, studies still show a high prevalence of smokers among health professionals [15–19], meaning they are not a good example for their patients [20, 21]. In some European countries, smoking prevalence among healthcare professionals is higher or at least equal to the prevalence in general population. For example, smoking prevalence among Italian physicians is 28%, this percentage among physicians in France is 34%, while there is 40% of Greek and Turkish physicians who smoke [22]. Also, studies have shown that nurses smoke more than physicians, especially the ones with the secondary level of education [23–28]. Bearing in mind that physicians and nurses are considered an example to community and colleagues [29], it is important that hospitals represent a place where the culture of health promotion and smoking cessation is developed [30].

The aim of this study was to investigate the prevalence of smoking among health care professionals, their smoking habit and personal attitudes toward smoking, in order to rise the responsibility of health care professionals in the prevention of smoking.

Methods

Study design

This study is designed as a descriptive cross-sectional survey.

Setting and sample

The study was carried out in 11 clinics, 8 departments and 4 Clinical Institutes of the University Hospital Centre Osijek. The total number of the examinees is 499, what makes up 23% of the total number of the health care professionals employed at the University Hospital Centre in 2015. A total of 620 surveys were distributed and 499 (80.4%) responded.

Ethical consideration

Prior to their participation in the research, examinees have been informed that the participation in the survey is voluntary and anonymous, also about what is expected from them and about the aim of the research, what has also been specified on the questionnaire. The approval from the University Clinical Hospital Centre Osijek's Ethical Committee was acquired before the conduction of the study.

Measurements/instruments

The study was conducted by means of an anonymous questionnaire which consists of general information, basic habits related to smoking, and personal attitudes related to smoking. The questionnaire was made on the basis of theoretical knowledge, literature review and prior experience. This questionnaire was not validated before this research.

The first part of the questionnaire contains 7 questions (sex, year of birth, occupation, years of work experience, respiratory tract difficulties). The second part of the questionnaire contains questions related to personal smoking habits – how long have you been smoking, how many cigarettes a day, do you smoke in your workplace, do you smoke in the presence of your patients. The third part of the questionnaire contains 14 questions related to personal attitudes toward smoking, at which point the examinees answered the questions using evaluation (from 1 to 5).

Statistical analysis

Numerical data was described by measures of centre and spread. The normality of the distribution of the observed numeric variables was tested using the Kolmogorov–Smirnov test. The categorical variables are described by absolute and relative frequencies. The differences between the categorical dependent variables were tested by chi-square (χ 2) test and by Fisher's exact test.

To evaluate the structure of the questionnaire about attitudes toward smoking we used the common factor analysis method with orthogonal rotation (Varimax). We have extracted two significant factors by Kaiser-Guttman and Cattell criterion. Those two factors explain the total of 53.99% variance, so we can conclude that the questionnaire has a valid structure (Table 1).

The level $p < 0.05$ was chosen for the statistical significance assessment of the obtained results. Statistics software package Statistica for Windows 2005 (version 7.1, StatSoft Inc., Tulsa, OK, USA) had been used).

Results

There were 499 examinees included in the research, 413 (82.8%) of which females. The average age of the examinees is 39.8 (±11.54) years. According to the workplace, the most numerous are nurses and medical technicians with secondary education - 253 (50.7%), followed by 97 (19.4%) nurses/technicians with an associate degree, significantly more females than males (χ^2 test, $p < .001$). Regarding years of service, 134 (26.9%) examinees had 11 to 20 years of service, and 73 (14.6%) examinees had more than 30 years of service.

Table 1 Common factor models after orthogonal rotation

	Factor	Factor
	1	2
osp3	.715	
osp2	.687	
osp4	.647	
osp7	.632	
osp1	.582	
osp5	.565	
osp14		.954
osp13		.848
osp15		.649
Characteristic values	2.61	2.25
% of Variance	29.02	24.98
Cumulative %	53.99	

Extraction Method: Principal Axis Factoring
Rotation Method: Varimax with Kaiser Normalization

The reliability of the questionnaire was verified by the Cronbach Alpha reliability coefficient. For the first factor the value is .82, and for the second is .88, suggesting both of them have relatively high internal consistency.

Out of the total number of examinees, there are 175 (35.1%) active smokers, 9 (5.8%) former smokers, and 295 (59.1%) non-smokers. There is no significant difference between wether someone is a smoker and which workplace they hold. The greatest number of smokers, 59 (11.8%), started smoking between 11 to 20 years ago, and 12 (2.4%) of the examinees smoke longer than 30 years. Concerning a number of cigarettes smoked, 86 (17.2%) examinees smoke 10 to 20 cigarettes per day while only 2 (0.4%) smoke over 30 cigarettes per day. In public areas smoke 99 (19.8%) examinees, significantly more females than males (Fisher's exact test, p = .023); 134 (26.9%) examinees smoke in their workplace, while only 1 (0.2%) examinee smokes in the presence of the patients.

There are 11 (2.2%) examinees who disagree with the claim that passive smoking is bad for the health, significantly more nurses/technicians (chi-square, p = .008) (Table 2). In addition, significantly more nurses/ technicians with secondary education consider that the recently introduced Smoking Ban Act is not fair to the smokers (Table 3). More nurses do not agree fully or partially about wether one should pay attention to smoking in the presence of non-smokers (Table 4).

There is no significant difference regarding whether smoking in front of patients in the work place is ethical, because most of the examinees, 399 (80.3%), consider that this is not ethical. Almost all examinees agree that health care professionals' ethical responsibility is to warn pregnant women of the harmful effects smoking has on the fetus (Table 5). There was no significant difference regarding the answers to questions wether the health care professionals have a greater responsibility when it comes to prevention of the harmful effects of smoking than other society members (Table 6).

The influence of gender, age, and workplace on the factors "attitudes toward smoking" and "opinion about

Table 2 Attitudes toward harmful effects of smoking

	Resident physicians	Specialist physicians	Trainee nurses	Nurses with secondary education	Nurses with associate degree	Total	p*
	N (%)	N (%)	N (%)	N (%)	N (%)	N (%)	
Smoking is harmful to health							
Strongly disagree	0 (0.0)	0 (0.0)	0 (0.0)	4 (1.6)	1 (1.0)	5 (1.0)	.004
Disagree	0 (0.0)	0 (0.0)	0 (0.0)	14 (5.5)	2 (2.1)	16 (3.2)	
Undecided	0 (0.0)	0 (0.0)	1 (2.6)	18 (7.1)	4 (4.1)	23 (4.6)	
Agree	0 (0.0)	5 (6.4)	8 (20.5)	35 (13.8)	11 (11.3)	59 (11.8)	
Strongly agree	32 (100)	73 (93.6)	30 (76.9)	182 (71.9)	79 (81.4)	396 (79.4)	
Second-hand smoking is harmful to health							
Strongly disagree	0 (0.0)	1 (1.3)	1 (2.6)	8 (3.2)	1 (1.0)	11 (2.2)	.008
Disagree	0 (0.0)	0 (0.0)	1 (2.6)	15 (5.9)	3 (3.1)	19 (3.8)	
Undecided	1 (3.1)	2 (2.6)	1 (2.6)	22 (8.8)	10 (10.3)	36 (7.2)	
Agree	4 (12.5)	12 (15.4)	10 (25.6)	63 (25.1)	14 (14.4)	103 (20.7)	
Strongly agree	27 (84.4)	63 (80.8)	26 (66.7)	143 (56.9)	69 (71.1)	328 (66.0)	

*chi-square

Table 3 Attitudes toward Smoking Ban Act

	Resident physicians	Spcialist physicians	Trainee nurses	Nurses with secondary education	Nurses with associate degree	Total	p*
	N (%)	N (%)	N (%)	N (%)	N (%)	N (%)	
Smoking Ban Act is fair to the non-smokers							
Strongly disagree	0 (0.0)	1 (1.3)	3 (7.7)	24 (9.6)	4 (4.2)	32 (6.5)	
Disagree	0 (0.0)	2 (2.6)	0 (0.0)	20 (8.0)	5 (5.2)	27 (5.5)	.021
Undecided	3 (9.4)	6 (7.8)	8 (20.5)	29 (11.6)	10 (10.4)	56 (11.3)	
Agree	108 (31.3)	14 (18.2)	5 (12.8)	51 (20.4)	21 (21.9)	101 (20.5)	
Strongly agree	19 (59.4)	54 (70.1)	23 (59.0)	126 (50.4)	56 (58.3)	278 (56.3)	
Smoking Ban Act is fair to the smokers							
Strongly disagree	3 (9.7)	6 (7.8)	5 (12.8)	52 (20.9)	19 (19.6)	85 (17.2)	.005
Disagree	3 (9.7)	9 (11.7)	3 (7.7)	43 (17.3)	9 (9.3)	67 (13.6)	
Undecided	7 (22.6)	9 (11.7)	13 (33.3)	45 (18.1)	19 (19.6)	93 (18.9)	
Agree	10 (32.3)	21 (27.3)	9 (23.1)	61 (24.5)	20 (20.6)	121 (24.5)	
Strongla agree	8 (25.8)	32 (41.6)	9 (23.1)	48 (19.3)	30 (30.9)	127 (25.8)	
Total	32 (100)	78 (100)	39 (100)	251(100)	97 (100)	497 (100)	

*chi-square

the role of healthcare provider in smoking" was tested through multivariate analysis of variance. We have three nominal variables and two continuous variables. Using multivariate analysis we found that there was no statistically significant influence of sex (Wilksov $\Lambda = 0.99$, F (2439) = 0.65, $p > 0.05$, $\eta2 = 0.003$) or age (Wilksov $\Lambda = 0.97$, F (8.880) = 1.53, $p > 0.05$, $\eta2 = 0.014$) on the attitude toward smoking and the opinion about the role of healthcare professionals in smoking. On the other hand, there was a statistically significant effect of the

Table 4 Attitudes toward smoking in front of non-smokers and children

	Resident physicians	Specialist physicians	Trainee nurses	Nurses with secondary education	Nurses with associate degree	Total	P*
	N (%)	N (%)	N (%)	N (%)	N (%)	N (%)	
One should pay attention to smoking in presence of non-smokers							
Strongly disagree	0 (0.0)	1 (1.3)	2 (5.1)	15 (5.9)	3 (3.1)	21 (4.2)	.012
Disagree	0 (0.0)	1 (1.3)	0 (0.0)	12 (4.8)	4 (4.2)	17 (3.4)	
Undecided	2 (6.2)	1 (1.3)	4 (10.3)	17 (6.7)	5 (5.2)	29 (5.8)	
Agree	7 (21.9)	7 (9.1)	9 (23.1)	55 (21.8)	10 (10.4)	88 (17.7)	
Strongly agree	23 (71.9)	67 (87.0)	24 (61.5)	153 (60.7)	74 (77.1)	341 (68.7)	
One should pay attention to smoking in presence of children							
Strongly disagree	1 (3.1)	4 (5.1)	1 (2.6)	7 (2.8)	4 (4.2)	17 (3.4)	.859
Disagree	0 (0.0)	0 (0.0)	1 (2.6)	3 (1.2)	0 (0.0)	4 (0.8)	
Undecided	0 (0.0)	2 (2.6)	0 (0.0)	3 (1.2)	2 (2.1)	7 (1.4)	
Agree	3 (9.4)	3 (3.9)	1 (2.6)	8 (3.2)	4 (4.2)	19 (3.8)	
Strongly agree	28 (87.5)	69 (88.5)	36 (92.3)	231 (91.7)	86 (89.6)	450 (90.5)	

*chi-square

Table 5 Attitude toward health care professionals' ethical responsibility to warn smokers and pregnant women who smoke about harmful effects of smoking

	Resident physicians	Specialist physicians	Trainee nurses	Nurses with secondary education	Nurses with associate degree	Total	p*
	N (%)	N (%)	N (%)	N (%)	N (%)	N (%)	
Health care professionals' ethical responsibility is to warn the smokers of the harmful effects of smoking							
Strongly agree	1 (3.1)	1 (3.1)	3 (7.9)	11 (4.4)	2 (2.1)	18 (3.6)	.044
Agree	0 (0.0)	2 (2.6)	0 (0.0)	5 (2.0)	1 (1.0)	8 (1.6)	
Undecided	0 (0.0)	2 (2.6)	8 (21.1)	27 (10.8)	9 (9.3)	46 (9.3)	
Agree	8 (25.0)	13 (16.7)	7 (18.4)	62 (24.7)	18 (18.6)	108 (21.8)	
Strongly agree	23 (71.9)	60 (76.9)	20 (52.6)	146 (58.2)	67 (69.1)	316 (63.7)	
Health care professionals' ethical responsibility is to warn pregnant women of the harmful effects smoking has on the fetus							
Strongly agree	0 (0.0)	1 (3.1)	0 (0.0)	8 (3.2)	2 (2.1)	11 (2.2)	.334
Agree	1 (3.1)	1 (3.1)	0 (0.0)	4 (1.6)	2 (2.1)	8 (1.6)	
Undecided	0 (0.0)	2 (2.6)	0 (0.0)	8 (3.2)	4 (4.2)	14 (2.8)	
Agree	5 (15.6)	5 (6.4)	6 (15.4)	49 (19.4)	10 (10.4)	75 (15.1)	
Strongly agree	26 (81.3)	69 (88.5)	33 (84.6)	183 (72.6)	78 (81.3)	389 (78.3)	
Total	32 (100)	78 (100)	39 (100)	251 (100)	97 (100)	497 (100)	

*chi-square

workplace on the attitude toward smoking and the opinion about the role of healthcare workers in smoking (Wilksov Λ = 0.93, F (10.880) = 3.86, $p < 0.01$, $\eta 2 = 0.034$). For better interpretation of results, one-way analysis of variance was performed with Bonferroni correction ($p < 0.025$), separately for each dependent variable, because the variable "workplace" had more than two factor levels. There was a statistically significant difference in the attitude toward smoking with regard to the level of workplace (F (5.477) = 9.76, $p < 0.01$, $\eta 2 = 0.076$). The difference was between physician specialists (M = 27.23, sd = 3.43), who have a high opinion that smoking is harmful, and nurses/technicians with the secondary level of education (M = 23.64, SD = 5.36). Furthermore, there was a statistically significant difference in the level of workplaces and the opinion about the role of healthcare workers in smoking (F (5.485) = 3.27, $p < 0.01$, $\eta 2 = 0.026$). The Bonferroni correction has confirmed that physician specialist (M = 12.64, SD = 3.06) averagely agree more with the claim that healthcare professionals are role models to the wider population, unlike nurses/technicians with secondary level of education (M = 11.34, SD = 3.55).

Discussion

Although the facts about the harmful effect of smoking are well-known, and health care providers are the first expected to be an example of awareness and consciousness, the data of this research shows a high prevalence of smokers among health care professionals, results similar to previous studies in Croatia [28, 31]. The higher smoking prevalence among health care professionals than that of the general population can potentially be explained by occupational stress, which is one of the key factors to addiction [32].

Occupational stress is mostly related to the nurses who finished secondary school, nursing shortage, nurses who have a large number of overtime working hours, also, nurses with the most shift working hours and the lowest level of education.

One of the key factors is the influence of cultural norms because not so long ago smoking was socially acceptable and highlighted as a specific status symbol.

Health care professionals are familiar with the harmful effects of smoking and passive smoking. The fact that only one of our examinees smokes in front of patients is very encouraging although it is not consistent with other studies where it was found that there are more health care professionals who smoke in front of patients [33]. Out of the total number of participants, 450 (90.5%) of them completely agrees on the issue that smokers should pay attention to smoking in the presence of children. Almost all of the examinees agree with the claim that the medical health professionals have an ethical

Table 6 Attitudes toward example and responsibility of health care professionals

	Resident physicians	Specialist physicians	Trainee nurses	Nurses with secondary education	Nurses with associate degree	Total	p*
	N (%)	N (%)	N (%)	N (%)	N (%)	N (%)	
Health care professionals are example to their patients							
Strongly disagree	2 (6.2)	5 (6.5)	2 (5.1)	24 (9.6)	4 (4.1)	37 (7.5)	.435
Disagree	2 (6.2)	2 (2.6)	1 (2.6)	10 (3.9)	2 (2.1)	17 (3.4)	
Undecided	4 (12.5)	5 (6.5)	6 (15.4)	41 (16.3)	15 (15.5)	71 (14.3)	
Agree	14 (43.7)	24 (31.2)	11 (28.2)	74 (29.5)	28 (28.8)	151 (30.4)	
Strongly agree	10 (31.2)	41 (53.2)	19 (48.7)	102 (40.7)	48 (49.5)	220 (44.3)	
Health care professionals are example to the society							
Strongly disagree	2 (6.2)	4 (5.2)	2 (5.1)	32 (12.7)	5 (5.1)	45 (9.0)	.088
Disagree	2 (6.2)	2 (2.6)	2 (5.1)	16 (6.3)	2 (2.1)	24 (4.8)	
Undecided	5 (15.6)	9 (11.7)	13 (33.3)	45 (17.9)	18 (18.6)	90 (18.1)	
Agree	11 (34.4)	26 (33.8)	8 (20.5)	70 (27.8)	26 (26.8)	141 (28.4)	
Strongly agree	12 (37.5)	36 (46.7)	14 (35.9)	89 (35.3)	46 (47.4)	197 (39.6)	
Health care professionals have a greater responsibility when it comes to prevention of the harmful effects of smoking than the other society members							
Strongly disagree	1 (3.1)	4 (5.2)	4 (10.3)	25 (10.0)	5 (5.1)	39 (7.9)	.074
Disagree	5 (15.6)	4 (5.2)	1 (2.6)	21 (8.4)	6 (6.2)	37 (7.5)	
Undecided	2 (6.2)	3 (3.9)	10 (25.6)	34 (13.6)	13 (13.4)	62 (12.5)	
Agree	10 (31.2)	19 (24.7)	11 (28.2)	65 (26.1)	22 (22.7)	127 (25.7)	
Strongly agree	14 (43.7)	47 (61.0)	13 (33.3)	104 (41.8)	51 (52.6)	229 (46.4)	
Total	32 (100)	78 (100)	39 (100)	251 (100)	97 (100)	497 (100)	

*chi-square

responsibility to warn pregnant women who smoke of the potentially harmful effects smoking can have on the fetus during pregnancy. Those are results similar to other studies where physicians showed willingness for a conversation with a pregnant woman about adverse effects of smoking and advising about cessation [34].

The great number of physicians completely agree that healthcare professionals have an ethical responsibility to warn smokers of the harmful effects of smoking. However, health care professionals who smoke feel discomfort in situations when they are supposed to counsel their patients about smoking cessation and the harmfulness of the tobacco smoke [35]. They have difficulties in creating transfer/countertransference relationship with patients in the smoking prevention [36]. Problems can also be caused by the lack of motivation of the health care professionals due to previous negative experiences when patients didn't accept the advice given by them regarding the use of tobacco products for cessation. On the other hand, health care professionals who have been additionally educated and acquainted with problems of smoking cessation, who understand their patients' problems, and have the will and desire to encourage them to stop smoking, personally feel more content [37].

Physicians and nurses, as a part of the health care system, play an equally important role in the prevention and education of patients about the harmfulness of smoking. Primary care physicians play a major role in the process of making the decision to stop smoking and should be the first one whom the patient turns to. The importance and responsibility of the visiting nurses are the key to promoting the healthy way of life and healthy behaviour. Their role in the community is significant because they participate in giving advice, encouraging people, supporting people and referring them to services which can help them with smoking cessation and pharmacological treatment [38]. Nurses that have been educated had more expertise and better results in interventions for smoking cessation. The studies show that the lack of time and education are the two main reasons that are preventing nurses in giving advice regarding the smoking cessation [39]. Nurses in our study showed disagreement with claims that passive smoking is harmful to health and that one should pay attention to smoking in the presence of non-smokers. Those findings confirm that inadequate knowledge about smoking and smoking cessation affect nurses' health promotion role. The main reasons for the high prevalence of smoking among nurses include occupational stress, nurse education, professional socialization and lack of support [40]. Although nurses fulfil important roles in health promotion, their potential is under-utilized due to poor knowledge, lack of confidence and a conflict of personal attitudes to smoking [41].

To improve the existing anti-tobacco strategies, the recommendations are to strengthen legislation for tobacco control in hospitals, and to expand current control efforts based on evidence of high-quality data, creating a smoke-free environment where social acceptability of smoking would be reduced. Also, regular surveillance of those programmes along with the dissemination of research findings would provide policy makers evidence that suggests the need for increasing tobacco control achievements [42].

Health care professionals who smoke have difficulty with insufficient education and insufficient motivation due to poor prior experiences when their patients have not accepted their advice on cessation of tobacco product consumption. In our society we need to raise the awareness of citizens and health workers about smoking hazards, so that every person can act responsibly. Health care professionals who are more informed and educated, are familiar with the problem of smoking cessation, understand the patient's problems, have a stronger will and desire to encourage smoking cessation.

Conclusions

The results of our research have shown that the prevalence of smokers among health care professionals is high, implying the ineffectiveness of the current anti-tobacco strategy. Health care professionals, who should inform others about the harmfulness of the tobacco smoke, are not fully aware to what extent smoking is harmful both to them and to people who surround them. It would be helpful to implement training programs for healthcare workers to improve their ability in smoking cessation counselling techniques to provide active support to their patients.

Acknowledgements
Not applicable.

Funding
Authors didn't have financial support in making this paper.

Authors' contributions
Conception and design of the study: BJ, ŽR, SV. Acquisition of data: MI, IB. Data analysis and interpretation: JJ, ŠM. Article draft: BJ, ŽR, JJ, ŠM. Critically advising article: SV, MI, IB. Approved the version to be published: BJ, ŽR, JJ, ŠM, SV, MI, IB. Agreed to be accountable for all aspects of the work: BJ, ŽR, JJ, ŠM, SV, MI, IB.

Competing interests
The authors declare that they have no competing interests in this manuscript.

Author details
[1]Faculty of Medicine, Josip Juraj Strossmayer University of Osijek, Cara Hadrijana 10/E, HR-31000 Osijek, Croatia. [2]Department of Culturology, Josip Juraj Strossmayer University of Osijek, Trg Svetog Trojstva 3, Osijek, Croatia. [3]Catholic Faculty of Theology in Đakovo, Josip Juraj Strossmayer University of Osijek, Petra Preradovića 17, Đakovo, Croatia. [4]Public Health Centre Osijek, Park kralja Petra Krešimira IV. 6, HR-31000 Osijek, Croatia.

References

1. Centers For Disease Control and Prevention. Smoking and tobacco use. Health effects. https://www.cdc.gov/tobacco/data_statistics/fact_sheets/health_effects/effects_cig_smoking/index.htm. Accessed 15 Oct 2015.
2. Smith SS, Beckley T, Fiore MC. Health care provider use of guideline-based smoking cessation interventions: results from the 2003 Wisconsin tobacco survey. WMJ. 2005;140:28–31.
3. Padjen I, Dabić M, Glivetić T, Biloglav Z, Biočina-Lukenda D, Lukenda J. The analysis of tobacco consumption in Croatia – are we successfully facing the epidemic? Cent Eur J Public Health. 2012;20(1):5–10.
4. World Health Organization. European strategy for tobacco control. Copenhagen: WHO Regional Office for Europe; 2002.
5. Joossens L, Raw M. The tobacco control scale: a new scale to measure country activity. Tob Control. 2006;15(3):247–53.
6. Bala M, Strzeszynski L, Cahill K. Mass media interventions for smoking cessation in adults. Cochrane Database Syst Rev. 2008;23(1):CD004704.
7. Thomas R, Perera R. School-based programmes for preventing smoking. Cochrane Database Syst Rev. 2006;3:CD001293.
8. Zakon o ograničavanju uporabe duhanskih proizvoda. Zagreb: Narodne novine d.d., 2009;119/09.
9. World Health Organization (WHO). The role of health professionals in tobacco control. Geneva: WHO. 2005.
10. Hussain SF, Tjeder-Burton S, Campbell IA, Davies PD. Attitudes to smoking and smoking habits among hospital staff. Thorax. 1993;48:174–5.
11. Smith DR, Leggat PA. An international review of tobacco smoking in the medical profession: 1974–2004. BMC Public Health. 2007;7:115.
12. Kottke TE, Battista RN, DeFriese GH, Brekke ML. Attributes of successful smoking cessation interventions in medical practice. A meta-analysis of 39 controlled trials. JAMA. 1988;259:2883–9.
13. Lancaster T, Stead LF. Self-help interventions for smoking cessation. Cochrane Database Syst Rev. 2005;3:CD001118.
14. Hollis JF, Lichtenstein E, Vogt TM, et al. Nurse-assisted counseling for smokers in primary care. Ann Intern Med. 1993;118:521–5.
15. Ferguson P, Small WP. Further study of the smoking habits of hospital nurses. Health Bull. 1985;43:13–8.
16. Olsen AD, Fugleholm AM, Rasmussen S, et al. Smoking behaviour and exposure to passive smoking among hospital employees 1992–1999. Ugeskr Laeger. 2000;162:5623–7.
17. Tapia-Conyer R, Cravioto P, de la Rosa B, et al. Cigarette smoking: knowledge and attitudes among Mexican physicians. Salud Publica Mex. 1997;39:507–12.
18. Kawakami M, Nakamura S, Fumimoto H, et al. Relation between smoking status of physicians and their enthusiasm to offer smoking cessation advice. Intern Med. 1997;36:162–5.
19. Nielsen PE, Falk J, Danielsen US. Smoking habits and attitudes towards

the tobacco issue among health professionals in Denmark in 1996. Ugeskrift. 2000;162:4140–4.
20. Davis RM. When doctors smoke. Tob Control. 1993;2:187–8.
21. Willaing I, Ladelund S. Smoking behavior among hospital staff still influences attitudes and counseling on smoking. Nicotine Tob Res. 2004;6:369–75.
22. Sotiropoulos A, Gikas A, Spanou E, Dimitrelos D, Karakostas F, Skliros E, Apostolou O, Politakis P, Pappas S. Smoking habits and associated factors amongGreek physicians. Public Health. 2007;121:333–40.
23. Glavaš D, Rumboldt M, Rumboldt Z. Smoking cessation with nicotine replacement therapy among health care workers: randomized Doubleblind study. CMJ. 2003;44:219–24.
24. Ravara SB, Calheiros JM, Aguiar P, Barata LT. Smoking behaviour predicts tobacco control attitudes in a high smoking prevalence hospital: a crosssectional study in a Portuguese teaching hospital prior to the national smoking ban. BMC Public Health. 2011;11:720.
25. Hodgetts G, Broesrs T, Godwin M. Smoking behaviour, knowledge and attitudes among family medicine physicians and nurses in Bosnia and Herzegovina. BMC Fam Pract. 2004;5:12.
26. Ramos MC, Vinagre S, Cardoso MF. Knowledge, behaviour and ethical responsibility of health professionals with regard to smoking. Rev Port Cardiol. 2010;29:923–46.
27. Fernandez Ruiz ML, Sanchez BM. Evolution of the prevalence of smoking among female physicians and nurses in the autonomous Community of Madrid. Gac Sanit. 2003;17:5–10.
28. Kumbrija S, Milaković SB, Jelinić JD, Matanić D, Marković BB, Simunović R. Health care professionals - attitudes towards their own health. Acta Med Croatica. 2007;61(1):105–10.
29. Nett LM. The physician's role in smoking cessation: a present and future agenda. Chest. 1990;97:28–32.
30. WHO – Integrating health promotion into hospitals and health services, 2007. http://www.euro.who.int/en/health-topics/Health-systems/public-healthservices/publications/2007/integrating-health-promotion-into-hospitals-and-health-services,-whoeurope-2007. Accessed 25 Oct 2015.
31. Gazdek D, Kovačić L. Smoking habits among health staff in the county of Koprivnica-Križevci - comparative study 1998 and 2002. Lijec Vjesn. 2004;126(1–2):6–10.
32. Ficarra MG, et al. Tobacco use prevalence, knowledge and attitudes among Italian hospital healthcare professionals. Eur J Pub Health. 2011;21(1):29–34.
33. Duaso M, Duncan D. Health impact of smoking and smoking cessation strategies: current evidence. Br J Community Nurs. 2012;17(8):356–63.
34. Glover M, Paynter J, Bullen C, Kristensen K. Supporting pregnant women to quit smoking: postal survey of New Zealand general practitioners and midwives' smoking cessation knowledge and practices. N Z Med J. 2008;121(1270):53–65.
35. Lancaster T, Fowler G. Training health professionals in smoking cessation. Cochrane Database Syst Rev. 2012. http://dx.doi.org/10.1002/14651858. CD000214. Accessed 25 Nov 2015.
36. Abdullah AS, Stillman FA, Yang L, Luo H, Zhiyong Z, Samet JM. Tobacco use and smoking cessation practices among physicians in developing countries: a literature review (1987–2010). Int J Environ Res Public Health. 2014;11:429–55.
37. Bostan PP, Demir CK, Elbek O, Akçay Ş. Association between pulmonologists' tobacco use and their effort in promoting smoking cessation in Turkey: a crosssectional study. BMC Pulm Med. 2015;15:143.
38. Sarna L, Bialous SA, Sinha K, Yang Q, Wewers ME. Are health care providers stil smoking? Data from the 2003 and 2006/2007 tobacco use supplement-Caurrent population surveys. Nicotine Tob Res. 2010;11:1167–71.
39. Li I, Lee SYD, Chen CY, Jeng YQ, Chen YC. Facilitators and Barriers to Effective Smoking Cessation: Counselling Services for Inpatients from Nurse-Counsellors' Perspectives — A Qualitative Study. Int J Environ Res Public Health. 2014;11(5):4782–98.
40. Strobol J, Latter S. Qualified nurse smokers attitudes towards a hospital smoking ban and its influence on their smoking behaviour. J Adv Nurs. 1998;27:179–88.
41. O'Donovan G. Smoking prevalence among qualified nurses in the Republic of Ireland and their role in smoking cessation. Int Nurs Rev. 2009;56:230–6.
42. Ljubicic D, Schneider NK, Vrazic H. Attitudes and knowledge of third year medical students in Croatia about tobacco control strategies: results of the Global Health professionals pilot survey in Croatia, 2005.

8

Is outdoor work associated with elevated rates of cerebrovascular disease mortality?A cohort study based on iron-ore mining

Ove Björ[1*], Håkan Jonsson[1], Lena Damber[1], Lage Burström[2] and Tohr Nilsson[2]

Abstract

Background: A cohort study that examined iron ore mining found negative associations between cumulative working time employed underground and several outcomes, including mortality of cerebrovascular diseases. In this cohort study, and using the same group of miners, we examined whether work in an outdoor environment could explain elevated cerebrovascular disease rates.

Methods: This study was based on a Swedish iron ore mining cohort consisting of 13,000 workers. Poisson regression models were used to generate smoothed estimates of standardized mortality ratios and adjusted rate ratios, both models by cumulative exposure time in outdoor work.

Results: The adjusted rate ratio between employment classified as outdoor work ≥25 years and outdoor work 0–4 years was 1.62 (95 % CI 1.07–2.42). The subgroup underground work ≥15 years deviated most in occurrence of cerebrovascular disease mortality compared with the external reference population: SMR (0.70 (95 % CI 0.56–0.85)).

Conclusions: Employment in outdoor environments was associated with elevated rates of cerebrovascular disease mortality. In contrast, work in tempered underground employment was associated with a protecting effect.

Keywords: Poisson regression, Occupation, Standardized mortality ratio, Mortality, Cohort study, Mining

Abbreviations: HWSE, Healthy worker survivor effect; ICD, International classification of disease; SMR, Standardized mortality ratio

Background

A cohort study of Swedish iron-ore miners reported that duration of employment time among blue collar workers, especially in underground mining, was associated with lower risks of mortality and incidental cancer [1]. Compared with other workers, mortality from cerebrovascular diseases was lower among long term underground mining blue-collar workers (Rate Ratio: 0.66 (95 % ci 0.49–0.89)). Three explanations for these inverse associations were suggested: a protecting effect from working in a tempered underground environment, a protecting effect from heavy physical workloads, or, a healthy worker survivor effect (HWSE).

The lower risks of cerebrovascular disease associated with duration of underground mining work could be explained by a protecting effect from the more tempered underground climate compared with the outdoor climate. Acute effects of cerebrovascular disease mortality have been explained by cold outdoor temperatures [2, 3]. Workers that remain in longer term employment underground could also be individuals that have better health because of lifestyle factors, beneficial effects from long-term employment or genetic factors. This selection phenomenon of healthier workers remaining in the workforce with a resulting inverse association between cumulative exposure and outcome is called the HWSE [4, 5]. A recent paper from the Kiruna- and Malmberget mines in Sweden showed that adjusting for the HWSE by g-estimation of accelerated failure-time modeling resulted in elevated risks of mortality from respirable dust [6]. Historically, high physical workloads have been associated with mining activities [7]. Several papers have suggested that physically active occupations and

* Correspondence: ove.bjor@vll.se
[1]Department of Radiation Sciences (Oncology), Umeå University, SE-901 85 Umeå, Sweden
Full list of author information is available at the end of the article

lifestyles protect from stroke [8, 9], and colon and rectal cancer [10, 11].

The aim of this study was, to examine if outdoor mining work was associated with elevated rates of cerebrovascular disease mortality. This study will also consider underground work, due to the results from the previous study on this cohort that found a negative association with cerebrovascular disease mortality [1].

Methods

The cohort

The Kiruna and Malmberget iron-ore mines are located in the northernmost part of Sweden. They have been in operation since the early 19th century. The mines have similar employment policies and safety routines, and use similar types of equipment. Malmberget has been an underground mine since it began operation. Kiruna was an open-pit mine until the 1950s, when the mining activities successively went underground. Employees were included in the study cohort if they had been employed for at least one year between 1923–1998 at the Kiruna mine, and between 1923–1996 at the Malmberget mine. The cohort has previously been described in detail [12, 13].

Cohort mortality was followed from 1952–2006. Data was collected from the Swedish national cause of death register. The mortality endpoint was cerebrovascular diseases (ICD10: I60–I69), subgroups' cerebral infarction (ICD10: I63–I64), and cerebral haemorrhage (ICD10: I61). Information on cerebral haemorrhage was only available from 1965. A unique Swedish personal identification number was used to link dates of events and ICD-codes for mortality to each cohort member. Subjects that were not found in the cause of death register or the national population register ($N = 584$) were excluded from the cohort because they had died before 1952 or had emigrated from Sweden. Time at emigration from Sweden after 1952 was censured in the statistical analysis ($N = 54$). Workers for whom information on occupational class (blue-collar worker, white-collar worker, miscellaneous), or work location (inside, outdoor, mining) was not available were excluded ($N = 130$). Work periods were categorized as working underground, working 50 % of the time underground, or other work. We used this work period variable to represent underground work, and the classification procedure has been previously described [12, 13]. Of the remaining workers, 493 of them were employed only in white collar work, and were excluded from the study. The final cohort consisted of 13,000 male workers.

Classification of work periods into outdoor work

Classification of work location was based on job title, workplace, and year. This information was collected from written and computerized company records. Work location categories were working outdoors, working inside, or working in the mines. Due to the successive change from open to underground mining, all pre-1954 Kiruna mine work periods that were not registered as working inside were classified as working outdoors. This method of classifying work periods into outdoor work implied a possible overlap between the previously defined underground work and this new variable, outdoor work. From 1954 to 1958, blue-collar mining work periods were increasingly classified as working underground with the following weights: 0.1, 0.3, 0.5, 0.7, and 0.9. Classification of work location was performed by three researchers in occupational medicine that were knowledgeable about mine conditions, guided by descriptions of mine history [7].

Statistical methods

Two log-linear Poisson regression models were calculated. One model was based on cohort data only. The other model also incorporated external rates from the reference population of northern Sweden (male population 1980: 460445).

The model limited to comparisons within the cohort was:

$$\log E(d_{kl}) = \log(n_{kl}) + \alpha + x_k\beta + z_l\beta^*$$

where

$E(d_{kl})$: predicted number of outcomes in the cohort per nuisance variable, k, and exposure level variable, l

n_{kl}: person years from the cohort per categories, k, and l

α: constant

$x_k\beta$: is a vector of nuisance variables attained age, calendar year, year of first employment, also having been employed as a white collar worker, mine, and cumulative employment time underground and β represents the corresponding parameter estimates.

$Z_l\beta^*$: is a vector representing cumulative time working outdoors and β is the corresponding parameter estimates.

The main predictor ($z_l\beta^*$) estimated the ratio between categories 5–14, 15–24, and ≥25 years of cumulative employment time outdoor and the reference category 0–4 years. All variables representing cumulative employment time, calendar year, attained age, cumulative employment time underground, and white collar worker (yes, from the first day of employment as a white collar worker and forward, or, no) were analyzed as time-dependent variables. Test of trend was performed by entering a single continuous covariate in this Poisson model, with values representing the mean duration of employment for each category. To evaluate if acute effects of outdoor work could explain elevated rates (deaths occurring close to being employed), a variable coded as 1 (employed) or 0 (not employed) for each time period was included in the model to be able to adjust for possible differences due to deaths that occurred while employed. All deaths within 20 days from the last date of employment were counted as death while employed.

The model that incorporated external rates was:

$$\log E(d_{ijl}) = \log\left(\exp_{ij}\right) + \alpha + f(z_l)$$

where

$E(d_{ijl})$: predicted number of outcomes in the cohort per year, i, age group, j and category of outdoor work

$\exp_{ij}$: expected number of outcomes in the cohort per year, i, age group, j. The expected values were derived from mortality and cancer incidence risks based on the reference population of northern Sweden

α: constant

$f(z_l)$: a cubic spline function of cumulative time in outdoor work

This model generated smoothed estimates [14] of standardized mortality ratios (SMR) by cumulative employment time categorized into outdoor work. The cubic spline function ($f(z_l)$) was based on 3 knots: at 0 years of exposure, at the median number of years of exposure, and at 35 years of exposure. The function was linear from year 35. To complement the adjusted Poisson model described earlier, and to give priority to precision of the estimated SMR, we chose not to include nuisance parameters in this model.

Because of the cohort inclusion criterion of a one year minimum employment time, first year of employment was not included in any statistical analysis as time at risk. The potential for overdispersion was accounted for during Poisson regression estimation of all confidence intervals.

By calculating SMR based on cerebrovascular disease mortality as the outcome, different subgroups of the cohort were compared with the population of northern Sweden. SMR was calculated from cell-specific external rates represented by calendar year in one year classes and age in five year classes (maximum age class, ≥85 years). Because of the wide upper category of ≥85 years in the reference rates, the analyses on subgroups were also performed limited to <85 years of age. 95 % confidence intervals were calculated by assuming that the number of deaths in the cohort followed a Poisson distribution.

Data were analyzed with the statistical software package R (version 3.1.1; R Development Core Team, R foundation for Statistical Computing, Vienna, Austria).

Results

The study cohort consisted of 13,000 workers representing 443,930 person years. The average age at death of all causes was 67.3 (standard deviation (SD), 14.3) years. The distribution for key variables based on mortality of cerebrovascular diseases as outcome is presented in Table 1.

Table 1 Mean (Standard Deviation), age at death and distribution of number of deaths of cerebrovascular diseases

		Cerebrovascular diseases
Mean (SD) age at outcome		72.0 (12.4)
Total number of outcomes		403
Number of outcomes per birth year	–1899	49
	1900–1909	106
	1910–1919	112
	1920–1929	85
	≥1930	51
Number of outcomes per year of first employment	≤1929	112
	1930–1939	60
	1940–1949	62
	1950–1959	137
	≥1960	32
Number of outcomes per cumulative employment time in years	0–4	51
	5–14	75
	15–29	111
	≥30	166
Number of outcomes per mine	Kiruna	246
	Malmberget	157

The distribution of time classified as outdoor and underground work

Nineteen percent of the person years, as employed, were classified as "outdoor workers", compared with 46 % "working inside", 31 % "mining", and 3 % "missing". Working outdoors was most common before 1960 because the Kiruna mine was an open pit mine prior to 1960 (Fig. 1). Of all person time classified as outdoor, 26 % was simultaneously classified as underground work. Of all person years representing employment, 43 % was neither classified as outdoor or underground work. The classification procedures were performed by different experts, and the transition between outdoor and underground work meant that the specific location could be interpreted as outdoor and underground, depending on the criteria for location.

Outdoor work and the association with cerebrovascular disease mortality

The adjusted rate ratio estimates for mortality from cerebrovascular diseases increased with cumulative outdoor employment time (Fig. 2 and Table 2). An expanded analysis that included an interaction term between year of first employment and cumulative outdoor employment indicated that rates for workers employed for the first time in later years (1930–1949) more clearly was associated with cumulative outdoor employment compared with earlier years (<1930). This interaction effect between year of first employment and cumulative employment time

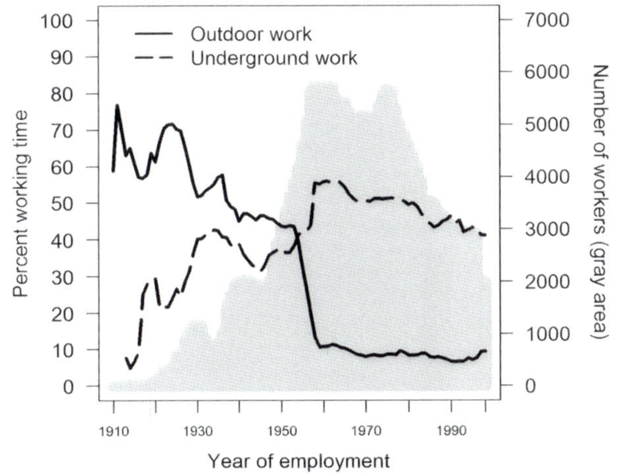

Fig. 1 Person year distribution of outdoor and underground work. Gray area represents the number of employed workers

outdoors did not significantly contribute to the model (p = 0.139, based on a likelihood ratio test for inclusion of the interaction effect). However, the rate ratio estimate for outdoor work ≥25 years compared with 0–4 years was 3.45 (95 % CI 1.55–7.65; 11 deaths: ≥25 years) for workers employed first time 1930–1949. The corresponding estimate was 1.16 (95 % CI 0.73–1.86; 37 deaths: ≥25 years) for workers that were employed first time before 1930. Because of the limited number of outcomes, it was not possible to calculate interaction term-estimates for later years of first employment. We also calculated adjusted rate ratio estimates from Poisson regression by delimiting outcomes to subgroups' cerebral haemorrhages and cerebral

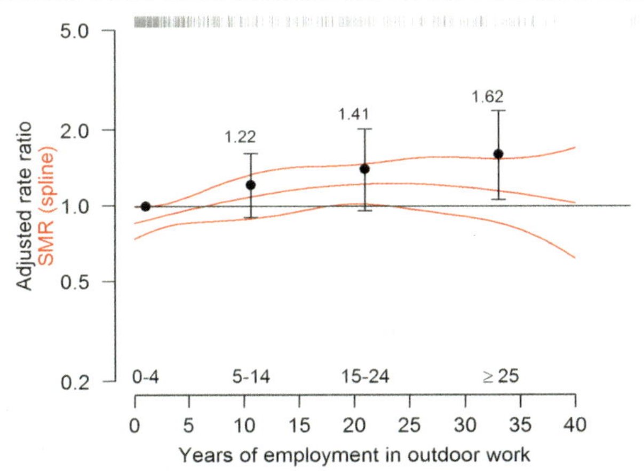

Fig. 2 Smoothed estimates of standardized mortality ratios (SMRs) with 95 % confidence intervals (lines) and adjusted point estimates of rate ratios in relation to cumulative time employed outdoors The categorical estimates in the figure are located at the mean employment time (1.0, 10.7, 21.0, 33.1 years). The location of the mortality outcomes in relation to cumulative time employed outdoors is marked on the top of the figure

infarctions. Due to the limited number of outcomes, long-term outdoor work was defined as outdoor work ≥15 years. For mortality of cerebral haemorrhages, the adjusted rate ratio for outdoor work 5–14 years (12 deaths) compared to outdoor work 0–4 years (46 deaths) was 1.21 (95 % CI 0.60–2.28) and the corresponding ratio for outdoor work ≥15 years (18 deaths) was 2.52 (95 % CI 1.23–5.04). For mortality of cerebral infarctions, the adjusted rate ratio for outdoor work 5–14 years (23 deaths) compared to outdoor work 0–4 years (71 deaths) was 1.38 (95 % CI 0.83–2.22) and the corresponding ratio for outdoor work ≥15 years (21 deaths) was 1.60 (95 % CI 0.88–2.81).

The results for SMR based on splines did not suggest as strong association between outdoor work and cerebrovascular disease mortality as suggested by the adjusted rate ratio estimates (Fig. 2). For short term outdoor work, the rates were lower than the corresponding expected rates derived from the reference population of northern Sweden which contributed to that the SMR, by design, was closer to unit for long term outdoor work compared to the category estimates.

Figure 3 shows the adjusted rate ratio estimates for cumulative outdoor work together with the corresponding estimates for underground work. The figure clearly illustrates the diverging trends when comparing the estimates of outside and underground work.

Delimiting the adjusted Poisson models to include only age ≥ 55 years did not change the interpretations of the results (Table 2). Adjusting for current employment status in the Poisson model had only small effects on the results (Table 2).

SMR based on subgroups from the cohort

The result for the estimated SMR of mortality from cerebrovascular disease revealed that the rates associated with underground work differed most from the expected rates (Fig. 4). Underground work ≥15 years represented 30 % lower rates: 0.70 (95 % CI 0.56–0.85). Corresponding SMR for outdoor work ≥15 years was 1.16 (95 % CI 0.94–1.40). Delimiting the calculations to include only ages < 85 years yielded similar conclusions, but with slightly lower levels of the estimates overall (data not shown).

Discussion

The results of this study suggested that there was an association between employments represented by temperature varying outdoor work environments and elevated rates of cerebrovascular disease mortality. The rate of cerebrovascular disease mortality representing cumulative outdoor employment time 25 years or more was 62 % higher (rate ratio: 1.62 (95 % CI 1.07–2.42)) compared with outdoor employment 0 to 4 years (Fig. 2 and Table 2). Moreover, diverging trends between outdoor work and underground work became evident when both variables were included

Table 2 Adjusted rate ratio estimates derived from Poisson regression models, with 95 % confidence intervals (CI)

	0–4 years		5–14 years			15–24 years			≥25 years			
	n[a]	Rate ratio	n[a]	Rate ratio	95 % CI	n[a]	Rate ratio	95 % CI	n[a]	Rate ratio	95 % CI	Test of trend, *p*-value
Cerebrovascular diseases	228	1	77	1.22	0.90–1.62	50	1.42	0.97–2.04	48	1.62	1.07–2.42	0.010
Cerebrovascular diseases limited to age ≥ 55	195	1	73	1.26	0.91–1.71	49	1.45	0.97–2.13	47	1.62	1.04–2.47	0.013
Cerebrovascular diseases adjusted for acute effects[b]	228	1	77	1.22	0.91–1.62	50	1.42	0.98–2.04	48	1.63	1.08–2.41	0.008

[a]Number of deaths. [b]Estimated from Poisson model, included a variable coded 1 if employed and 0 otherwise to control for death occurring while employed

in the same adjusted Poisson model (Fig. 3). There was an indication that the elevated rates for outdoor work were most pronounced for long term outdoor workers employed first time 1930–1949, compared with corresponding workers employed first time before 1930. The adjusted categorical rate ratios for long term outdoor work were noticeably more elevated than the corresponding SMRs based on the reference population (Fig. 2). The rates for short term outdoor work were clearly lower than the reference population of northern Sweden, whereas, the lower limit of the point estimated rate ratio is by design, equal to one. For outdoor work ≥15 years, the rate of cerebral haemorrhages (i.e., the delimiting outcomes for cerebral haemorrhages and cerebral infarctions) was statistically significantly higher than outdoor work 0–4 years – 2.52 (95 % CI 1.23–5.04). The corresponding rate of cerebral infarctions was also elevated, but not statistically significant – 1.60 (95 % CI 0.88–2.81).

The results of the cohort subgroup comparisons of the observed rates and expected rates of cerebrovascular disease mortality derived from the reference population showed that cumulative employment time underground most clearly deviated from the expected rates (Fig. 4). However, the causal link explaining these results could have been connected to both outdoor and underground work. Although adjustments were made for year of employment, attained age, and calendar year in the analysis, outdoor and underground work represented different time-windows of exposure (Fig. 1) as mining methods changed and safety precautions improved. However, the emphasis of the analysis was on earlier years of employment in both groups as the largest proportion of deaths as the result of cerebrovascular diseases occurred among workers who had been employed before 1960 (>90 % in both groups). The relatively smaller deviation in SMR from the reference population for outdoor workers compared with underground workers (Fig. 4) may have been diluted by the 26 % overlap with underground work in the classification procedure. The overlapping work-periods may be explained by the crude classification of outdoor mining, which was defined as all mining in Kiruna before the late 1950s. Moreover, the classification was affected by the fact that some of the mining performed in the earlier periods in Kiruna was drift mining

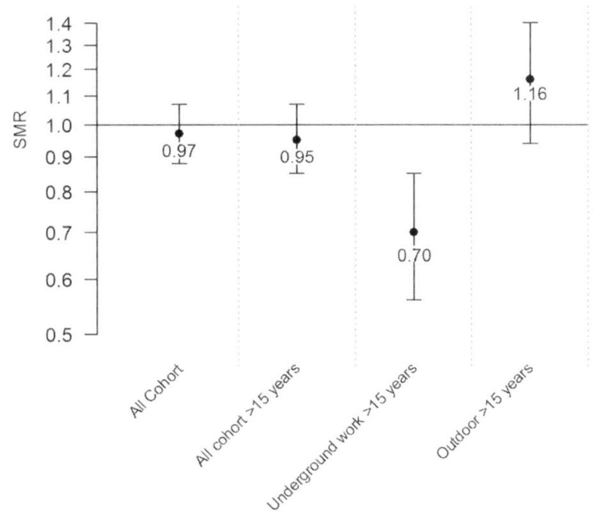

Fig. 3 Adjusted rate ratio estimate for cumulative outdoor and underground employment time based on Poisson regression. The estimates are derived from the same model based on the same category levels and the points are located at the mean employment time per category

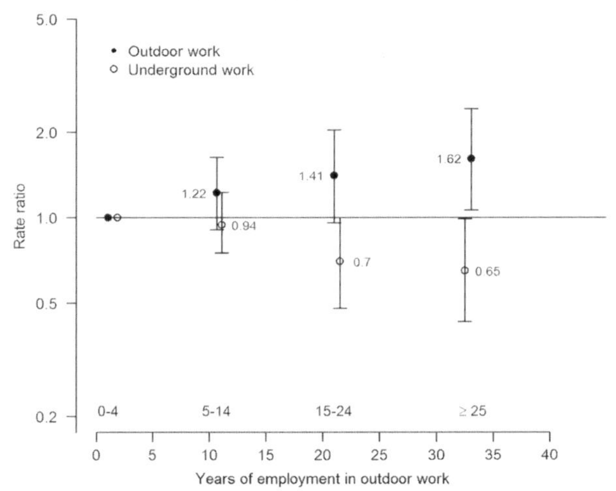

Fig. 4 Standardized mortality ratios (SMRs) for cerebrovascular disease based on northern Sweden as reference population. The numbers within the graph are the estimated SMRs

that could be described as a sub-underground mining method.

Cold winter-time temperatures and large seasonal variations in sun light are characteristic of outdoor work in the northernmost part of Sweden. Exposure to cold temperature has been shown to increase blood pressure [15], with several potential mechanisms leading to cerebrovascular disease [16]. However, cold temperatures that result in elevated mortality from cerebrovascular disease act mainly through acute or subacute effects [2]. The monthly distribution of the 304 deaths during one season showed that the three months with the highest frequency of deaths were December, January, and February (31 % of all deaths). Although, adjusting for current status (employed or not employed) did not weaken the association between outdoor work and mortality (Table 2), which implies that outdoor-work employments could have a preserving effect on mortality. We believe that temperature caused hypertension is the risk factor from work that likely best explains these results even if this explanation does require that work has a preserving effect on hypertension.

Smoking increases the risk of cerebrovascular diseases and the associations are strongest in younger ages [9]. The different working conditions and regulations of outdoor and underground work could contribute to different smoking habits by making smoking more or less accessible. We did not have data to adjust for smoking in the analysis. However, a previous study on this cohort showed a SIR of 1.74 (95 % CI 1.52–1.99) for lung cancer among underground workers [1]. The corresponding SIR for outdoor workers was 1.86 (95 % CI 1.53–2.23), a comparable SIR to underground workers. Smoking is a considerably stronger risk factor for lung cancer than it is for cerebrovascular diseases, which indirectly supports that smoking is not a strong confounder in this study. Also, a previous study on workers in the Malmberget mines, which used data on smoking for 2310 workers, found that 75 % of the smokers (1972–1992) had worked underground compared to 71 % of the non-smokers [13], indicating that a possible prohibition on smoking on underground workers did not result in smoking being less common among underground workers. Other known risk factors not possible to adjust for in this study include diabetes, atrial fibrillation, dyslipidemia, asymptomatic carotid stenosis, heredity, and an unhealthy lifestyle factors such as alcohol consumption [9]; these risk factors are harder to causally link with working outdoor or underground (but could still be possible confounders). The hypothesis that excess sunlight could be a cause of mortality from cerebrovascular disease has not been not supported by the literature [17].

A weakness of using cause-specific mortality as a measure has been that the causes of death register contains misclassification errors. In a validation study based on the Swedish cause of death register for 1094 deaths registered in 1995, 0.68 % (95 % CI 0.60–0.77) of all deaths from cerebrovascular underlying causes was correctly classified [18].

The healthy worker survivor effect

A healthy worker survivor effect (HWSE) [4, 5] could contribute to the reduced mortality rates associated with underground work found in the previous study of this cohort [1]. For cerebrovascular disease, we observed simultaneously elevated rates with outdoor work and reduced rates with underground work, as was found in the previous study. If the HWSE explains this inverse association with underground mining work, it would mirror a shift from underground mining to other categories of employment in the mines that is correlated with increased cerebrovascular disease mortality. The pattern of lower risks for several diseases with longer employment as a blue collar worker, especially underground, that was reported in the previous paper [1], elucidates the need to account for the HWSE when performing studies that focus on cumulative exposures in occupational cohorts.

Validity of this study

This study was based on iron ore miners from the Kiruna and Malmberget mines and consisted of a relatively large cohort with 443,930 person years and 13,000 workers. The cohort data are of very high quality because of the accuracy of the records of the mining company and because the exposure assessments were performed by occupational health researchers with knowledge about the mines. A study based on workers located in the far reaches of Sweden could be expected to represent a relatively homogeneous population in terms of socio-economic and lifestyle factors, potentially reducing bias from residual confounding. We only included workers who had a valid Swedish unique personal identification number. That is, only Swedish citizens are in the cohort as immigration to Sweden from outside Europe was limited before the 1980s. We did not have any information on the workers' ethnicity, but a study by Sjölander [19] found that the risk of cardiovascular diseases among the Swedish Sami was slightly lower than the majority population, a finding explained by the active reindeer herding lifestyle. A weakness could have been misclassification of both exposures and for outcomes. As in most epidemiological studies, unmeasured confounding could have influenced the results. Information on hypertension, physical activity, and lifestyle factors other than work would have increased study validity.

Conclusions

The results of this cohort study revealed that rates of cerebrovascular disease mortality increased with time of employment categorized as outdoor work. This association was also in contrast with the previous observation that work performed in a tempered underground environment has a protecting effect on cerebrovascular disease mortality. However, compared with the northern Sweden reference population, rates for long term outdoor employment were only marginally elevated.

Acknowledgements
Not applicable.

Funding
This document was been produced with financial assistance from the European Union (Kolarctic ENPI CBC Project 02/2011/043/KO303- MineHealth). The contents of this document are the sole responsibility of Umeå University and under no circumstances can be regarded as reflecting the position of the European Union. The funding body has had no role in the collection, analysis, interpretation of data or in writing the manuscript.

Authors' contributions
All authors (OB, HJ, LD, LB and TN) have contributed according to the following criteria: Substantial contributions to the conception or design of the work; or the acquisition, analysis, or interpretation of data for the work; Drafting the work or revising it critically for important intellectual content; Final approval of the version to be published.

Competing interests
The authors declare that they have no competing interests.

Author details
[1]Department of Radiation Sciences (Oncology), Umeå University, SE-901 85 Umeå, Sweden. [2]Department of Public Health & Clinical Medicine, Occupational and Environmental Medicine, Umeå University, SE-901 85 Umeå, Sweden.

References
1. Bjor O, Jonsson H, Damber L, Wahlstrom J, Nilsson T. Reduced mortality rates in a cohort of long-term underground iron-ore miners. Am J Ind Med. 2013;56(5):531–40. doi:10.1002/ajim.22168.
2. Analitis A, Katsouyanni K, Biggeri A, Baccini M, Forsberg B, Bisanti L, et al. Effects of cold weather on mortality: results from 15 European cities within the PHEWE project. Am J Epidemiol. 2008;168(12):1397–408. doi:10.1093/aje/kwn266.
3. Rocklov J, Ebi K, Forsberg B. Mortality related to temperature and persistent extreme temperatures: a study of cause-specific and age-stratified mortality. Occup Environ Med. 2011;68(7):531–6. doi:10.1136/oem.2010.058818.
4. Arrighi HM, Hertz-Picciotto I. The evolving concept of the healthy worker survivor effect. Epidemiology. 1994;5(2):189–96.
5. Kolstad HA, Olsen J. Why do short term workers have high mortality? Am J Epidemiol. 1999;149(4):347–52.
6. Björ O, Damber L, Jonsson H, Nilsson T. A comparison between standard methods and structural nested modeling when bias from a healthy worker survivor effect is suspected: an iron-ore mining cohort study. Occup Environ Med. 2015;72(7):536–42. doi:10.1136/oem.2014.102251.
7. Eriksson U. Gruva och arbete: Kiirunavaara 1890–1990. Uppala: Uppsala University; 1991.
8. Wendel-Vos GC, Schuit AJ, Feskens EJ, Boshuizen HC, Verschuren WM, Saris WH, et al. Physical activity and stroke. A meta-analysis of observational data. Int J Epidemiol. 2004;33(4):787–98. doi:10.1093/ije/dyh168dyh168.
9. Goldstein LB, Bushnell CD, Adams RJ, Appel LJ, Braun LT, Chaturvedi S, et al. Guidelines for the primary prevention of stroke: a guideline for healthcare professionals from the American Heart Association/American Stroke Association. Stroke. 2011;42(2):517–84. doi:10.1161/STR.0b013e3181fcb238.
10. Friedenreich CM, Neilson HK, Lynch BM. State of the epidemiological evidence on physical activity and cancer prevention. Eur J Cancer. 2010; 46(14):2593–604. doi:10.1016/j.ejca.2010.07.028.
11. Moradi T, Gridley G, Bjork J, Dosemeci M, Ji BT, Berkel HJ, et al. Occupational physical activity and risk for cancer of the colon and rectum in Sweden among men and women by anatomic subsite. Eur J Cancer Prev. 2008;17(3):201–8. doi:10.1097/CEJ.0b013e3282b6fd78.
12. Bergdahl IA, Jonsson H, Eriksson K, Damber L, Jarvholm B. Lung cancer and exposure to quartz and diesel exhaust in Swedish iron ore miners with concurrent exposure to radon. Occup Environ Med. 2010;67(8):513–8. doi:10.1136/oem.2009.047456.
13. Jonsson H, Bergdahl IA, Akerblom G, Eriksson K, Andersson K, Kagstrom L, et al. Lung cancer risk and radon exposure in a cohort of iron ore miners in Malmberget, Sweden. Occup Environ Med. 2010;67(8):519–25. doi:10.1136/oem.2009.047449.
14. Wood SN. Generalized Additive Models. An Introduction with R. 1st ed. Boca Raton: Chapman & Hall/CRC; 2006.
15. Halonen JI, Zanobetti A, Sparrow D, Vokonas PS, Schwartz J. Relationship between outdoor temperature and blood pressure. Occup Environ Med. 2011;68(4):296–301. doi:10.1136/oem.2010.056507.
16. Brickman AM, Reitz C, Luchsinger JA, Manly JJ, Schupf N, Muraskin J, et al. Long-term blood pressure fluctuation and cerebrovascular disease in an elderly cohort. Arch Neurol. 2010;67(5):564–9. doi:10.1001/archneurol.2010.70.
17. Kent ST, McClure LA, Judd SE, Howard VJ, Crosson WL, Al-Hamdan MZ, et al. Short- and long-term sunlight radiation and stroke incidence. Ann Neurol. 2013;73(1):32–7. doi:10.1002/ana.23737.
18. Johansson LA, Bjorkenstam C, Westerling R. Unexplained differences between hospital and mortality data indicated mistakes in death certification: an investigation of 1,094 deaths in Sweden during 1995. J Clin Epidemiol. 2009;62(11):1202–9. doi:10.1016/j.jclinepi.2009.01.010.
19. Sjolander P. What is known about the health and living conditions of the indigenous people of northern Scandinavia, the Sami? Glob Health Action. 2011;4. doi:10.3402/gha.v4i0.8457.

Health utilities for chronic low back pain

Anna Lene Seidler[1,2], Constanze Rethberg[3], Jochen Schmitt[1,3], Albert Nienhaus[4,5] and Andreas Seidler[1*]

Abstract

Background: Chronic low back pain (LBP) is a common health problem, with a large potential for primary prevention. Health utilities (HU) reflect which proportion of their expected remaining life time individuals would hypothetically trade to be alleviated of a health condition of interest. A value of 0 means "prefer to die immediately", a value of 1 means "not willing to trade any life time". The aim of this cross-sectional study was to assess HU for LBP patients and for healthy participants and to examine whether HU for LBP are useful indicators to substantiate preventive and therapeutic decision making.

Methods: Healthy participants ($n = 126$) and LBP patients ($n = 32$) were recruited mainly among the employees of a tertiary care hospital in Germany. Standardized LBP scenarios were presented to all participants and HU values were assessed using the time-trade-off method.

Results: Median HU for LBP were 0.90 (IQR 0.31) for participants and 0.93 (IQR 0.10) for LBP patients. Measurements were consistent across illness severity ratings with HU and with a visual analogue scale (VAS); in the healthy sample the intraclass correlation coefficient (ICC) was 0.61 (95% CI 0.23–1.00, $F(1125) = 190$, $p < .001$), in the patient sample the ICC was 0.66 (95% CI = 0.24–1.00, $F(1,31) = 62$, $p < .001$). 8% of participants reported HU of 1. There was no statistically significant relation between HU and age, income, or gender.

Conclusion: On average, participants chose a 7 to 10% shorter life expectancy to avoid LBP, but almost 1 in 10 participants were not willing to trade any life years. The results indicate a certain stability of HU due to the comparability of HU ratings across patients and healthy participants, the measurement consistency when comparing VAS and HU ratings, and the lack of association between demographic variables and HU. This underlines the usefulness of HU for measuring illness severity in comparative health economics evaluations of preventive and therapeutic measures that address chronic LBP or other pain-characterized diseases. Future studies should focus on different LBP intensities and derive stratified HU that reflect the distribution of pain intensity in the population.

Keywords: Chronic Low back pain, Health utilities, Health economics, Time-trade-off

Background

Chronic low back pain (LBP) is a common health problem. The global 1-month prevalence of LBP has been estimated to be 23.2 ± 2.9% [1]. Assessing and addressing chronic LBP – commonly defined as LBP of more than 12 weeks duration [2] – is highly relevant not only to general medicine and orthopedics, but also to occupational medicine [3, 4]. Chronic LBP is a leading cause of work absence worldwide which puts a massive economic burden on both the society and individuals [5–7]. It is related to the working conditions in many different job sectors, since it is associated with physically straining work-tasks (e.g. heavy lifting, forward bending, whole-body vibration) and psychosocial work factors (e.g. high demand and low control) [8]. A review of occupational LBP and preventive approaches found that there is high potential for work-related primary prevention of chronic LBP [9]. Decision making concerning occupational prevention measures and treatments for chronic LBP requires health economic evaluations and cost-utility analyses. A systematic review of previous cost utility studies for LBP identified a need for additional studies [10].

Health utilities (HU) are a measure of illness severity that are widely used to facilitate cost-effectiveness analyses and health-related policy making [11]. HU assessed with the time-trade-off method provide a measure of health-related quality of life based on decision-making theory: a value of 0 would mean "prefer to die

* Correspondence: ArbSozPH@mailbox.tu-dresden.de
[1]Institute and Policlinic of Occupational and Social Medicine (IPAS), Faculty of Medicine, Technische Universität Dresden, Dresden, Germany
Full list of author information is available at the end of the article

immediately", a value of 1 would mean "not willing to trade any life time". HU scores reflect which proportion of their life time affected patients and non-affected healthy individuals would hypothetically trade to be aileviated of a respective condition [12]. For instance, a score of 0.6 indicates that an individual would choose to live 60% of their (hypothetical) remaining life time in perfect health over living their full remaining life time with the respective condition. HU can be used to assess trade-offs relevant for resource allocation [13] and they allow for a direct comparison of disease outcomes across different health conditions [14]. HU for chronic LBP could provide a tool to conduct cost-utility analyses for treatments and occupational prevention measures and to compare the cost-utility of occupational health promotion targeting chronic LBP to occupational health promotion addressing different diseases such as mental illnesses [15–17].

A previous study assessing patient utilities for LBP found an average utility of 0.93 for mild, 0.65 for moderate, and 0.18 for severe back pain [18]. However, the sample was highly selective; it consisted of 41 LBP patients in a tertiary care hospital. The derived HU are likely to not represent generalizable views on chronic LBP and might thus not be suitable for work-related as well as lifestyle-related primary preventive interventions for healthy individuals. Due to the high potential of occupational preventative approaches targeting healthy individuals, it is important to assess health utility values in this healthy target group. Another previous study examined HU in a healthy sample for chronic pain in general but not chronic LBP specifically [19]. The authors found mean HU of 0.84 for mild, 0.72 for moderate, 0.04 for severe and −0.15 for very severe chronic pain; the negative value indicates that participants would prefer death to suffering these pain. However, the usefulness of HU varies across disease type [20]. While the cited study gives important information on healthy individuals' ratings of chronic pain and shows that the HU are sensitive to severity of pain, it remains unclear whether these general values are transferable to chronic LBP.

The primary aim of the current study was to assess HU for chronic LBP in a sample of LBP patients and a healthy sample. The secondary aim was to examine whether HU for chronic LBP are useful indicators to substantiate decision making generally and in preventive (e.g. occupational) medicine specifically by assessing: how HU compare to a standard measure of pain severity (VAS-scale) and other severity measures; whether there are many individuals not willing to trade any life years; and whether HU derived with the time-trade-off method are influenced by other variables (age, gender, and own level of pain).

Methods

Participants

The data for this cross-sectional study were collected between October 2011 and August 2015 at the Institute and Policlinic of Occupational and Social Medicine and the Center for Evidence-Based Healthcare, Faculty of Medicine of the TU Dresden. The study population included two groups of participants: 126 healthy participants and 32 patients with chronic LBP. Eligible for inclusion were only participants that: were at least 18 years old; were affiliated with University Hospital and Faculty of Medicine Dresden; and that gave informed consent to participate in the study. Exclusion criteria were: lack of willingness to co-operate and lack of understanding of the study questions. Individuals were eligible for inclusion as patients if an ICD-10 code M54.5 was specified by a careful medical examination and anamnesis and if they reported a LBP duration of more than 3 months, which is in accordance with a widely accepted definition of chronic LBP [2, 9]. Patients with specific lumbar spine diseases (e.g. disc herniation, lumbago with sciatica) were excluded. The healthy participants were working in health-related sectors, to ensure the ability to make informed judgements about LBP. The healthy sample was considered the primary study population to derive HU for healthy individuals as recommended for health economic analyses [17]. The patient group was interviewed to specifically assess the influence of being personally affected by chronic LBP on HU.

The sample was recruited from the employees at the University Hospital and Faculty of Medicine Dresden, and through the social media presence and the intranet of the University Hospital and Faculty of Medicine. The study protocol was approved by the responsible ethics committee of the University Clinic Dresden. This manuscript follows the STROBE Statement for cross-sectional studies [21].

Data collection and measures

Data were collected through a standardized computer-assisted interview. Firstly, participants' age, sex, and income group were assessed. For employees of the University Hospital no direct information on income was available, their income was thus estimated based on their occupational role. After assessing this demographic information, a standardized scenario for chronic LBP was presented to all participants to assess HU using the time-trade-off method (see Table 1). Participants were given the choice between living for their remaining life expectancy (calculated by the software based on participants' age and sex) with the described chronic LBP or for a shorter duration in perfect health. The shorter duration in perfect health was a randomly chosen

Table 1 Health state scenario

	Unspecified chronic low back pain
Disease Duration	>3 months
Affected Regions	Low back, one-or-two sided, can radiated to other body regions
Pain Sensations	Pain, sensory disturbances, sometimes numbness and tingling sensations in the legs
Causes/Detoriation	Overstraining, lack of exercise, relieving postures, psychosocial factors, being overweight, smoking
Treatment	Symptom-oriented: Physical activity (e.g. physiotherapy), possibly analgesics
Impact on Life	Occupational impacts, limitations everyday activities and interpersonal relationships

duration based on a normal distribution with mean (± SD) = participant's remaining life expectancy × 0.8 (±0.05) to avoid a starting point bias [22]. The duration of life in perfect health was then altered until the individual's preferences were equal. HU were calculated by taking the ratio between the duration of life in perfect health and the duration of life with chronic LBP. Additionally, participants were asked to rate the severity of the standardized LBP scenario on a visual analogue scale (VAS) with 0 reflecting perfect health and 100 reflecting worst imaginable condition. Willingness to pay (WTP) was assessed by asking participants how much they would be willing to pay monthly to not suffer from chronic LBP, and how much they think health insurances should spend monthly so people do not have to suffer from chronic LBP.

The patient group suffering from chronic LBP rated their current pain with the time-trade-off method and on a VAS scale; their level of disability was assessed using the Roland Morris disability index [23]. Impairment and productivity were assessed using the Work Productivity and Activity Impairment (WPAI) questionnaire [24]. Furthermore, patients completed the Center for Epidemiological Studies Depression Scale (CES-D) [25] to measure depressive symptoms that may systematically influence HU ratings [26].

We conducted a sample size calculation assuming a standard deviation of 0.1 for the patient sample and of 0.2 for the healthy sample. A sample size of 32 LBP patients and 126 healthy individuals was necessary to obtain 95% confidence intervals with a width of 0.1.

Statistical analysis

Descriptive statistics were calculated for all variables. Arithmetic means with standard deviations, and medians with interquartile range were calculated to derive average disease severity values for HU, VAS and WTP. The key variables were not normally distributed. Thus, robust Spearman correlation analysis and robust regression analysis were applied to assess relations between the disease severity measures and third variables. Measurement consistency between HU and VAS values was tested by calculating two-way random effect intraclass correlation coefficients (ICCs). T-tests were performed to assess group differences. Welsh t-tests were applied when Levene Tests revealed that the variances were not homogenous. All analyses were performed using the open-source software R [27].

Results

Sociodemographic and disease specific characteristics of study participants are shown in Table 2. There were no missing data for any individuals or variables. The mean age of patients with chronic LBP was 41 years (SD = 13), they were thus considerably older than the group of healthy participants (mean age: 30 years, SD = 9). Furthermore, a slightly higher percentage of LBP patients were in the lower income groups compared to the healthy participants (see Table 2). Chronic LBP was a well-known disease in the group of healthy participants (that were mainly health professionals) not suffering from LBP: The vast majority (94%) had a good idea of what chronic LBP is, and 62% had friends or relatives suffering from LBP.

For the group suffering from chronic LBP, the mean disease duration was 15.48 (SD = 9.48; range 1–40) years. According to the Roland Morris Disability index, the degree of disability was light for 72% ($n = 23$), moderate for 25% ($n = 8$), and severe for 3% ($n = 1$) of the patients. This relatively light impairment for most LBP patients is also reflected in the HU for their current pain assessed with the time-trade-off method (median = 0.96, IQR = 0.06), and in the ratings of current pain on a VAS scale (mean = 22.25, SD = 21.60). The mean VAS of LBP patients with a light degree of disability (according to the Roland Morris Disability index) was 14.78 (median 11.0), the mean VAS of patients with a moderate degree of disability was 39.75 (median 32.5), the only patient with a severe degree of disability had a VAS of 54.

HU values for healthy participants and LBP patients

Median HU for the standardized chronic LBP scenario were 0.90 ($IQR = 0.31$) as rated by healthy participants and 0.93 ($IQR = 0.10$) as rated by LBP patients. They were thus comparable between the groups. The mean difference between healthy individuals ($M = 0.81$, $SD = 0.19$) and LBP patients ($M = 0.88$, $SD = 0.14$) was statistically significant ($t(63.64) = -2.48$, $p = 0.02$). However, the less pronounced median difference indicates that the mean difference is related to more extreme ratings in the healthy group (see Table 3 and Fig. 1).

Table 2 Sociodemographics and disease-specific characteristics of study participants

Variable	Healthy participants $n = 126$	Patients with chronic low back pain $n = 32$
Sex (% female)	54%	59%
Age in years (mean, SD)	29.95 (9.25)	41.03 (12.85)
Income group (%)		
<1000 €/month	10%	16%
1000–2000 €/month	2%	13%
2000–3000 €/month	56%	48%
3000–4000 €/month	30%	19%
>4000 €/month	2%	3%
Having idea of what low back pain is (%)	94%	100%
Friends/family members with low back pain (%)	62%	66%
Family history of LBP (positive, %)	-	56%
Disease duration in years (mean, SD)	-	15.48 (9.48)
Roland Morris disability index		
light (%)	-	72%
moderate (%)	-	25%
severe (%)	-	3%
Degree health affected productivity while working (0 to 1) (WPAI) (mean, SD)	-	0.18 (0.18)
Degree health affected regular activities (0 to 1) (WPAI) (mean, SD)	-	0.28 (0.24)
Depressive Symptoms (CES-D) (mean, SD)	-	12.06 (7.52)
HU own disease (0 to 1) (mean, SD)	-	0.93 (0.13)
Pain own disease (100 mm VAS) (mean, SD)	-	22.25 (21.60)

SD Standard Deviation, *WPAI* Work Productivity and Activity Impairment Questionnaire, *CES-D* Center for Epidemiological Studies Depression Scale, *VAS* Visual Analogue Scale, – not applicable

Relation of HU to VAS and other severity measures

Mean, standard deviation, median and interquartile range for the HU, VAS, and WTP scores for the standardized scenarios are shown in Table 3. There was a good reliability across VAS and HU, the two-way random effects ICC was .61 (95% CI = 0.23–1.00, F(1125) = 190, $p < .001$) for the healthy sample, and .66 (95% CI = 0.24–1.00, F(1,31) = 62, $p < .001$) for the patient sample. Correlations between the different measures of rated illness severity are shown in Table 4. HU and VAS are moderately correlated, interestingly, the correlation between HU and VAS is stronger for the group of healthy participants ($r = -.53$, $p < .001$) than for the patient group ($r = -.31$, $p = .09$). VAS and HU show a stronger correlation and thus seem to be more related constructs than VAS and WTP or HU and WTP.

Individuals not willing to trade any life years

As shown in Fig. 1, ten of the healthy participants (8%), were not willing to hypothetically trade any life years to be relieved of the presented standardized scenario of chronic LBP (and thus received HU of 1). In comparison, no healthy participant rated chronic LBP as equal to perfect health on a VAS scale, and only one healthy participant was not willing to pay any money to be relieved of LBP. Similarly, three of the LBP patients (9%)

Table 3 HU and VAS values for standardized chronic low back pain scenario for different groups

Group	HU		VAS		WTP own money		WTP health insurance	
	Mean (SD)	Median (IQR)	Mean (SD)	Median (IQR)	Mean (SD)	Median (IQR)	Mean (SD)	Median (IQR)
Healthy ($n = 126$)	0.81 (0.19)	0.90 (0.31)	44.34 (20.84)	48.00 (34.00)	236.03 (314.98)	150.00 (200.00)	664.93 (945.21)	300.00 (500.00)
Low Back Pain ($n = 32$)	0.88 (0.14)	0.93 (0.10)	40.91 (19.64)	47.00 (30.50)	180.78 (269.78)	100.00 (150.00)	785.31 (1234.48)	300.00 (410.00)
Total ($n = 156$)	0.83 (0.18)	0.91 (0.25)	43.65 (20.59)	47.00 (33.75)	224.84 (306.36)	150.00 (170.00)	689.94 (1008.83)	300.00 (528.75)

HU Health Utilities, *VAS* 100 mm Visual Analogue Scale Values, *WTP* Willingness to Pay Monthly in Euros, *SD* Standard Deviation, *IQR* Interquartile Range

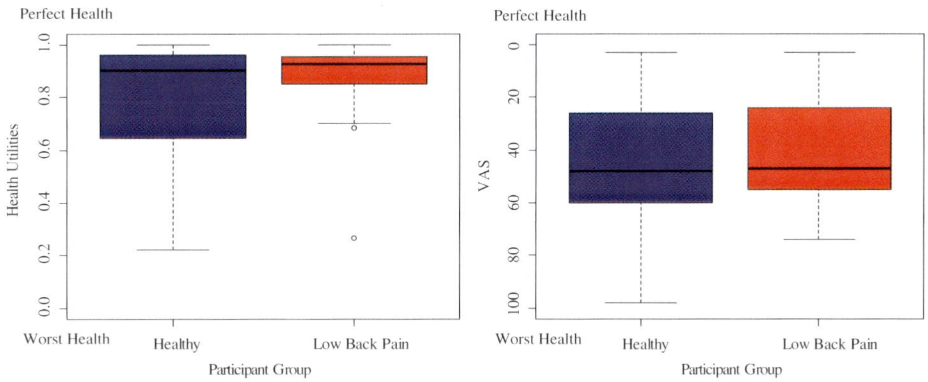

Fig. 1 Median and interquartile range of Health Utilities and VAS values by participant group

had HU values of 1, but no LBP patient rated the disease as equal to perfect health on a VAS scale, and no patient was not willing to pay any money to be relieved of LBP.

Demographic factors, own pain, and HU

In the sample, younger people were willing to trade a higher proportion of life years (since they reported lower HU), however, this association was not statistically significant ($r(156) = .10$, $p = .24$). VAS and age do not seem to be related in the sample, if anything, younger people rated chronic LBP as less severe ($r = .05$, $p = .55$). Males were willing to trade slightly more life years ($M_{male} = 0.81$, $SD_{male} = 0.19$, $M_{female} = 0.83$, $SD_{female} = 0.18$), but again this difference was not statistically significant ($t(156) = -0.67$, $p = .50$). There was no sex difference for VAS ($M_{male} = 44.24$, $SD_{male} = 21.38$, $M_{female} = 43.16$, $SD_{female} = 20.02$, $t(156) = 0.33$, $p = .74$). There was a tendency (albeit not statistically significant) for individuals in the higher income group to report higher HU ($r = .12$, $p = .14$), while income group did not influence VAS ratings ($r = -.01$, $p = .92$). As shown in Fig. 2, there was a positive relation for chronic LBP patients between HU for their own LBP, and HU for the standardized description of LBP ($r = .57$, $p < .001$).

Discussion

This study derived HU values with the time-trade-off method for a sample of patients with chronic LBP and a sample of healthy participants. Median HU for chronic LBP in the healthy sample were 0.90, while median HU in the LBP patient sample were 0.93. HU derived with the time-trade-off method were related to other severity measures and particularly VAS, and there was good measurement consistency when comparing HU and VAS. This indicates that HU for chronic LBP reflect a fairly direct severity rating of LBP and are thus a useful indicator of illness severity. The usefulness of HU is also supported by the lack of statistically significant associations between HU and demographic variables (age, gender, and income). However, almost one in ten participants (in both the healthy and the patient sample) was not willing to trade any life years to be relieved of chronic LBP, while no participant rated chronic LBP as equivalent to being perfectly healthy on a VAS scale.

This observed ceiling effect that exists in HU derived with the time-trade-off method but not in other severity measures has previously been reported for other diseases but not for chronic LBP [20]. On the one hand, this effect impairs the interpretability of HU, as it is not possible to differentiate between 'perfect health' and 'condition not worse enough to trade life years'. It also impairs the direct comparability between HU and other measures of disease severity [20]. On the other hand, the ceiling effect provides useful information for the planning of prevention and intervention measures: It indicates that measures against chronic LBP including the risk of a reduced life expectancy or of other adverse side effects would not be accepted by some individuals since

Table 4 Spearman correlation coefficients for different measures of illness severity for different groups

Group	HU ↔ VAS	HU ↔ Own WTP	HU ↔ Insurance WTP	VAS ↔ Own WTP	VAS ↔ Insurance WTP	Own WTP ↔ Insurance WTP
Healthy (*n* = 126)	−.53***	−.29***	−.15	.22*	.20*	.67***
Low Back Pain (*n* = 32)	−.31+	−.20	−.10	−.11	−.04	.73***
Total (*n* = 156)	−.50***	−.30***	−.15+	.18*	.16*	.68***

HU Health Utilities, *VAS* 100 mm Visual Analogue Scale Values, *WTP* Willingness to Pay, + = $p < .01$, * = $p < .05$, ** = $p < .01$, *** = $p < .001$

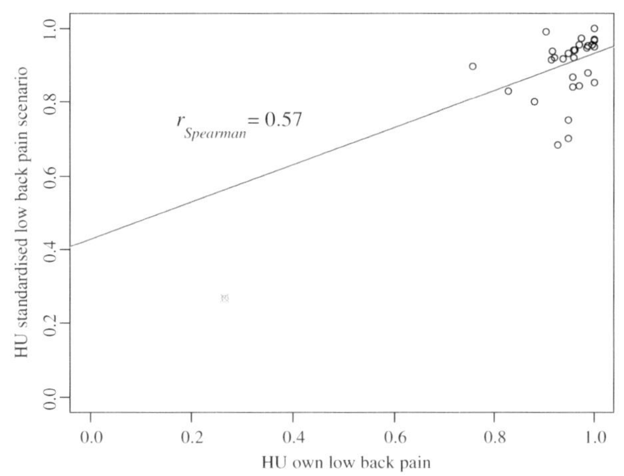

Fig. 2 Association between Health Utilities rating of own LBP and Health Utilities rating of standardized LBP scenario

some individuals would not trade any life years to not suffer LBP.

The assessed associations between HU and potential influencing factors (e.g. age or sex) were stronger than the assessed associations between VAS and these factors. While none of these associations were statistically significant, this may have been due to the small sample size, since previous studies did find significant associations: Dolan & Roberts [20] used the time-trade-off method to assess health preferences for different health states (but not LBP) and found that age, sex and marital status influenced the derived values. HU increased up to the age of 45 and then started to fall until the age of 70. Men, and married or cohabiting individuals showed higher HU compared to women and individuals living alone. Additionally, mental health states such as depression have previously been shown to influence HU for cancer patients [26]. It is likely, that mental health states also influence HU for chronic LBP, since depression changes people's outlooks on life and death (which the extreme case of suicidality illustrates).

Generally, death is a very vague concept and may mean something different to each individual. The perception of life and death possibly largely influences whether an individual would be willing to trade life years and if so how many to be relieved from a disease. A reason for this may be that people with depression place a lower value on life, while it may not reflect perceived severity of the illness. This is related to the finding that there are inconsistencies in HU values that can be attributed to loss aversion, the idea that people are more sensitive to losses than to gains [28]. There is strong evidence showing a higher prevalence of depression among chronic LPB patients [29, 30], it is thus possible that co-morbid depression might also influence HU ratings. These findings pose two difficulties. Firstly, it is difficult to interpret whether differences between population groups result from differing evaluations of the respective health state or of differing evaluations of the value of a life year. For instance, a married or cohabiting person may live a happier life and thus be less likely to trade these happy life years, despite judging the respective health state similarly severe as a person living alone. Secondly, HU being influenced by individual characteristics makes them less informative for cost-effectiveness analyses that concern the general population since it reduces their generalizability.

The HU for chronic LBP found with the time-trade-off method in this study are comparable to the mean HU of 0.93 for mild LBP found in a previous study with a patient sample [18], and they are slightly higher than HU assessed in a healthy sample for general mild chronic pain that were on average 0.84 [19]. This indicates that the LBP scenario used in this study to describe chronic LBP was perceived as a fairly mild type of pain. This is in line with a study comparing the perceived severity of different illnesses, showing that LBP is perceived as comparably moderate [31].

A strength of this study is that HU were assessed for both healthy participants and patients with chronic LBP. Looking at those two different samples is particularly useful for this particular disease: chronic LBP is often addressed in preventive health promotion programs. Because healthy individuals are the target of these programs, it is their rating that is relevant to inform decision makers, while for therapeutic interventions patient ratings are more relevant. Furthermore, this design allows a comparison between these two groups allowing for a judgement on the influence of perspective on HU. There were no drop-outs or missing values for any of the core variables (HU, VAS, WTP, age, gender). The risk of interviewer bias was minimized since all the interviews were conducted by the same well-trained interviewer, and the interviews were computer-assisted to standardize the testing procedure. The concept of chronic LBP was well known to the vast majority of healthy participants, reducing the risk of arbitrary values.

A major limitation to this study is that the sample is not representative of the general population. The average Roland Morris disability index of the current sample was lower (5.34) than that of a population-representative sample of LBP patients in a Greek survey (average Roland Morris disability index 10.01) [32]. This principally impacts the generalizability of the results. However, the mentioned Greek study gives the mean Roland Morris disability index of all individuals that suffered from LBP at the time of the survey, whereas the present sample also includes patients with chronic LBP that are currently free of pain (or almost free of pain). If only looking at individuals in our sample that are currently suffering from LBP (defined as pain levels of at least 20 out of 100 on a VAS scale), the mean Roland Morris disability index of this subsample was 9.09, and is thus comparable to the population-representative Greek study. Moreover, we found similar values for healthy participants and patients, this indicates a certain stability of the derived HU.

Furthermore, the use of a restricted sample of mainly health professionals ensures that healthy participants were informed about chronic LBP. Pain is a hard concept to grasp for someone not suffering from it, since it is invisible and hard to describe. Health professionals are likely to have better insight to this illness since they encounter people suffering from it and are likely to have factual knowledge on chronic LBP and its implications. They are therefore likely to be able to make more informed judgements. The sample size was too small to precisely assess the influence of potential covariates on HU ratings. Future studies should use larger and population-based samples. There was an age difference of 11 years between healthy participants and patients which may have introduced systematic differences to the HU ratings of the two groups. However, this concern is slightly alleviated by the finding that there was no statistically significant association between age and HU ratings.

For health economic evaluations of (primarily) preventable disorders like chronic LBP a reflection of the disease expression in the general population is of particular importance. In the chronic LBP description used in this study, we did not give explicit indications of pain intensity. However, the description seems to reflect moderate pain intensity since the mean VAS as rated by all LBP patients for the standardized chronic LBP scenario was 40.91 which is comparable to the mean VAS of 39.75 that LBP patients with a moderate degree of disability attributed to their own complaints. The advantage of not giving explicit indications of pain intensity is that it reflects how the intensity of chronic LBP varies in the population. The disadvantage of this approach is that it impedes the concrete description of an illness that is primarily pain based. This problem becomes clear when comparing the patient and the population group in our sample: On average, healthy participants rated chronic LBP as more severe than patients with chronic LBP did (note that most chronic LBP patients in our sample reported only light pain intensities). Furthermore, patients with more severe LBP rated the standardized chronic LBP scenario as more severe than patients with less severe LBP (Fig. 2). Consequently, future studies should incorporate explicit descriptions of a range of different pain intensities in their chronic LBP scenarios and derive HU for different levels of pain intensity. HU could then be weighted with respect to the distribution of pain intensities in the general population to derive values that can be used for a health economic evaluation of primary prevention programs. Pain-intensity stratified HU could also be useful for the health economics evaluations of therapeutic treatments, since often chronic LBP cannot be cured completely, but it can be eased. Ideally, these stratified values would be supplemented by HU for a pain reduction from strong to moderate and from moderate to light to optimize the evaluation of curative measures. Overall, deriving HU stratified by pain intensity should be the next step to improve the applicability of HU values to evaluate preventive and pain reduction measures for chronic LBP.

Conclusion

The present study shows that on average chronic LBP patients chose a 7% shorter life expectancy and healthy participants chose a 10% shorter life expectancy to avoid chronic LBP, but almost 1 in 10 participants were not willing to trade any life years. Since LBP is one of the most common diseases in the population and has high preventive potential, these HU can give decision makers in preventive health promotion and health care valuable insight to how patients and healthy individuals perceive chronic LBP. Furthermore, the results indicate a certain stability of HU due to the comparability of HU ratings across patients and healthy participants, the measurement consistency and association between VAS and HU, and the lack of association between demographic variables and HU. The results point towards an applicability of HU for assessing illness severity of LBP specifically and the applicability of HU for diseases that are mainly characterized through pain in general. Future studies looking at pain-characterised diseases should include explicit descriptions of pain intensities in their disease scenarios and independently assess HU for these different pain intensities ideally in a sample that is representative of the population of interest.

Abbreviations

CES-D Scale: Center for Epidemiological Studies Depression Scale; HU: Health Utilities; ICC: Intraclass Correlation Coefficient; IQR: Interquartile Range; LBP: Low Back Pain; M_{female}: Mean Among Females; M_{male}: Mean Among Males; r: Correlation Coefficient; SD: Standard Deviation; VAS: Visual Analogue Scale; WPAI Scale: Work Productivity and Activity Impairment Scale; WTP: Willingness to Pay

Acknowledgments

Not applicable.

Funding

The study was supported by the German Social Accident Insurance Institution for the Health and Welfare Service (BGW). We acknowledge support by the German Research Foundation and the Open Access Publication Funds of the TU Dresden.

Authors' contributions
ALS analyzed and interpreted the data and drafted the manuscript. CR performed the data elevation. JS participated in the development of the epidemiological concept and in the interpretation of the study results. AN participated in the interpretation of the study results. AS coordinated the study and participated in the development of the epidemiological concept and the drafting of the manuscript. All authors read and approved the final manuscript.

Authors' information
Not applicable.

Competing interests
The authors declare that they have no competing interests.

Author details
[1]Institute and Policlinic of Occupational and Social Medicine (IPAS), Faculty of Medicine, Technische Universität Dresden, Dresden, Germany. [2]NHMRC Clinical Trials Centre, Systematic Reviews & Health Technology Assessment, University of Sydney, Sydney, Australia. [3]Center for Evidence-Based Healthcare, University Hospital and Medical Faculty Carl Gustav Carus, TU Dresden, Dresden, Germany. [4]German Social Accident Insurance Institution for the Health and Welfare Service, Hamburg, Germany. [5]Institute for Health Services Research in Dermatology and Nursing, University Medical Center Hamburg-Eppendorf, Hamburg, Germany.

References

1. Hoy D, Bain C, Williams G, March L, Brooks P, Blyth F, Woolf A, Vos T, Buchbinder R. A systematic review of the global prevalence of low back pain. Arthritis Rheum. 2012;64(6):2028–37.
2. Violante FS, Mattioli S, Bonfiglioli R. Low-back pain. Handb Clin Neurol. 2015; 131:397–410.
3. Hoy D, Brooks P, Blyth F, Buchbinder R. The Epidemiology of low back pain. Best Pract Res Clin Rheumatol. 2010;24(6):769–81.
4. Steenstra I, Verbeek J, Heymans M, Bongers P. Prognostic factors for duration of sick leave in patients sick listed with acute low back pain: a systematic review of the literature. Occup Environ Med. 2005;62(12):851–60.
5. Guo H-R, Tanaka S, Halperin WE, Cameron LL. Back pain prevalence in US industry and estimates of lost workdays. Am J Public Health. 1999;89(7):1029–35.
6. Maetzel A, Li L. The economic burden of low back pain: a review of studies published between 1996 and 2001. Best Pract Res Clin Rheumatol. 2002; 16(1):23–30.
7. Wynne-Jones G, Cowen J, Jordan JL, Uthman O, Main CJ, Glozier N, van der Windt D. Absence from work and return to work in people with back pain: a systematic review and meta-analysis. Occup Environ Med. 2014;71(6):448–56.
8. Sterud T, Tynes T. Work-related psychosocial and mechanical risk factors for low back pain: a 3-year follow-up study of the general working population in Norway. Occup Environ Med. 2013;70(5):296–302.
9. Seidler A, Liebers F, Latza U. Prävention von Low-Back-Pain im beruflichen Kontext. Bundesgesundheitsblatt Gesundheitsforschung Gesundheitsschutz. 2008;51(3):322–33.
10. Dagenais S, Roffey DM, Wai EK, Haldeman S, Caro J. Can cost utility evaluations inform decision making about interventions for low back pain? Spine J. 2009;9(11):944–57.
11. Longworth L, Yang Y, Young T, Mulhern B, Hernández Alava M, Mukuria C, et al. Use of generic and condition-specific measures of health-related quality of life in NICE decision-making: a systematic review, statistical modelling and survey. Health Technol Assess. 2014;18(9).
12. Torrance GW, Feeny D. Utilities and quality-adjusted life years. Int J Technol Assess Health Care. 1989;5(04):559–75.
13. Gold M, Siegel J, Russell L, Weinstein M. Cost-effectiveness in health and medicine. New York: Oxford Univ Press; 1996.
14. Doth AH, Hansson PT, Jensen MP, Taylor RS. The burden of neuropathic pain: a systematic review and meta-analysis of health utilities. Pain®. 2010; 149(2):338–44.
15. Seidler A, Thinschmidt M, Deckert S, Then F, Hegewald J, Nieuwenhuijsen K, Riedel-Heller SG. The role of psychosocial working conditions on burnout and its core component emotional exhaustion–a systematic review. J Occupat Med Toxicol. 2014;9(1):10.
16. Russell LB, Gold MR, Siegel JE, Daniels N, Weinstein MC. The role of cost-effectiveness analysis in health and medicine. JAMA. 1996;276(14):1172–7.
17. Drummond MF, Sculpher MJ, Claxton K, Stoddart GL, Torrance GW: Methods for the economic evaluation of health care programmes. Oxford, UK: Oxford University Press; 2015.
18. Lai KC, Provenzale JM, Delong D, Mukundan S. Assessing patient utilities for varying degrees of low back pain. Acad Radiol. 2005;12(4):467–74.
19. Eldabe S, Lloyd A, Verdian L, Meguro M, Maclaine G, Dewilde S. Eliciting health state utilities from the general public for severe chronic pain. Eur J Health Econ. 2010;11(3):323–30.
20. Robinson A, Dolan P, Williams A. Valuing health status using VAS and TTO: What lies behind the numbers? Soc Sci Med. 1997;45(8):1289–97.
21. Vandenbroucke JP, Von Elm E, Altman DG, Gøtzsche PC, Mulrow CD, Pocock SJ, Poole C, Schlesselman JJ, Egger M, Initiative S. Strengthening the Reporting of Observational Studies in Epidemiology (STROBE): explanation and elaboration. PLoS Med. 2007;4(10):e297.
22. Schmitt J, Meurer M, Klon M, Frick K. Assessment of health state utilities of controlled and uncontrolled psoriasis and atopic eczema: a population-based study. Br J Dermatol. 2008;158(2):351–9.
23. Roland M, Fairbank J. The Roland–Morris disability questionnaire and the Oswestry disability questionnaire. Spine. 2000;25(24):3115–24.
24. Reilly MC, Zbrozek AS, Dukes EM. The validity and reproducibility of a work productivity and activity impairment instrument. PharmacoEconomics. 1993; 4(5):353–65.
25. Radloff LS. The CES-D scale a self-report depression scale for research in the general population. Appl Psychol Meas. 1977;1(3):385–401.
26. Fujisawa D, Inoguchi H. Impact of depression on health utility value in cancer patients. Psycho-Oncology. 2016;25(5):491–495.
27. R Core Team: R: A language and environment for statistical computing. Vienna: R Foundation for Statistical Computing. 2017. https://www.R-project.org/.
28. Bleichrodt H, Pinto JL, Maria Abellan-Perpiñan J. A consistency test of the time trade-off. J Health Econ. 2003;22(6):1037–52.
29. Pinheiro MB, Ferreira ML, Refshauge K, Maher CG, Ordoñana JR, Andrade TB, Tsathas A, Ferreira PH. Symptoms of depression as a prognostic factor for low back pain: a systematic review. Spine J. 2016;16(1):105–16.
30. Sagheer MA, Khan MF, Sharif S. Association between chronic low back pain, anxiety and depression in patients at a tertiary care centre. J Pak Med Assoc. 2013;63(6):688–90.
31. Mo F, Choi BC, Li FC, Merrick J. Using Health Utility Index (HUI) for measuring the impact on health-related quality of life (HRQL) among individuals with chronic diseases. Sci World J. 2004;4:746–57.
32. Billis E, Koutsojannis C, Matzaroglou C, Gliatis J, Fousekis K, Gioftsos G, Tsepis E. Association of low back pain on physical, sociodemographic and lifestyle factors across a general population sample within Greece. J Back Musculoskelet Rehab. 2017;30(2):279–290.

Using IFN-gamma release assay to confirm tuberculin skin test improves the screening of latent tuberculosis infection

Raffaela Olivieri[1], Sara Scarnera[2], Annalisa Ciabattini[1], Giulia De Vuono[2], Pietro Manzi[3], Gianni Pozzi[1], Giuseppe Battista[2] and Donata Medaglini[1*]

Abstract

Background: Healthcare workers (HCWs) represent a tuberculosis (TB) risk group for a wide range of tasks in healthcare, even in countries with low TB incidence, like Italy. Latent Tuberculosis Infection (LTBI) screening programs are an important tool for TB prevention in these setting.

Methods: A retrospective study under a LTBI screening program among HCWs at the Siena University Hospital (Italy), was conducted between September 2011 and July 2015. Tuberculin Skin Test (TST) was used as a first level examination; all TST-positive cases were tested with QuantiFERON-TB Gold In-Tube (QFT-GIT) test, together with a group of TST-negative subjects.

Results: Among the 2136 HCWs screened, 144 (6.7 %) were TST-positive and therefore tested with QFT-GIT, confirming a positive result in 36 cases (25 %). Agreement between two tests was poor ($k = 0.092$; 95 %, Confidence Interval [CI]- 0.048–0.136, $p = 0.002$). Among TST-positive cases, discordant results occurred more frequently in BCG vaccinated than unvaccinated HCWs (86.3 %, $p < 0.001$). The probability of a QFT-GIT-positive result increased according to the TST diameter ($p = 0.001$). No putative risk factor was associated with LTBI occurrence.

Conclusions: The use of QFT-GIT test as a second step in TST-positive cases offers an appropriate tool for LTBI detection, especially among BCG-vaccinated HCWs.

Keywords: LTBI, Tuberculosis, Interferon-gamma release assays, Healthcare workers

Background

Healthcare workers (HCWs) are an important group at increased risk for exposure to various infectious agents including *Mycobacterium tuberculosis*. Probability of exposure to tuberculosis (TB) infection depends on the specific tasks and settings; for this reason HCWs are stratified in different risk levels and should be included in TB screening programs [1, 2].

Systematic testing for diagnosis of Latent Tuberculosis Infection (LTBI) is an important component of infection control strategies among HCWs [3]. LTBI is a state of immune response to stimulation by *M. tuberculosis* antigens without evidence of clinically manifested active TB [3]. The lifetime risk of TB reactivation in case of LTBI is estimated to be 5–10 %, decreasing over the years depending on several factors, the most important one being the immunological status of the host [3, 4]. In many high-income countries, periodic screening of HCWs and contacts of confirmed TB patients for LTBI is a routine component of TB control, including routinely repeated screening or tracing after accidental contact with infected patients or materials.

Until the introduction of Interferon Gamma Release Assays (IGRAs), the only method for LTBI detection was Tuberculin Skin Test (TST). TST is based on an intradermal injection of a purified protein derivative (PPD)

* Correspondence: donata.medaglini@unisi.it
[1]Laboratorio di Microbiologia Molecolare e Biotecnologia, Dipartimento di Biotecnologie Mediche, Università degli Studi di Siena, Siena, Italy
Full list of author information is available at the end of the article

from *M. bovis* to elicit T-cell mediated delayed-type hypersensitivity reaction if the person has been previously infected with *M. tuberculosis*. However, TST assay has several intrinsic limitations: i) low sensitivity; ii) subjective interpretation of results; iii) cross reaction with Bacillus Calmette-Guerin (BCG) vaccination and non-tuberculous mycobacteria (NTM) infections iv) booster phenomenon [5–8]. The interpretation of TST results in the serial testing of HCWs is a major issue: findings show TST reversions or unclear conversions resulting from either random variability (e.g., differences in administration, reading or biologic response), boosting effect or an actual new infection [9–12].

IGRAs overcome some of these shortcomings and have emerged as an alternative to TST. IGRAs are indeed ex-vivo blood-based tests, are not affected by BCG vaccination status and by most infections with environmental NTM, can be repeated any number of times without sensitization or boosting, require only one patient visit and the result is available within 24 h.

To date, there are two commercial IGRAs, the QuantiFERON®-TB Gold In-Tube (QFT-GIT, QIAGEN, Hilden, Germany) test that measures by ELISA assay the amount of IFN-γ released by circulating T cells and the T-SPOT®.*TB* assay (Oxford Immunotec Ltd, Abingdon, UK) which assesses by enzyme-linked immunospot (ELISPOT) the number of blood cells releasing IFN-γ. The antigens used in QFT-GIT (ESAT-6, CFP-10 and TB7.7), are present in *M. tuberculosis* but absent from the BCG vaccine strain and from most NTM, except for *M. kansasii, M. marinum, M. szulgai, M. flavescens*, and *M. gastrii*. Thus, the proteins used as test antigens offer greater specificity compared to TST [13, 14].

Different protocols for LTBI diagnosis combining TST and IGRAs are currently used worldwide but the optimal screening strategy is still debated. In the United States, the Centers for Disease Control and Prevention (CDC, Atlanta, GA) have suggested that IGRAs can be used in place of TST for detection of TB infection [1]. However, there are only limited data on the reproducibility of IGRAs during serial testing. Studies have documented conversions and reversions during repeated IGRAs and there is no consensus on how to define and interpret these phenomena [6, 15–17]. In the United Kingdom, the National Institute for Health and Clinical Excellence (NICE) guidelines recommend a two-step strategy for LTBI diagnosis based on the initial screening with TST followed by an IGRA in TST-positive cases [18, 19].

With an overall TB incidence of 5.7 per 100,000 inhabitants, Italy is considered among those countries at low TB incidence. WHO guidelines indicate that in high-income and upper middle-income countries, with low TB incidence, systematic testing of LTBI, using IGRAs or TST, should be considered for HCWs [3]. However, in countries like Italy where until recently BCG vaccination has been widely used in HCWs, surveillance of TB infection has been hampered by the low specificity of TST. Current Italian guidelines for LTBI screening among HCWs recommend TST as primary assay, that can be integrated with IGRAs in the case of TST positive result [20].

The present work is a retrospective study under a LTBI screening program among HCWs at the Siena University Hospital (Italy) based on the initial screening with TST followed by QFT-GIT assay in TST-positive cases. The agreement between the two tests, the LTBI prevalence among Siena's hospital HCWs and the identification of putative risk factors for LTBI, were analyzed.

Methods

A screening program for TB was carried out from September 2011 at the Siena University Hospital that is a low TB risk level hospital. According to this program, all HCWs and students with access to the health profession school, undergo TST as first step examination, followed by QFT-GIT in the case of TST-positive result. TST is repeated yearly in HCWs serving high risk wards, such as Infectious Diseases ward and Microbiology Laboratories.

A total of 2136 HCWs were screened from September 2011 to July 2015 by TST. All TST-positive individuals ($n = 144$), as well as a control group of randomly selected subjects with negative TST ($n = 25$), performed QFT-GIT and were enrolled in this retrospective analysis ($n = 169$) (Fig. 1). A group of 142 HCWs was excluded from the study since they were screened only by IGRA because TST was refused ($n = 64$, 45.1 %), contraindicated ($n = 59$, 41.5 %) or avoided for other motivations ($n = 19$, 13.4 %). The time elapsed between TST and blood draw for QFT-GIT was variable. In 30 cases blood for IGRA testing was drawn within 15 days, in 38 cases within 6 months and in 17 within 1 year. In the cases with known positivity to TST in the past, the time elapsed was longer than 1 year. The Fisher exact test showed that there was not a statistically significant correlation between time intervals (TST and blood draw for QFT-GIT) and the probability of a positive QFT-GIT result ($p = 0.282$).

The subjects with positivity for TST and IGRA underwent a chest X-ray to exclude an active TB disease. In the absence of clinical and radiographic signs of active TB, they were considered to have a LTBI and underwent a clinical follow up at 6, 12 and 24 months after diagnosis. An infectious diseases consultant evaluated all LTBI cases and the decision of prescribing prophylaxis was taken case by case.

TST was performed by trained personnel following standard procedures. Intradermal injection of 0.1 ml of PPD (TUBERTEST®, Sanofi Pasteur MSD, France) containing 5 tuberculin units was performed into the volar surface of the forearm. The reaction to TST was assessed

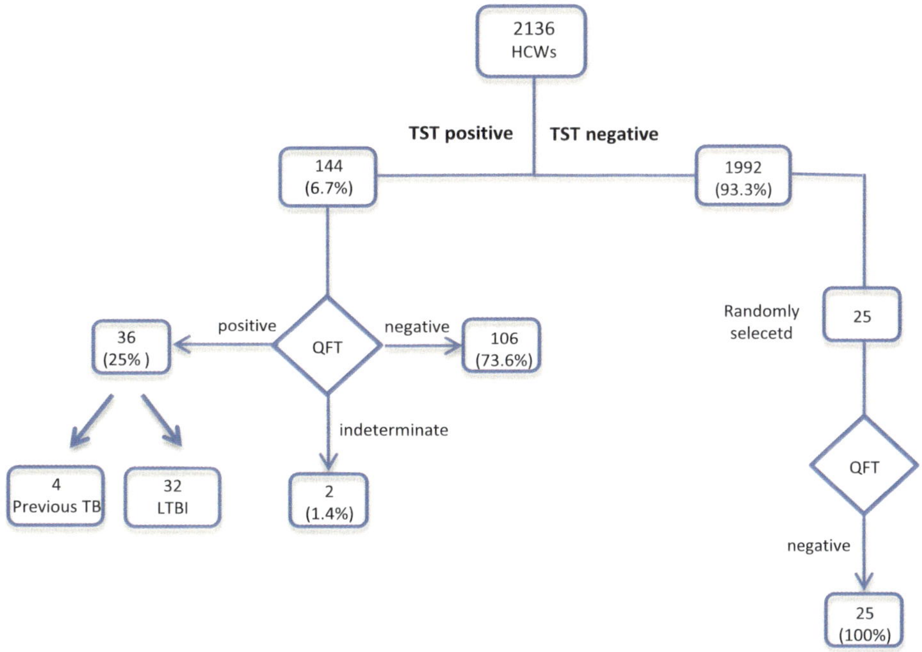

Fig. 1 Study population flow chart. HCWs: Healthcare Workers; TST: Tuberculin Skin Test; QFT: Quantiferon; TB: Tuberculosis; LTBI: Latent Tuberculosis Infection

after 48 to 72 h from the injection by health-care workers trained to read TST results, while self-reporting of results was not allowed. Induration of 10 mm or more was considered a positive result in persons who had increased risk factors to TB exposure such as HCWs according to CDC's interpretation criteria [1]. A diameter of 5 mm or more was considered positive in HCWs after accidental contact with infectious patients or materials (identified as "contacts").

The QuantiFERON®-TB Gold In-Tube test was performed in accordance with the manufactures's instructions. Briefly, 1 mL of blood was sampled in each of the three tubes containing no antigen (Nil Control tube), TB-specific antigens (ESAT-6, CFP-10 and TB7.7; TB Antigen tube), and positive control (Mitogen Control tube), respectively. Tubes were incubated at 37 °C for 16–24 h before centrifugation, and IFN-γ concentration (IU/ml) was measured by ELISA following the manufacturer's protocol. The test was considered positive when IFN-γ concentration was ≥ 0.35 IU/ml after correction for the negative control.

For each individual, information on age, gender, place of birth, job category, workplace, previous exposure to TB, family history of TB, prior TST results and BCG vaccination was collected by clinical chart review and vaccination records. BCG vaccination was mandatory in Italy for HCWs until 2001, when it was restricted to contacts and HCWs exposed to multidrug resistant strains with a negative TST at first screening.

According to the retrospective observational nature of the present study and to the authorizations signed by the HCWs related to personal data management including scientific research, formal ethical approval by local Ethics Committee is not requested. Personal information on the subjects included in the study was protected according to Italian law [Italian Law decree n. 196, 30 June 2003 (article 24): http://www.camera.it/parlam/leggi/deleghe/03196dl.htm.].

Statistical analysis

The concordance between the TST and QFT-GIT results was measured by kappa (k) statistics. A k value ≤ 0.4 was regarded as poor, > 0.8 as excellent, and in between as fair to good agreement according to the Landis and Koch scale. The Fisher exact test was used to compare the frequencies of test results among different groups of participants. Descriptive statistics were reported as mean values ± standard deviations for quantitative variables and as frequencies and percentages for qualitative variables. A p value ≤ 0.05 was considered statistically significant. All statistical analysis were performed by using GraphPad 6 software.

Results

Of the 2136 screened subjects, 1992 resulted TST-negative (93.3 %) and 144 TST-positive (6.7 %) using the established cut-off values. QFT-GIT was performed in all TST-positive subjects, as well as in 25 randomly selected HCWs with a negative TST. Of the 144 TST-positive HCWs, 36 were QFT-GIT positive (25 %), 106 negative (73.6 %) and two indeterminate (1.4 %) therefore excluded from our analysis (Fig. 1). Selected subjects with negative TST were all negative to the QFT-GIT test (Fig. 1). Among the 36 cases of TST+/QFT-GIT+, 4 had radiological signs of previous TB disease (0.2 % of the total HCWs evaluated) while 32 were diagnosed as LTBI (1.5 % of the total HCWs evaluated). Chest X-rays excluded an active TB disease in all cases of positivity for both TST and IGRA. All LTBI cases were evaluated by an infectious diseases consultant but in any case a chemoprophylaxis was indicated. None of the TST positive cases developed active TB in the following months/years.

Overall agreement between IGRA and TST was poor ($k = 0.092$; 95 % Confidence Interval [CI]- 0.048–0.136, $p = 0.002$) (Table 1). Discordance between the two tests was significantly higher among BCG-vaccinated (86.3 %) than unvaccinated subjects (52.8 %) ($p < 0.001$), regardless of time since vaccination (Table 2). As shown in Table 2, more than 50 % of the HCWs had reported a history of BCG vaccination, while 25.3 % had never received BCG. Nevertheless, a clear history of BCG vaccination could not be retrieved in 23.3 % of the studied population.

No association between other occupational and demographic factors and test results was observed. Indeed, gender (68.3 % were female), age (median age 44.4 years), birth in high (9.8 %) or low (90.2 %) endemic places, working in high TB risk wards (10.6 %), previous exposure to TB infectious patients or materials (22.5 %), and job category (most of HCWs were nurses) did not represent putative risk factors for a positive QFT-GIT test (Table 2).

The probability of a QFT-GIT positive result increased with the TST diameter ($p = 0.001$; Table 3). Indeed, HCWs with a TST <10 mm were all QFT-GIT negative, while in those with a TST between 10 and 15 mm the probability was 24.0 % and in those with TST diameter >15 mm, it was 27.5 % (Table 3).

Discussion

Screening programs for LTBI among HCWs together with TB infection-control measures represent an important tool to reduce the risk of TB transmission in healthcare settings. These screening strategies are also recommended in low TB incidence countries, such as Italy, where an annual TB incidence of 5.7 per 100,000 inhabitants has been estimated [3]. Only a few studies have been conducted to assess the outcome of a two-step LTBI screening strategy (TST plus IGRA) among healthcare workers in Italy [21, 22]. The present work shows the results of a two-step LTBI screening among HCWs in Siena University Hospital and provides an updated epidemiology of LTBI among Italian

Table 1 TST and IGRA results

TST	IGRA Negative n. (%)	Positive n. (%)	Total n. (%)	*k*	*p*-value
Negative	25 (15.0)	-	25 (15.0)	0.092[b]	0.002
Positive	106 (63.5)	36 (21.6)	142 (85.0)[a]		
All	131 (78.4)	36 (21.6)	167 (100)		

[a]Two IGRA-indeterminate subjects were excluded
[b]95 % CI- 0.048–0.136

Table 2 Association of TST and QFT-GIT results with demographic and occupational characteristics of TST-positive HCWs population

Characteristics	Total n. (%)	TST/IGRA +/+ n. (%)	+/− n. (%)	*p*-value
Female	97 (68.3)	22 (22.7)	75 (77.3)	0.304
Male	45 (31.7)	14 (31.1)	31 (68.9)	
Age, years				
19–29	2 (1.4)	0 (0.0)	2 (100.0)	0.272
30–39	40 (28.2)	8 (20.0)	32 (80.0)	
40–49	50 (35.2)	10 (20.0)	40 (80.0)	
50–59	43 (30.3)	15 (34.9)	28 (65.1)	
≥ 60	7 (4.9)	3 (42.9)	4 (57.1)	
Place of birth				
High endemic	14 (9.8)	4 (28.6)	10 (71.4)	0.752
Low endemic	128 (90.2)	32 (25.0)	96 (75.0)	
BCG vaccination				
yes	73 (51.4)	10 (13.7)	63 (86.3)	<0.001
no	36 (25.3)	17 (47.2)	19 (52.8)	
unknown	33 (23.3)	9 (22.3)	24 (72.7)	
Time since BCG vaccination, years				
< 10	3 (4.1)	1 (33.3)	2 (66.7)	0.184
10–14	13 (17.8)	3 (23.1)	10 (76.9)	
≥ 15	57 (40.1)	6 (10.5)	51 (89.5)	
Previous TST				
yes	95 (66.9)	23 (24.2)	72 (75.8)	0.685
no	47 (33.1)	13 (27.6)	34 (72.4)	
TB contacts				
yes	32 (22.5)	7 (21.8)	25 (78.2)	0.817
no	110 (77.5)	29 (26.4)	81 (73.6)	
Job category				
Physician	15 (10.6)	4 (26.7)	11 (73.3)	0.555
Nurse	66 (46.5)	13 (19.7)	53 (80.3)	
Nurse assistant	29 (20.4)	8 (28.6)	20 (71.4)	
Student	12 (8.5)	4 (33.3)	8 (66.7)	
other	20 (14.0)	7 (35.0)	13 (65.0)	
Ward				
High TB risk	15 (10.6)	3 (20.0)	12 (80.0)	0.760
Low TB risk	127 (89.4)	33 (26.0)	94 (74.0)	

Table 3 Correlation between TST diameter (mm) and QFT-GIT results*

	IGRA				*p*-value
	Negative		Positive		
	n.	%	n.	%	
TST diameter (n.)					
0–9 (29)	29	100.0	-	-	0.001
10–15 (75)	57	76.0	18	24.0	
> 15 (51)	37	72.5	14	27.5	

**p*-value refers to the Fisher exact test to compare the frequency distribution of positive and negative QFT-GIT for three increasing diameter ranges

HCWs. In our setting, a global prevalence of LTBI of 1.5 % was observed, consistent with other studies performed among HCWs in areas with a low TB incidence (mean value of 1 %, range 0.2–12 %) [8, 11, 23]. These data are justified by the low circulation of *M. tuberculosis* in hospitals of low TB prevalence countries that reduces the risk of contact with infected patients.

In our study, 144 subjects were positive to the tuberculin test, corresponding to the 6.7 %. In line with data reported by other Italian and European studies [24–26], only the 22.2 % of TST positive HCWs also had a positive QFT-GIT result. Our data also show that the probability of a QFT-GIT positive result increased with TST diameter and this correlation was already reported in previous studies among HCWs [24, 27, 28].

A poor agreement was observed between the two tests and discordant results (TST+/QFT-GIT-) occurred primarily among BCG vaccinated subjects in line with what was reported in other studies conducted in low TB prevalence countries [25, 29]. This is particularly relevant for countries like Italy where BCG vaccination was mandatory for HCWs until 2001, when it was restricted to defined high TB risk categories only, based on risk assessment at hospital level [30]. Of course, since the sensitivity of QFT-GIT in infected individuals is not 100 %, caution should be taken into account when interpreting discordant results (TST+/QFT-GIT-) occurring in high risk HCWs [14, 18]. Another putative cause of TST+/QFT-GIT- results could be the exposure to NTM [31]. These data strongly support the added value of using both clinical tests, rather than TST alone, for LTBI diagnosis.

Conclusion

Our data strongly support the added value of using QFT-GIT test in TST-positive HCWs for LTBI diagnosis, especially in settings with a high rate of BCG vaccination. TST is widely used as a first LTBI screening tool but the introduction of IGRA as a second step assay in TST-positive HCWs reduces the potential occurrence of "false positives" due to BCG vaccination or atypical mycobacteria infections and improves the clinical management of LTBI cases. In fact, the introduction of QFT-GIT test could reduce the number of unnecessary chest X-ray and avoid the costs and toxicity associated with unnecessary treatment. Despite the monocentric and observational nature of the study, our results could help to better understand factors influencing screening results and the optimal strategy for LTBI diagnosis among HCWs. Absence of a true gold standard test for LTBI represents a major challenge for determining the accuracy of new LTBI tests, therefore the choice of using a two-step strategy is also aimed at increasing the accuracy level of the diagnostic workup, providing additional information for management and clinical follow-up of LTBI cases.

Abbreviations

BCG, Bacillus Calmette-Guerin; HCWs, healthcare workers; IGRAs, Interferon gamma release assays; LTBI, latent tuberculosis infection; NTM, non-tuberculous mycobacteria; PPD, purified protein derivative; QFT-GIT -GIT, QuantiFERON-TB Gold In-Tube test; TB, tuberculosis; TST, tuberculin skin test

Acknowledgments

The authors thank Prof. Gabriele Cevenini for support in statistical analysis.

Authors' contributions

RO performed QFT-GIT studies, collected and analyzed QFT-GIT data, performed the statistical analysis, contributed to the study design, interpretation of the results and drafted the manuscript. SS performed TST and collected TST data, contributed to the study design and interpretation of the results. AC contributed to the study design, collection and analysis of data, interpretation of the results and helped to draft the manuscript. GDV performed TST and contributed to the analysis of TST data. PM contributed to the design of the study and critically revised the manuscript. GP contributed to the design of the study and critically revised the manuscript. GB contributed to the design of the study and critically revised the manuscript. DM conceived the study, participated in its design and coordination; contributed to the analysis of QFT-GIT data and writing of the manuscript. All authors read and approved the final manuscript.

Competing interests

The authors declare that they have no competing interests.

Author details

[1]Laboratorio di Microbiologia Molecolare e Biotecnologia, Dipartimento di Biotecnologie Mediche, Università degli Studi di Siena, Siena, Italy. [2]Medicina Preventiva e Sorveglianza Sanitaria, Dipartimento di Biotecnologie Mediche, Universita' degli Studi di Siena, Siena, Italy. [3]Direzione Medica di Presidio, Azienda Ospedaliera Universitaria Senese, Siena, Italy.

References

1. Jensen PA, Lambert LA, Iademarco MF, Ridzon R. Guidelines for preventing the transmission of *Mycobacterium tuberculosis* in health-care settings. MMWR RecommRep. 2005;54(RR-17):1–141.
2. Nienhaus A, Ringshausen FC, Costa JT, Schablon A, Tripodi D. IFN-gamma release assay versus tuberculin skin test for monitoring TB infection in healthcare workers. Expert Rev Anti Infect Ther. 2013;11(1):37–48. doi:10.1586/eri.12.150.
3. World Health Organization. Guidelines on the management of latent tuberculosis infection. 2015.
4. Mack U, Migliori GB, Sester M, Rieder HL, Ehlers S, Goletti D, et al. LTBI: latent tuberculosis infection or lasting immune responses to *M. tuberculosis*? A TBNET consensus statement. Eur Respir J. 2009;33(5):956–73. doi:10.1183/09031936.00120908.
5. Singh D, Sutton C, Woodcock A. Repeat tuberculin testing in BCG-vaccinated subjects in the United Kingdom. The booster effect varies with

the time of reading. Am J Respir Crit Care Med. 2001;164(6):962–4. doi:10.1164/ajrccm.164.6.2102076.

6. Dorman SE, Belknap R, Graviss EA, Reves R, Schluger N, Weinfurter P, et al. Interferon-gamma release assays and tuberculin skin testing for diagnosis of latent tuberculosis infection in healthcare workers in the United States. Am J Respir Crit Care Med. 2014;189(1):77–87. doi:10.1164/rccm.201302-0365OC.
7. Camacho GDR, Perea-Milla E, Gonzalez JR, Frias JP. Interpretation of a serial Mantoux test taking into account the annual risk of tuberculous infection. Int J Tuberc Lung Dis. 2009;13(2):196–200.
8. Menzies D, Joshi R, Pai M. Risk of tuberculosis infection and disease associated with work in health care settings. Int J Tuberc Lung Dis. 2007; 11(6):593–605.
9. Sauzullo I, Massetti AP, Mengoni F, Rossi R, Lichtner M, Ajassa C, et al. Influence of previous tuberculin skin test on serial IFN-gamma release assays. Tuberculosis. 2011;91(4):322–6. doi:10.1016/j.tube.2011.05.004.
10. Zwerling A, van den Hof S, Scholten J, Cobelens F, Menzies D, Pai M. Interferon-gamma release assays for tuberculosis screening of healthcare workers: a systematic review. Thorax. 2012;67(1):62–70. doi:10.1136/thx.2010.143180.
11. Baussano I, Nunn P, Williams B, Pivetta E, Bugiani M, Scano F. Tuberculosis among health care workers. Emerg Infect Dis. 2011;17(3):488–94. doi:10.3201/eid1703.100947.
12. Menzies D. Interpretation of repeated tuberculin tests. Boosting, conversion, and reversion. Am J Respir Crit Care Med. 1999;159(1):15–21. doi:10.1164/ajrccm.159.1.9801120.
13. Moon HW, Hur M. Interferon-gamma release assays for the diagnosis of latent tuberculosis infection: an updated review. Ann Clin Lab Sci. 2013; 43(2):221–9.
14. Diel R, Goletti D, Ferrara G, Bothamley G, Cirillo D, Kampmann B, et al. Interferon-gamma release assays for the diagnosis of latent *Mycobacterium tuberculosis* infection: a systematic review and meta-analysis. Eur Respir J. 2011;37(1):88–99. doi:10.1183/09031936.00115110.
15. Pai M, O'Brien R. Serial testing for tuberculosis: can we make sense of T cell assay conversions and reversions? PLoS Med. 2007;4(6):e208. doi:10.1371/journal.pmed.0040208.
16. Pai M, Joshi R, Dogra S, Mendiratta DK, Narang P, Kalantri S, et al. Serial testing of health care workers for tuberculosis using interferon-gamma assay. Am J Respir Crit Care Med. 2006;174(3):349–55. doi:10.1164/rccm.200604-472OC.
17. Slater ML, Welland G, Pai M, Parsonnet J, Banaei N. Challenges with QuantiFERON-TB Gold assay for large-scale, routine screening of U.S. healthcare workers. Am J Respir Crit Care Med. 2013;188(8):1005–10. doi:10.1164/rccm.201305-0831OC.
18. Mazurek GH, Jereb J, Vernon A, LoBue P, Goldberg S, Castro K. Updated guidelines for using interferon gamma release assays to detect *Mycobacterium Tuberculosis* infection — united states. MMWR. 2010;59(RR-5):1–25.
19. National Institute for Health and Care Excellence. Clinical diagnosis and management of tuberculosis and measures for its prevention a006Ed control. Clinical Guidelines, CG117. London, UK: NICE;2011.
20. Italian Ministry of Health. Prevenzione della tubercolosi negli operatori sanitari e soggetti ad essi equiparati. Roma: 2013. http://www.salute.gov.it/imgs/C_17_pubblicazioni_1901_allegato.pdf.
21. Ciaschetti A, Franchi A, Richeldi L, Rumpianesi F, Meacci M, Valente A, et al. Screening of latent tuberculosis infection in health care workers by QuantiFERON-TB and tuberculin skin test. G Ital Med Lav Ergon. 2007;29(3 Suppl):406–7.
22. Girardi E, Angeletti C, Puro V, Sorrentino R, Magnavita N, Vincenti D, et al. Estimating diagnostic accuracy of tests for latent tuberculosis infection without a gold standard among healthcare workers. Euro Surveill. 2009;14(43): pii=19373.
23. Durando P, Alicino C, Orsi A, Barberis I, Paganino C, Dini G, et al. Latent tuberculosis infection among a large cohort of medical students at a teaching hospital in Italy. Biomed Res Int. 2015;2015:746895. doi:10.1155/2015/746895.
24. Moucaut A, Nienhaus A, Courtois B, Nael V, Longuenesse C, Ripault B, et al. The effect of introducing IGRA to screen French healthcare workers for tuberculosis and potential conclusions for the work organisation. J Occup Med Toxicol. 2013;8:12. doi:10.1186/1745-6673-8-12.
25. Torres CJ, Sa R, Cardoso MJ, Silva R, Ferreira J, Ribeiro C, et al. Tuberculosis screening in Portuguese healthcare workers using the tuberculin skin test and the interferon-gamma release assay. Eur Respir J. 2009;34(6):1423–8. doi:10.1183/09031936.00053809.
26. Lamberti M, Muoio M, Monaco MG, Uccello R, Sannolo N, Mazzarella G, et al. Prevalence of latent tuberculosis infection and associated risk factors among 3,374 healthcare students in Italy. J OccupMed Toxicol. 2014;9(1):34. doi:10.1186/s12995-014-0034-5.
27. Charisis A, Tatsioni A, Gartzonika C, Gogali A, Archimandriti D, Katsanos C, et al. Value of adding an IGRA to the TST to screen for latent tuberculous infection in Greek health care workers. Int J Tuberc Lung Dis. 2014;18(9): 1040–6. doi:10.5588/ijtld.14.0018.
28. Alvarez-Leon EE, Espinosa-Vega E, Santana-Rodriguez E, Molina-Cabrillana JM, Perez-Arellano JL, Caminero JA, et al. Screening for tuberculosis infection in spanish healthcare workers: comparison of the QuantiFERON-TB gold in-tube test with the tuberculin skin test. Infect Control Hosp Epidemiol. 2009;30(9):876–83. doi:10.1086/598519.
29. Babayigit C, Ozer B, Ozer C, Inandi T, Duran N, Gocmen O. Performance of QuantiFERON-TB gold in-tube test and tuberculin skin test for diagnosis of latent tuberculosis infection in BCG vaccinated health care workers. Med Sci Monit. 2014;20:521–9. doi:10.12659/MSM.889943.
30. Italian Law Decree n.465, 7 Novembre 2001. Regolamento che stabilisce le condizioni nelle quali è obbligatoria la vaccinazione antitubercolare, a norma dell'articolo 93, comma 2, della legge 23 Dicembre 2000, n.388.
31. von Reyn CF, Horsburgh CR, Olivier KN, Barnes PF, Waddell R, Warren C, et al. Skin test reactions to *Mycobacterium tuberculosis* purified protein derivative and *Mycobacterium avium* sensitin among health care workers and medical students in the United States. Int J Tuberc Lung Dis. 2001;5(12):1122–8.

11

Burnout among young physicians and its association with physicians' wishes to leave

Birte Pantenburg[1*], Melanie Luppa[1], Hans-Helmut König[2] and Steffi G. Riedel-Heller[1]

Abstract

Background: Concerns about burnout, and its consequences, among German physicians are rising. However, data on burnout among German physicians are scarce. Also, a suspected association between burnout and German physicians' wishes to leave remains to be studied. Therefore, the extent of burnout, and the association between burnout and wishes to leave clinical practice or to go abroad for clinical work was studied in a sample of young physicians in Saxony.

Methods: In a cross-sectional survey, all physicians ≤40 years and registered with the State Chamber of Physicians of Saxony, Germany ($n = 5956$) received a paper-pencil questionnaire inquiring about socio-demographics, job satisfaction, and wishes to leave clinical practice or to go abroad for clinical work. Response rate was 40 % ($n = 2357$). Burnout was measured with the German version of the Maslach Burnout Inventory - Human Services Survey (MBI) consisting of the subscales *emotional exhaustion* (feeling emotionally drained), *depersonalization* (feelings of cynicsm) and *personal accomplishment* (feelings of personal achievement in job). Variables associated with burnout, and the association between burnout and wishes to leave were assessed in multivariate logistic regression analyses.

Results: For *emotional exhaustion* participants reached a mean of 21.3 [standard deviation = 9.74], for *depersonalization* a mean of 9.9 [5.92], and for *personal accomplishment* a mean of 36.3 [6.77]. Men exhibited significantly higher depersonalization than women (11.3 [6.11] versus 9 [5.62], $p < 0.001$). Eleven percent of participants showed a high degree of burnout on all subscales, while 35 % did not show a high degree of burnout on any subscale. Confirming that one would become a physician again, and higher satisfaction with the components "work environment" and "humaneness", were associated with a lower chance for a high degree of burnout on all subscales. Higher *emotional exhaustion* and lower *personal accomplishment* were associated with an increased chance of wishing to leave clinical practice. Higher *emotional exhaustion* and higher *depersonalization* were associated with an increased chance of wishing to go abroad for clinical work.

Conclusions: Preventing physician burnout may not only benefit the affected individual. It may also benefit the health care system by potentially preventing physicians from leaving clinical practice or from going abroad for clinical work.

Keywords: Burnout, Maslach Burnout Inventory, Physician attrition, Physicians' wishes to leave

* Correspondence: Birte.Pantenburg@medizin.uni-leipzig.de
[1]Institute of Social Medicine, Occupational Health and Public Health, University of Leipzig, Philipp-Rosenthal-Str. 55, 04103 Leipzig, Germany
Full list of author information is available at the end of the article

Background

The issue of burnout is of high concern in the current debate in Germany [1, 2]. In Germany, sick leave due to burnout has increased from 0.7 days/100 insured live years in 2004 to 9.1 days/100 insured live years in 2011 [3]. In a study from the USA, physicians were more likely to have symptoms of burnout, as measured with the Maslach Burnout Inventory (MBI), than the working general population [4]. In a national sample of US physicians 46 % and among family physicians in 12 European countries nearly 65 % of participants showed signs of high burnout [4, 5].

There have been several studies of burnout among German physicians within specific specialties. However, they are scarce and employ various measuring instruments. One of the most widely used instruments is the Maslach Burnout Inventory (MBI). It consists of the three subscales *emotional exhaustion, depersonalization* and *personal accomplishment* [6]. *Emotional exhaustion* reflects "feelings of being emotionally overextended" [6]. *Depersonalization* relates to an "impersonal response towards recipients of one's service" [6]. *Personal accomplishment* stands for "feelings of competence and successful achievement in one's work with people" [6], which turns into the opposite in a burnout situation.

Instruments other than the MBI are also in use and results are therefore difficult to compare: Klein et al. [7] used the Copenhagen Burnout Inventory and estimated that 49 % of participating surgeons met the burnout criteria. Employing the same instrument, Heinke et al. [8] revealed that 40 % of anesthetists were at high risk for burnout. Using the MBI, Böhle et al. [9] estimated that of participating German urologists 40, 37, and 11 % showed high *emotional exhaustion*, high *depersonalization* and low *personal accomplishment*, respectively. With the same instrument, Pajonk et al. [10] estimated that 4 % of emergency physicians met the criteria of burnout and 11 % were at risk for developing burnout. In a study by Voltmer et al. [11] employing the Work-related Behavior and Experience Patterns questionnaire (AVEM), 22 % of physicians of various specialties in medical practice were at risk of burnout. Richter et al. [12] performed a study employing the MBI with hospital physicians of various specialties but did not categorize the results into "low", "medium" and "high" symptoms of burnout. Larger German studies covering a broad range of medical specialties and including both physicians working in inpatient and outpatient settings are, to the best of our knowledge, missing.

Mental distress among physicians has been associated with, among others, substance abuse, depression and family conflicts [13]. In several studies using varying instruments to measure burnout, the consequences of physician burnout were investigated. Apart from the negative effect on an individual's health, burnout may negatively impact the healthcare system as a whole by lowering quality of patient care [14], decreasing physician productivity [15], and leading to significant costs for the healthcare system due to early retirement and reduction in clinical hours [16].

Importantly, burnout among physicians has also been associated with increased rates of job turnover intentions [17, 18], and the intent to leave the medical profession [19].

In Germany, there is an ongoing debate about a potential shortage of physicians, among other reasons, due to physicians leaving clinical practice and/or going abroad for clinical work [20–23]. To the best of our knowledge, however, there are no studies from Germany investigating the association between burnout and physicians' wishes to leave.

To address these gaps in knowledge, we aimed to assess the following questions within a study on wishes to leave among young physicians in Saxony, Germany:

1. To what extent are symptoms of burnout present among the study population?
2. Is there an association between burnout symptoms and physicians' wishes to leave clinical practice or to go abroad for clinical work?

Methods

Study population and study design

The study was designed as a cross-sectional study. In a comprehensive survey, all physicians up to 40 years of age and registered with the State Chamber of Physicians of Saxony (SLÄK) ($n = 5956$) were sent a paper-pencil questionnaire. Registration with the SLÄK is obligatory for all licensed physicians practicing medicine in Saxony or, if not practicing medicine, having their main residence in Saxony. Two thousand three hundred fifty-seven questionnaires were returned from September 2012 to February 2013, equaling a response rate of 40 %. Compared to the population of physicians in Saxony, the sample contained more women (58 % versus 66 %, $p < 0.001$) and participants were slightly younger (33.2 years versus 32.9 years, $p < 0.001$). The letter accompanying the paper-pencil questionnaire stated that sending back the filled out questionnaire was regarded as giving consent to participating in the study. All questionnaires were anonymous and at no point could a filled out questionnaire be related to the respective respondent. The study was approved of by the Ethics committee of the University of Leipzig (Ethik-Kommission an der Medizinischen Fakultät der Universität Leipzig).

Questionnaire and instruments

The anonymous paper-pencil questionnaire was developed based on a literature review, existing, mostly

German-language, instruments, and self-generated questions: It contained questions on general socio-demographics [24, 25]; self-generated questions on wishes to leave clinical practice, and respective reasons (based on [20, 23, 24, 26]), and wishes to go abroad for clinical work, and respective reasons (based on [23, 24]) (English translation: "How much do you currently wish you could go abroad for clinical work?" and "How much do you currently wish you could leave clinical practice?". Possible answers were: „not at all" (1), "rather not (2), "don't know (3), "rather yes" (4), "absolutely" (5)); questions addressing job satisfaction, mainly based on the job satisfaction questionnaire developed by Bovier and Perneger [26], which was slightly modified by eliminating one question and adjusting the wording to fit the German context, while adding questions on working climate and career opportunities (based on [20]), job security and relationship with superiors (based on [27]) and a question on gender equality. Thus, to measure job satisfaction, participants were asked to rate their satisfaction with the job situation as a whole as well as on 20 aspects on a 5-point Likert scale ranging from 1 = very dissatisfied to 5 = very satisfied. Kaiser criterion of eigenvalues >1 was applied and items with factor loadings ≥0.5 were included. Factor analysis (principal component analysis) with promax rotation revealed 5 underlying factors: factor 1: "work environment" (intellectual stimulation at work, relationship with superiors, relationship and professional exchange with colleagues, work enjoyment, working atmosphere); factor 2: "work load" (work load, time for family, friends and leisure activities, stress level at work); factor 3: "patient care" (possibility to treat patients as you deem optimal, possibility to refer patients to specialists whenever you deem it necessary, quality of the medical care you provide); factor 4: "structural aspects" (career opportunities, current income, job security, equality of women and men) and factor 5: "humaneness" (relationship with non-medical staff, relationship with patients).

Symptoms of burnout were measured with the German version of the Maslach Burnout Inventory - Human Services Survey (MBI) [6]. The MBI's three subscales were analysed separately as suggested by Maslach et al. [6]: *emotional exhaustion* (ranging from 0 to 54 points), *depersonalization* (ranging from 0 to 30 points) and *personal accomplishment* (ranging from 0 to 48 points). Higher scores on the subscales *emotional exhaustion* and *depersonalization* indicate a higher degree of burnout, while a higher score on the subscale *personal accomplishment* indicates a lower degree of burnout.

Means were calculated and subscales were categorized into "low", "average", and "high" degrees of burnout using the cut off values suggested by Maslach et al. [6]: For the subscale *emotional exhaustion* this translates into ≤18, 19–26, and ≥27 points, respectively; for the subscale *depersonalization* into ≤5, 6–9, and ≥10 points, respectively; and for the subscale *personal accomplishment* into ≥40, 39–34, and ≤33 points, respectively. Before employing it in the study, the questionnaire was pretested by physicians for comprehensibility and usability. The questionnaire is available from the authors upon request.

Data analysis

Of the 2357 questionnaires returned, 9 questionnaires were excluded from the analysis: 3 persons were older than 40 years, 1 person worked abroad and 5 questionnaires were incomplete. For the purpose of studying burnout, only questionnaires of physicians working in patient care who fully completed the MBI were analysed ($n = 1784$). Means on MBI subscales were compared with t-test, and proportions were compared with χ^2 -test.

In multivariate logistic regression analyses, variables associated with a high degree of burnout were assessed for each subscale. Participants' age (in years), clinical work experience (in years), and satisfaction with the factors "work environment", "work load", "patient care", "structural aspects", and "humaneness" were introduced as continuous variables. Female sex (reference category [rc]: male), being in a relationship (rc: no relationship), having children (rc: no children), having German citizenship (rc: no German citizenship), being a specialist (rc: no specialization), would become a physician again (rc: would not become a physician again or indecisive), working full-time (rc: part-time), working in an urban setting (rc: rural setting), working in an inpatient setting (rc: outpatient setting), having a leading position/having their own practice (rc: non-leading position/employee in a practice) were dummy coded before introducing them into the regression models. Participants with missing values on variables were excluded from the analyses.

Multivariate logistic regression analyses were also performed to study the association between burnout symptoms and wishing to leave. Dependent variables were wishing to leave clinical practice and wishing to go abroad for clinical work. Scores on the subscales *emotional exhaustion*, *depersonalization* and *personal accomplishment*, as well as age, were introduced as continuous independent variables. Female sex (rc: male), being in a relationship (rc: no relationship), and having children (rc: no children) were dummy coded before introducing them into the regression models. Participants with missing values on variables were excluded from the analyses.

As not all participants fully completed all questions, the percentages in the results section correspond to the number of actual answers given. Data analysis was performed with Stata 12.0 for Windows.

Results

Characteristics of the study population

The characteristics of the study population are detailed in Table 1. Eighty-three percent ($n = 1457$) of the physicians worked in an inpatient setting and of these 85 % ($n = 1222$) worked in a hospital with more than 100 beds. Fifty percent ($n = 138$) of the physicians working in an outpatient setting worked as primary care physicians.

Degree of burnout

The degree of experienced burnout was assessed with the Maslach Burnout Inventory - Human Services Survey (MBI). The means of each subscale are presented in Table 2. Men reached a significantly higher score than women on the subscale *depersonalization* (mean: 11.3 [standard deviation: 6.11] versus 9 [5.62], p <0.001). Subscales were also categorized into low, middle and high degrees of burnout (Table 2). Again, distribution differed significantly between men and women on the subscale *depersonalization*, with a higher proportion of men showing a high degree of burnout.

Extent of high degree of burnout

To assess the overall extent of burnout symptoms, the percentage of participants showing a high degree of burnout over all of the scales was analysed.

Eleven percent of participants showed a high degree of burnout on all subscales, while 34 % of participants did not show a high degree of burnout on any subscale (Table 3). A higher proportion of men (12 % of men versus 11 % of women, $p < 0.01$), of participants working full-time (12 % of participants working full-time versus 6 % of participants working part-time, $p < 0.05$), and of participants working in an inpatient setting (12 % of participants working in an inpatient versus 8 % of participants working in an outpatient setting, $p = 0.001$) showed a high degree of burnout on all subscales (Table 3).

Table 1 Characteristics of the study population ($n = 1784$)

Female [% (n)]	61 (1086)
Age (years) [mean (SD; range)]	32.8 (4; 25 – 40)
German nationality [% (n)]	91 (1611)
In a relationship [% (n)]	84 (1489)
Children [% (n)]	52 (935)
Length of work experience (years) [mean (SD; range)]	5.6 (3.8; 0 – 17)
Specialist [% (n)]	38 (671)
Works full-time [% (n)]	84 (1501)
Works in an inpatient setting [% (n)]	83 (1457)

Percentages were calculated with the number of answers actually given and may differ from calculations based on a denominator without missing values. SD = standard deviation

Finally, a higher proportion of participants wishing to leave showed a high degree of burnout on all subscales (14 % of participants wishing to go abroad for clinical work versus 10 % of participants not wishing to go abroad for clinical work; and 24 % of participants wishing to leave clinical practice versus 7 % of participants not wishing to leave clinical practice, $p < 0.001$) (Table 4).

Parameters associated with a high degree of burnout

To identify parameters associated with a high degree of burnout, multivariate logistic regressions were performed. The results are detailed in Table 5. Confirming that one would become a physician again, as well as higher satisfaction with the components "work environment" and "humaneness", were associated with a lower chance for a high degree of burnout on all subscales. Higher satisfaction with the component "work load" was associated with a lower chance for a high degree of burnout on the subscales *emotional exhaustion* and *depersonalization*. Women were less likely to exhibit a high degree of burnout on the subscale *depersonalization*.

Association between burnout symptoms and wishes to leave

A higher score on the subscale *emotional exhaustion* and a lower score on the subscale *personal accomplishment* were associated with an increased chance of wishing to leave clinical practice (Table 6). Higher scores on the subscales *emotional exhaustion* and *depersonalization* were associated with an increased chance of wishing to go abroad for clinical work. In contrast, female sex, being in a relationship and having children were associated with a lower chance of wishing to go abroad (Table 6).

Discussion

This study investigated the extent of burnout symptoms among a large sample of young physicians in Saxony, Germany. The achieved mean scores on the MBI subscales (*emotional exhaustion*: 21.3, *depersonalization*: 9.9, and *personal accomplishment*: 36.3) were similar to those detected among European family doctors (*emotional exhaustion*: 24, *depersonalization*: 7, and *personal accomplishment*: 37) and among hospital physicians in Hamburg, Germany (*emotional exhaustion*: 21.8, *depersonalization*: 9.7, and *personal accomplishment*: 34.1) [5, 12]. Likewise, in the present study, the percentage of participants showing high burnout symptoms on all subscales (approximately 11 %) was comparable to that among European family doctors (12 %) [5]. In both studies only a third of participants (34 and 35 %) did not show high symptoms of burnout on any of the subscales [5]. As several instruments are in use to measure burnout, estimates need to be interpreted and compared with caution across different studies.

Table 2 Burnout symptoms

	All ($n = 1784$) Mean [SD]	Women ($n = 1086$) Mean [SD]	Men ($n = 698$) Mean [SD]	p value
Emotional exhaustion	21.3 [9.74]	21.5 [9.67]	20.9 [9.84]	ns
Depersonalization	9.9 [5.92]	9 [5.62]	11.3 [6.11]	<0.001
Personal accomplishment	36.3 [6.77]	36.1 [6.77]	36.5 [6.77]	ns
Degree of burnout	% (n)	% (n)	% (n)	
Emotional exhaustion				ns
Low	42 (741)	40 (437)	44 (304)	
Average	28 (505)	29 (312)	28 (193)	
High	30 (538)	31 (337)	29 (201)	
Depersonalization				<0.001
Low	25 (452)	29 (318)	19 (134)	
Average	27 (481)	29 (320)	23 (161)	
High	48 (851)	41 (448)	58 (403)	
Personal accomplishment				ns
Low	36 (641)	35 (377)	38 (264)	
Average	33 (591)	34 (364)	33 (227)	
High	31 (552)	32 (345)	30 (207)	

Means were calculated for each subscale of the MBI, and compared between women and men using the t-test. MBI subscales were categorized into low, average and high degree of burnout, and distribution compared between women and men using $\chi 2$ -test. SD = standard deviation, ns = not significant

However, the above named studies all employed the MBI. Thus, the present sample of physicians in Saxony does not seem to present more symptoms of burnout than other physician samples. However, burnout does exist in this sample and it should be addressed.

In the present sample, a higher percentage of men exhibited high symptoms of burnout in bivariate analyses. Men also showed higher degrees of *depersonalization*, an "impersonal response towards recipients of one's service" [6], widely described as cynicism. Consistently, in multivariate analysis, female sex was associated with a lower chance for *depersonalization*. A possible explanation may be that the German society expects less of men than of women to be empathic and to show emotions, but rather to be strong and not to show weakness. Thus, the social context may promote men to experience, but also to express, feelings of depersonalization. Similarly, in a meta-analysis by Purvanova et al. [28] including studies covering a range of professions, men showed higher degrees of *depersonalization*, whereas women showed higher *emotional exhaustion*. Purvanova and colleagues argue that women rather report *emotional exhaustion* as the main symptom of burnout, whereas men tend to present with increased levels of *depersonalization* as the main symptom of burnout [28].

In bivariate analysis, physicians who work in an inpatient setting exhibited more burnout. In multivariate analysis, however, inpatient work was associated with a lower chance for high *emotional exhaustion*. This is consistent with a meta-analysis of worldwide studies: Outpatient-based physicians showed a higher degree of

Table 3 Extent of high degree of burnout

High degree on	All % (n)	Women % (n)	Men % (n)	Full-time % (n)	Part-time % (n)	Outpatient % (n)	Inpatient % (n)
No subscale	34 (611)	37 (407)	29 (204)	34 (506)	37 (105)	44 (129)	32 (467)
1 subscale	34 (600)	31 (342)	37 (258)	33 (499)	36 (101)	32 (94)	34 (497)
2 subscales	21 (378)	21 (223)	22 (155)	21 (318)	21 (60)	16 (48)	22 (323)
3 subscales	11 (195)	11 (114)	12 (81)	12 (178)	6 (17)	8 (23)	12 (170)
Total	100 (1784)	100 (1086)	100 (698)	100 (1501)	100 (283)	100 (294)	100 (1457)

The percentage of participants showing a high degree of burnout on none, one, two or all of the MBI subscales was calculated. Using $\chi 2$ -test results were compared between women and men ($p < 0.01$); participants working full- or part-time ($p < 0.05$); and participants working in an in- or outpatient setting ($p = 0.001$)

Table 4 Extent of high degree of burnout

High degree on	Wish to go abroad		Wish to leave clinical practice	
	No	Yes	No	Yes
	% (n)	% (n)	% (n)	% (n)
No subscale	39 (473)	24 (130)	40 (542)	16 (67)
1 subscale	33 (400)	36 (193)	35 (474)	29 (119)
2 subscales	19 (231)	26 (143)	18 (251)	30 (125)
3 subscales	10 (117)	14 (75)	7 (93)	24 (100)
Total	101 (1221)	100 (541)	100 (1360)	99 (411)

The percentage of participants showing a high degree of burnout on none, one, two or all of the MBI subscales was calculated. Using the χ2-test, results were compared between participants wishing to go abroad for clinical work and those who do not ($p < 0.001$); and participants wishing to leave clinical practice and those who do not ($p < 0.001$). Percentages may not add up to 100 % due to rounding

emotional exhaustion [29]. In contrast, in a recent study from the USA, internal medicine hospitalists and outpatient general internists did not differ regarding *emotional exhaustion* and *depersonalization.* However, lower *personal accomplishment* was more common among hospitalists [30]. In cross-sectional studies, such as the present one, no conclusions can be drawn on causality. It is therefore both conceivable that the work setting may promote burnout, or that burned out individuals chose a certain work setting. The inconsistent findings across studies may be due to differing burnout-promoting and –preventing features of inpatient and outpatient work settings depending on the location and the respective health system.

Among a sample of French physicians, low quality of teamwork was associated with burnout and highly associated with intentions to leave the medical profession [19]. Likewise, in multivariate analysis, higher satisfaction with the aspects "work environment" (including the elements relationship with superiors, relationship and professional exchange with colleagues) and "humaneness" (including relationship with non-medical staff, relationship with patients) were associated with a lower chance for burnout on all subscales. The component "work environment" also comprised the element "intellectual stimulation at work". Consistently, in a sample of Swiss physicians, lower exposure to continuing education was associated with a higher risk for *depersonalization* [31].

Long-term studies are needed to define predictors of burnout instead of mere associations. It is conceivable that burnout may prevent good teamwork and prevent from perceiving the work environment as intellectually stimulating. However, it would make even more sense if good teamwork and an intellectually stimulating

Table 5 Variables associated with a high degree of burnout on the subscales *emotional exhaustion, depersonalization* and *personal accomplishment*

	Emotional exhaustion			Depersonalization			Personal accomplishment		
Independent variable	OR [SE]	CI 95 %	*p*	OR [SE]	CI 95 %	*p*	OR [SE]	CI 95 %	*p*
Female sex	1.21 [0.17]	0.92–1.59	0.165	0.48 [0.06]	0.38–0.60	<0.001	1.06 [0.14]	0.82–1.37	0.642
Age	1.01 [0.03]	0.95–1.08	0.730	0.95 [0.03]	0.90–1.01	0.079	1.02 [0.03]	0.96–1.08	0.608
In a relationship	0.89 [0.16]	0.63–1.26	0.507	0.98 [0.15]	0.72–1.32	0.871	0.82 [0.13]	0.59–1.13	0.218
Having children	0.83 [0.13]	0.62–1.13	0.240	1.09 [0.14]	0.84–1.41	0.511	1.11 [0.16]	0.84–1.47	0.474
German citizenship	0.67 [0.14]	0.44–1.02	0.060	0.69 [0.13]	0.48–1.01	0.056	0.67 [0.13]	0.45–0.98	0.041
Clinical work experience	0.99 [0.04]	0.92–1.07	0.786	1.02 [0.03]	0.95–1.08	0.600	0.96 [0.03]	0.90–1.03	0.271
Specialist qualification	0.77 [0.16]	0.51–1.16	0.214	0.85 [0.15]	0.60–1.20	0.356	1.27 [0.24]	0.87–1.85	0.214
Would become a physician again	0.55 [0.08]	0.42–0.72	<0.001	0.77 [0.10]	0.60–0.98	0.036	0.50 [0.06]	0.39–0.65	<0.001
Full-time employment	1.16 [0.23]	0.79–1.72	0.452	0.87 [0.14]	0.63–1.20	0.400	1.16 [0.21]	0.82–1.65	0.405
Urban setting	0.88 [0.13]	0.66–1.18	0.410	1.21 [0.16]	0.94–1.56	0.133	0.94 [0.13]	0.71–1.23	0.640
Inpatient setting	0.65 [0.13]	0.43–0.96	0.031	0.88 [0.14]	0.64–1.22	0.446	1.27 [0.24]	0.88–1.84	0.204
Leading position/own practice	1.35 [0.31]	0.87–2.11	0.180	1.29 [0.25]	0.89–1.88	0.181	0.55 [0.12]	0.36–0.85	0.008
Satisfaction with									
- work environment	0.54 [0.06]	0.43–0.67	<0.001	0.75 [0.07]	0.61 – 0.90	0.003	0.71 [0.07]	0.58–0.87	0.001
- work load	0.30 [0.03]	0.25–0.37	<0.001	0.79 [0.06]	0.68–0.91	0.002	0.97 [0.08]	0.82–1.14	0.712
- patient care	0.92 [0.10]	0.75–1.12	0.402	0.76 [0.07]	0.63 – 0.91	0.002	0.58 [0.06]	0.48–0.70	<0.001
- structural aspects	1.10 [0.11]	0.91–1.33	0.339	1.05 [0.09]	0.89–1.24	0.564	0.95 [0.09]	0.80–1.14	0.584
- humaneness	0.79 [0.09]	0.63–0.99	0.043	0.54 [0.06]	0.44–0.67	<0.001	0.52 [0.06]	0.42–0.65	<0.001

Multivariate logistic regression analysis was performed to determine variables associated with a high degree of burnout on the subscales *emotional exhaustion* ($R^2 = 0.2223$), *depersonalization* ($R^2 = 0.0955$) and *personal accomplishment* ($R^2 = 0.1324$). Analysis was performed with the data of 1656 participants. OR = odds ratio; SE = standard error, CI 95 % = 95 % confidence interval

Table 6 Association between burnout symptoms and physicians' wishes to leave

	Wish to go abroad for clinical work			Wish to leave clinical practice		
Independent variables	OR [SE]	CI 95 %	*p*	OR [SE]	CI 95 %	*p*
Female sex	0.70 [0.08]	0.56 – 0.87	0.002	1.09 [0.14]	0.84 – 1.42	0.500
Age	1.02 [0.02]	0.99 – 1.05	0.172	1.00 [0.02]	0.97 – 1.04	0.858
In a relationship	0.71 [0.10]	0.53 – 0.95	0.019	1.14 [0.20]	0.80 – 1.62	0.462
Having children	0.44 [0.06]	0.34 – 0.57	<0.001	1.21 [0.18]	0.90 – 1.61	0.200
Score *emotional exhaustion*	1.03 [0.01]	1.01 – 1.04	<0.001	1.09 [0.01]	1.07 – 1.10	<0.001
Score *depersonalization*	1.02 [0.01]	1.00 – 1.04	0.036	1.01 [0.01]	0.98 – 1.03	0.512
Score *personal accomplishment*	1.00 [0.01]	0.98 – 1.01	0.759	0.96 [0.01]	0.94 – 0.98	<0.001

Multivariate logistic regression analysis was performed to determine variables associated with the wish to go abroad for clinical work ($R^2 = 0.0614$) and the wish to leave clinical practice ($R^2 = 0.1307$). Analysis was performed with the data of 1748 and 1757 participants, respectively. OR = odds ratio; SE = standard error; CI 95 % = 95 % confidence interval

work environment contributed to mental well-being, reduced work-related stress, and also to the prevention of burnout. Moreover, quality of teamwork and training *can* be addressed and improved by specific measures in an effort to improve the work environment and to prevent burnout – in contrast to the work setting, as in- and outpatient settings most likely will always be needed in a health care system.

While neither being in a relationship nor having children were associated with a high degree of burnout, higher satisfaction with the factor "work load" (comprising the elements time for family, friends and leisure activities, stress level at work) was associated with a lower chance for high *emotional exhaustion* and *depersonalization.* In the context of this study, qualitative aspects related to private life seem to be more important than quantitative facts. German hospital physicians exhibit a higher degree of "work interfering with family" conflicts when compared to the general public [32]. Work-family conflict has been identified as an important risk factor for burnout among physician populations in Germany [32, 33]. These data support study results from the USA and France revealing an association between work-life conflicts and burnout [19, 34]. A previous analysis among the same physician population revealed that difficulties in reconciling work and private life were an important reason for wishing to leave clinical practice [22]. These data confirm an earlier study among German physicians where a higher degree of "work interfering with family" conflict was positively correlated with intentions to quit the job [32].

There is an ongoing discussion in Germany about whether physicians may leave clinical practice or go abroad for clinical work [20–23]. Therefore, we investigated whether burnout may be associated with wishing to leave clinical practice or to go abroad for clinical work. In the setting of this study, higher symptoms of burnout were indeed associated with wishing to leave: Interestingly, higher *emotional exhaustion* and lower *personal accomplishment* were associated with the wish to leave clinical practice. Higher *emotional exhaustion* and higher *depersonalization* were associated with the wish to go abroad for clinical work.

Emotional exhaustion, the core symptom of burnout, was associated with both the wish to leave clinical practice and the wish to go abroad for clinical work. We can only speculate why, in the setting of this study, lower *personal accomplishment* was associated with the wish to leave clinical practice but higher *depersonalization* with the wish to go abroad. Perhaps participants scoring low on *personal accomplishment* rather focus on professional success and hope for better achievements by changing the occupational field. In contrast, participants scoring high on *depersonalization* may consider a change of health care systems to allow for more, or less, contact with patients, with the additional benefit of the adventure of going abroad. To elucidate this, further research would be warranted on burned out physicians' expectations associated with leaving clinical practice or going abroad.

It should be taken into account that also factors not measured in the context of this study may contribute to the development of wishing to leave, such as available career opportunities, financial investments, etc. In the setting of this study, female sex, being in a relationship and having children were associated with a lower chance of wishing to go abroad. Participants with a partner and/or children may be more rooted in their current living situation in Germany and not consider moving abroad attractive due to the difficulties of finding a job for the partner and day care or school for the children.

The present results are consistent with a recent study among French physicians in which burnout increased the risk for intentions to leave the medical profession [19]. Similarly, studies among physicians in Spain and in China revealed that burnout might be associated with job turnover intentions (thoughts of leaving, looking for new jobs within a year, willing to accept other better job opportunities) [17, 18]. To the best of our knowledge, our study is the first revealing an association between symptoms of burnout and physicians' wishing to leave the country and work abroad in clinical care.

These findings raise the question of how to prevent or to reduce burnout among physicians. Two recent randomized controlled trials from Spain and the USA indicate that mindfulness-based interventions in a group setting may decrease physician burnout at the individual level [35, 36]. These data are backed by a meta-analysis including randomized controlled trials and pre-post studies among physicians in Spain, Argentina, Norway, and the USA [37]. The authors conclude that "cognitive-, behavioral-, and mindfulness-based approaches" may be useful tools in decreasing physician burnout [37]. Reports on organizational approaches are scarce. A hospital in the USA attempted a "culture change" by switching the focus from physician burnout to physician wellness [38]. Measures included team building, creating a supportive work environment, and regular self-assessments with the MBI, along with providing sources of help [38]. Also in the USA, a primary care group rated physician well-being as important as quality of care [39]. The intervention targeted "influence over work environment", efficiency, and "satisfaction with clinical and human aspects of patient care" [39]. During the study period, physicians' *emotional exhaustion* decreased significantly [39].

It remains to be evaluated whether similar approaches may be effective in reducing or preventing burnout among physician populations in Germany. A recent systematic review by Seidler et al. points out that multidimensional approaches are needed as burnout is most likely multifactorial, and which work related factors are perceived as strain depends on the individual [40].

Preventing or reducing symptoms of burnout among physicians will not only improve individual health and decrease personal suffering. It may also be beneficial for the health care system as a whole in terms of lower costs, e.g. by avoiding costly treatment of burned-out physicians as well as avoiding early physician retirement and decreased physician productivity due to burnout [15, 16]. Preventing or reducing symptoms of burnout among physicians may also lead to better quality of care [14]. Importantly, preventing or reducing burnout may potentially also prevent physicians from leaving the (German) health care system.

Limitations

Although we investigated a large sample of physicians, the results cannot be generalized to the population of physicians in Saxony: The sample is younger than the population and the proportion of women is larger in the sample. Due to the anonymised nature of the survey, non-responders could not be followed up and reasons for non-participation could not be elucidated. It is possible that only those participants who felt that the topics applied to them, and might exhibit higher symptoms of burnout, responded. Thus, prevalence of burnout would be overestimated. However, it is also conceivable that those physicians with higher burnout symptoms did not respond to the survey, which would lead to an underestimation of the prevalence of burnout. Importantly, participants could not be followed up and therefore it is not possible to trace whether wishes to leave were actually put into practice. Among family practitioners in England, intention to leave predicted actually leaving [41]. Among US physicians not all physicians put their intentions to leave into practice [42]. However, the percentage of physicians who actually left was higher among those who had intentions to quit clinical practice than those who did not have these intentions [42]. Thus, also for the sample of the present study, it is likely that at least some of the physicians wishing to leave will put these wishes into practice.

The study was a cross sectional study and no conclusions regarding causality can be drawn.

Conclusions

The sample of physicians in the present study was not more burdened by burnout than previous physician samples. Still, the extent of burnout among these young physicians in Saxony is of concern. Higher satisfaction with the components "work environment" and "humaneness" were associated with a lower chance for burnout on all subscales. This may be a starting point for developing measures to reduce or prevent burnout in this study population. Several recent studies suggest that interventions on the individual or organizational level may improve symptoms of burnout among physicians. Future projects should concentrate on adapting preventive measures to the reality of physicians in Germany.

Furthermore, higher *emotional exhaustion* was associated with a higher probability for wishing to leave clinical practice or to go abroad for clinical work. While the link between burnout and intentions to quit the job or the profession has been established in previous studies, to the best of our knowledge, this is the first study to investigate the association between burnout and the wish to leave the country and practice medicine abroad. Future studies are warranted to evaluate burned out physicians' expectations associated with leaving clinical practice or going abroad for clinical work.

Preventing or reducing burnout among physicians will not only improve individual health and decrease personal suffering. Importantly, preventing or reducing burnout may potentially also prevent the German health care system from losing physicians.

Competing interests
The authors declare that they have no competing interests.

Authors' contributions
BP participated in study design, acquired and analysed the data, and drafted the manuscript. ML participated in study design, helped to analyse the data and draft the manuscript, and revised the manuscript critically for important intellectual content. HHK participated in data analysis and revised the manuscript critically for important intellectual content. SRH conceived of the study, participated in study design and revised the manuscript critically for important intellectual content. All authors contributed to data interpretation. All authors read and approved the final manuscript.

Acknowledgements
We thank the State Chamber of Physicians of Saxony, especially the president Prof. Dr. Schulze, for their support in conducting the study. We are also grateful to the AOK Bundesverband for financing the study.

Author details
[1]Institute of Social Medicine, Occupational Health and Public Health, University of Leipzig, Philipp-Rosenthal-Str. 55, 04103 Leipzig, Germany. [2]Department of Health Economics and Health Services Research, University Medical Center Hamburg-Eppendorf, Martinistr. 52, 20246 Hamburg, Germany.

References
1. Angermeyer MC, Schomerus G, Carta MG, Moro MF, Toumi M, Millier A, et al. Burnout: a German phenomenon? Psychiatr Prax. 2013;40:425–9. doi:10.1055/s-0033-1343199.
2. Maske UE, Riedel-Heller SG, Seiffert I, Jacobi F, Hapke U. Prevalence and Comorbidity of Self-Reported Diagnosis of Burnout Syndrome in the General Population. Psychiatr Prax. 2014. doi:10.1055/s-0034-1387201.
3. Bundespsychotherapeutenkammer. BPtK-Studie zur Arbeitsunfähigkeit - Psychische Erkrankungen und Burnout. 2012. http://www.bptk.de/fileadmin/user_upload/Publikationen/BPtK-Studien/Arbeitsunf%C3%A4higkeit_aufgrund_psychischer_Belastungen/20120606_BPtK-Studie_Arbeitsunfaehigkeit_2012.pdf. Accessed 13 Apr 2015.
4. Shanafelt TD, Boone S, Tan L, Dyrbye LN, Sotile W, Satele D, et al. Burnout and satisfaction with work-life balance among US physicians relative to the general US population. Arch Intern Med. 2012;172:1377–85. doi:10.1001/archinternmed.2012.3199.
5. Soler JK, Yaman H, Esteva M, Dobbs F, Asenova RS, Katic M, et al. Burnout in European family doctors: the EGPRN study. Fam Pract. 2008;25:245–65. doi:10.1093/fampra/cmn038.
6. Maslach C, Jackson SE, Leiter MP. Maslach Burnout Inventory Manual. Third edition 1996.
7. Klein J, Grosse Frie K, Blum K, von dem Knesebeck O. Burnout and perceived quality of care among German clinicians in surgery. Int J Qual Health Care. 2010;22:525–30. doi:10.1093/intqhc/mzq056.
8. Heinke W, Dunkel P, Brähler E, Nübling M, Riedel-Heller S, Kaisers UX. Burnout in anesthesiology and intensive care: is there a problem in Germany? Anaesthesist. 2011;60:1109–18. doi:10.1007/s00101-011-1947-3.
9. Böhle A, Baumgärtel M, Götz ML, Müller EH, Jocham D. Burn-out of urologists in the county of Schleswig-Holstein, Germany: a comparison of hospital and private practice urologists. J Urol. 2001;165:1158–61.
10. Pajonk FB, Cransac P, Müller V, Teichmann A, Meyer W. Trauma and stress-related disorders in German emergency physicians: the predictive role of personality factors. Int J Emerg Ment Health. 2012;14:257–68.
11. Voltmer E, Schwappach DLB, Frank E, Wirsching M, Spahn C. Work-related behavior and experience patterns and predictors of mental health in German physicians in medical practice. Fam Med. 2010;42:433–9.
12. Richter A, Kostova P, Baur X, Wegner R. Less work: more burnout? A comparison of working conditions and the risk of burnout by German physicians before and after the implementation of the EU Working Time Directive. Int Arch Occup Environ Health. 2014;87:205–15. doi:10.1007/s00420-013-0849-x.
13. Shanafelt TD, Sloan JA, Habermann TM. The well-being of physicians. Am J Med. 2003;114:513–9.
14. Shirom A, Nirel N, Vinokur AD. Overload, autonomy, and burnout as predictors of physicians' quality of care. J Occup Health Psychol. 2006;11:328–42. doi:10.1037/1076-8998.11.4.328.
15. Dewa CS, Loong D, Bonato S, Thanh NX, Jacobs P. How does burnout affect physician productivity? A systematic literature review. BMC Health Serv Res. 2014;14:325. doi:10.1186/1472-6963-14-325.
16. Dewa CS, Jacobs P, Thanh NX, Loong D. An estimate of the cost of burnout on early retirement and reduction in clinical hours of practicing physicians in Canada. BMC Health Serv Res. 2014;14:254. doi:10.1186/1472-6963-14-254.
17. Moreno-Jiménez B, Gálvez-Herrer M, Rodríguez-Carvajal R, Sanz Vergel AI. A study of physicians' intention to quit: the role of burnout, commitment and difficult doctor-patient interactions. Psicothema. 2012;24:263–70.
18. Zhang Y, Feng X. The relationship between job satisfaction, burnout, and turnover intention among physicians from urban state-owned medical institutions in Hubei, China: a cross-sectional study. BMC Health Serv Res. 2011;11:235. doi:10.1186/1472-6963-11-235.
19. Estryn-Behar M, Fry C, Guetarni K, Aune I, Machet G, Doppia MA, et al. Work week duration, work-family balance and difficulties encountered by female and male physicians: results from the French SESMAT study. Work. 2011;40 Suppl 1:S83–100. doi:10.3233/WOR-2011-1270.
20. Köhler S, Kaiser R. Junge Ärzte – Ausstieg aus der Patientenversorgung? Hessisches Ärzteblatt. 2003;9:462–4.
21. Kopetsch T. Dem deutschen Gesundheitswesen gehen die Ärzte aus! - Studie zur Altersstruktur- und Arztzahlentwicklung. 2010. http://www.kbv.de/media/sp/Arztzahlstudie_2010.pdf. Accessed 13 Apr 2015.
22. Pantenburg B, Luppa M, König H, Riedel-Heller SG. Young physicians' thoughts about leaving patient care–results of a survey in Saxony, Germany. Gesundheitswesen. 2014;76:406–12. doi:10.1055/s-0034-1381986.
23. Ramboll Management. Gutachten zum Ausstieg aus der kurativen ärztlichen Berufstätigkeit in Deutschland. 2004. http://www.bundesgesundheitsministerium.de/fileadmin/dateien/Publikationen/Gesundheit/Sonstiges/Abschlussbericht_Gutachten_zum_Ausstieg_aus_der_kurativen_aerztlichen_Berufstaetigkeit_in_Deutschland.pdf. Accessed 13 Apr 2015.
24. Gesellschaft für Forschung und Beratung im Gesundheits- und Sozialbereich im Auftrag des Sächsischen Staatsministeriums für Soziales. Studie zur Erfassung, Analyse und Auswertung von Daten über nicht ärztlich tätige Ärztinnen und Ärzte im Freistaat Sachsen unter Gender Mainstreaming Gesichtspunkten mit dem Ziel der Erarbeitung von (Wieder-) Einstiegsprogrammen für diese Ärztinnen und Ärzte. 2006. http://www.soziales.sachsen.de/download/gleichstellung/Abschlussbericht_Aerzte_Sachsen_27_10_06_mit_Lesezeichen_pdf.pdf. Accessed 13 Apr 2015.
25. Günther OH, Kürstein B, Riedel-Heller SG, König H. The role of monetary and nonmonetary incentives on the choice of practice establishment: a stated preference study of young physicians in Germany. Health Serv Res. 2010;45:212–29. doi:10.1111/j.1475-6773.2009.01045.x.
26. Bovier PA, Perneger TV. Predictors of work satisfaction among physicians. Eur J Public Health. 2003;13:299–305.
27. Janus K, Amelung VE, Gaitanides M, Schwartz FW. German physicians "on strike"–shedding light on the roots of physician dissatisfaction. Health Policy. 2007;82:357–65. doi:10.1016/j.healthpol.2006.11.003.
28. Purvanova RK, Muros JP. Gender differences in burnout: A meta-analysis. J Vocat Behav. 2010;77:168–85. doi:10.1016/j.jvb.2010.04.006.
29. Roberts DL, Cannon KJ, Wellik KE, Wu Q, Budavari AI. Burnout in inpatient-based versus outpatient-based physicians: a systematic review and meta-analysis. J Hosp Med. 2013;8:653–64. doi:10.1002/jhm.2093.
30. Roberts DL, Shanafelt TD, Dyrbye LN, West CP. A national comparison of burnout and work-life balance among internal medicine hospitalists and outpatient general internists. J Hosp Med. 2014;9:176–81. doi:10.1002/jhm.2146.
31. Arigoni F, Bovier PA, Mermillod B, Waltz P, Sappino A. Prevalence of burnout among Swiss cancer clinicians, paediatricians and general practitioners: who are most at risk? Support Care Cancer. 2009;17:75–81. doi:10.1007/s00520-008-0465-6.
32. Fuss I, Nübling M, Hasselhorn H, Schwappach D, Rieger MA. Working conditions and Work-Family Conflict in German hospital physicians: psychosocial and organisational predictors and consequences. BMC Public Health. 2008;8:353. doi:10.1186/1471-2458-8-353.
33. Nitzsche A, Driller E, Kowalski C, Ansmann L, Pfaff H. The conflict between work and private life and its relationship with burnout - results of a physician survey in breast cancer centers in North Rhine-Westphalia. Gesundheitswesen. 2013;75:301–6. doi:10.1055/s-0033-1337996.

34. Dyrbye LN, Sotile W, Boone S, West CP, Tan L, Satele D, et al. A survey of U. S. physicians and their partners regarding the impact of work-home conflict. J Gen Intern Med. 2014;29:155–61. doi:10.1007/s11606-013-2581-3.
35. Asuero AM, Queraltó JM, Pujol-Ribera E, Berenguera A, Rodriguez-Blanco T, Epstein RM. Effectiveness of a mindfulness education program in primary health care professionals: a pragmatic controlled trial. J Contin Educ Health Prof. 2014;34:4–12. doi:10.1002/chp.21211.
36. West CP, Dyrbye LN, Rabatin JT, Call TG, Davidson JH, Multari A, et al. Intervention to promote physician well-being, job satisfaction, and professionalism: a randomized clinical trial. JAMA Intern Med. 2014;174:527–33. doi:10.1001/jamainternmed.2013.14387.
37. Regehr C, Glancy D, Pitts A, LeBlanc VR. Interventions to reduce the consequences of stress in physicians: a review and meta-analysis. J Nerv Ment Dis. 2014;202:353–9. doi:10.1097/NMD.0000000000000130.
38. Eckleberry-Hunt J, van Dyke A, Lick D, Tucciarone J. Changing the Conversation From Burnout to Wellness: Physician Well-being in Residency Training Programs. J Grad Med Educ. 2009;1:225–30. doi:10.4300/JGME-D-09-00026.1.
39. Dunn PM, Arnetz BB, Christensen JF, Homer L. Meeting the imperative to improve physician well-being: assessment of an innovative program. J Gen Intern Med. 2007;22:1544–52. doi:10.1007/s11606-007-0363-5.
40. Seidler A, Thinschmidt M, Deckert S, Then F, Hegewald J, Nieuwenhuijsen K, et al. The role of psychosocial working conditions on burnout and its core component emotional exhaustion - a systematic review. J Occup Med Toxicol. 2014;9:10. doi:10.1186/1745-6673-9-10.
41. Hann M, Reeves D, Sibbald B. Relationships between job satisfaction, intentions to leave family practice and actually leaving among family physicians in England. Eur J Public Health. 2011;21:499–503. doi:10.1093/eurpub/ckq005.
42. Rittenhouse DR, Mertz E, Keane D, Grumbach K. No exit: an evaluation of measures of physician attrition. Health Serv Res. 2004;39:1571–88.

12

"It's still a great adventure" – exploring offshore employees' working conditions in a qualitative study

Janika Mette*, Marcial Velasco Garrido, Volker Harth, Alexandra M. Preisser and Stefanie Mache

Abstract

Background: Despite the particular demands inherent to offshore work, little is known about the working conditions of employees in the German offshore wind industry. To date, neither offshore employees' job demands and resources, nor their needs for improving the working conditions have been explored. Therefore, the aim of this study was to conduct a qualitative analysis to gain further insight into these topics.

Methods: Forty-two semi-structured telephone interviews with German offshore employees ($n = 21$) and offshore experts ($n = 21$) were conducted. Employees and experts were interviewed with regard to their perceptions of their working conditions offshore. In addition, employees were asked to identify areas with potential need for improvement. The interviews were analysed in a deductive-inductive process according to Mayring's qualitative content analysis.

Results: Employees and experts reported various demands of offshore work, including challenging physical labour, long shifts, inactive waiting times, and recurrent absences from home. In contrast, the high personal meaning of the work, regular work schedule (14 days offshore, 14 days onshore), and strong comradeship were highlighted as job resources. Interviewees' working conditions varied considerably, e.g. regarding their work tasks and accommodations. Most of the job demands were perceived in terms of the work organization and living conditions offshore. Likewise, employees expressed the majority of needs for improvement in these areas.

Conclusions: Our study offers important insight into the working conditions of employees in the German offshore wind industry. The results can provide a basis for further quantitative research in order to generalize the findings. Moreover, they can be utilized to develop needs-based interventions to improve the working conditions offshore.

Keywords: Offshore wind industry, Working conditions, Job demands, Job resources, Qualitative analysis

Background

Offshore wind is a relatively new technology that has become competitive with other forms of energy in Europe [1]. Among European countries, Germany is considered one of the pioneers in the offshore wind energy sector. In recent years, the German offshore wind industry has increased rapidly [2], leading to a substantial growth in employment figures. In 2015, approximately 20,500 persons worked in the German offshore wind industry [3]. According to rough estimates, the number of direct and indirect workers in this sector is expected to increase to 33,000 by 2021 [4].

* Correspondence: j.mette@uke.de
Institute for Occupational and Maritime Medicine, University Medical Centre Hamburg-Eppendorf, Hamburg, Seewartenstr. 10, 20459 Hamburg, Germany

Working conditions offshore

It has been described that working in the German offshore wind industry places high demands on its employees, in terms of personal, technical, and safety-related qualifications [5, 6]. Offshore employees in Germany perform their work in the hazardous work environment of the high seas. Their work schedule generally consists of 2 weeks offshore work, followed by 2 weeks free time onshore (i.e. 14/14-work schedule). During their offshore assignments, employees typically work for 12 hours a day [7–11]. They must often perform their tasks under time pressure [9] and are exposed to unfavourable weather conditions that might pose risks to themselves and cause work delays or interruptions [7, 8, 10]. Working at heights or on the deck of the platforms often places the workers in physically demanding and potentially dangerous situations [6, 7, 10]. Furthermore, the workers' transportation from the platforms to the offshore wind farms has been described as challenging [8, 10], and the remote location of the wind parks represents an obstacle in case of emergencies [7, 9, 10]. Depending on the type of offshore environment, employees must work in confined spaces, share double cabins, and may experience limited privacy [7–9, 11]. Moreover, they might be subjected to a restricted social environment and must deal with recurrent periods of absence from home [7, 9, 11].

Despite these considerations for German offshore workers being outlined in single reports and statements, empirical data on the topic is still missing. To our knowledge, no empirical research studies have been carried out that systematically examine the working conditions of employees in the growing German offshore wind branch. However, closing this research gap and gaining a deeper understanding of their perceived work situation is highly relevant, especially since offshore work has been described as particularly challenging and stressful [12, 13].

Research studies from related branches, e.g. the international wind industry, offshore oil and gas industry, and seafaring branch [7, 14], have also revealed high job demands for their workers, including high quantitative demands [15, 16], perceived risks at work [17], harsh environmental conditions [18], and long absences from home [17, 19–22]. Nonetheless, transferring the findings from these industries to the German offshore wind branch is not permissible; despite sharing certain similarities, there remain distinctive differences between the industries, e.g. regarding the workflows, rules and regulations [7]. This makes an in-depth investigation of the working conditions in the German offshore wind branch necessary. Due to the lack of available data, a qualitative research approach was chosen to gain first explorative insights into the topic.

Theoretical background

When exploring offshore employees' working conditions, the Job Demands-Resources model [JD-R model] by Demerouti and Bakker [23, 24] provides an adequate theoretical framework. The JD-R model was introduced as a further development to other relevant models, such as the Job Demands-Control model [25] and the Effort-Reward-Imbalance model [26]. It incorporates a broad range of working conditions for which it describes two key categories: job demands (aspects of the job that require physical or mental effort and are associated with certain physiological and psychological costs) and job resources (aspects of the job that may assist in achieving work goals, reduce job demands and the associated costs, and stimulate personal growth) [23, 24].

Study aims

The aim of our study was to conduct a qualitative analysis to gain further insight into offshore employees' perceived working conditions, and to identify both hindering and conducive factors of offshore work from their perspective. Furthermore, we intended to compare and contrast the perceptions of offshore employees and experts, and to investigate offshore employees' needs for improvement regarding their work. We addressed the following research questions:

1. *What are offshore employees' and experts' perceptions of demands and resources of offshore work?*
2. *What are offshore employees' specific needs for improvement regarding their working conditions?*

Methods

Participants

Data were gathered through 42 semi-structured telephone interviews with offshore workers ($n = 21$) and offshore experts ($n = 21$) during July and August 2016. The qualitative interview approach was chosen as it seemed most suitable to acquire initial knowledge on the topic. Due to practicability and logistical issues, all interviews were conducted via telephone. To be eligible, both offshore workers and experts had to be over the age of 18 and had to be fluent in German. Furthermore, the offshore employees had to work in a regular 14/14-work schedule. The sample of offshore experts was restricted to persons with professional expertise, work experience, and managerial responsibility (e.g. health and safety specialists, occupational physicians, offshore managers, and managers of offshore service providers). Participation in the study was on a voluntary basis. For announcing the interview study, invitation emails were sent and leaflets were distributed to human resources departments and company physicians of offshore wind energy operators via mail, asking them to promote the interview study and recruit suitable participants. Additionally, we presented the study in health and safety trainings for offshore workers, encouraging the workers to participate in the study and to inform their colleagues and supervisors. Prior to the interviews, a written informed consent was sent to and signed by all participants. The telephone interviews were carried out by the first author who had prior experiences with conducting qualitative interviews. A pre-test interview was performed, and feedback to the interviewer was provided by supervisors and fellow members. Interview length ranged from 24 min (expert) to 1 hour (employee). All interviews were conducted in German and were tape recorded.

Interview guideline

The interviews were conducted using two slightly varying versions of a semi-structured interview guideline (one for the employees and one for the experts). The guideline was developed in accordance with the research questions and was based on the theoretical framework (JD-R model [23, 24]). The interview topic list is depicted in Table 1 in the order in which the topics are presented in the guideline. Different questions regarding employees' and experts' perceptions of their working conditions and employees' needs for improvement were integrated. The interview guideline was piloted with the help of an offshore worker and minor revisions were made based on the worker's recommendations.

Analysis

Audio recordings from the interviews were transcribed and anonymized. The transcripts were analysed by the first author in a deductive-inductive process according to Mayring's qualitative content analysis, using the software MAXQDA Analytics Pro (version 12, VERBI GmbH, 2016). Different codes, categories, and sub-categories were systematically identified and refined in an iterative process to fit the data. The results were discussed thoroughly in several meetings with all co-authors. Precisely, discrepancies were reviewed and differences were resolved by in-depth discussions until consensus was reached. Reflexivity (e.g. regarding the researchers' personal values, objectives and preconceptions, and how they might affect the research) was enhanced at every step of the research process. For the purpose of publication, interviewees' quotes were translated into English with the support of an English native speaker.

Results

Participants

Of the 21 offshore employees we interviewed, 19 (90.5%) were male and 2 (9.5%) were female (Table 2). With respect to the offshore experts, 17 (81.0%) were male and 4 (19.0%) were female. Employees' average experience in the offshore wind industry was 3.4 years (range 7 months – 8 years), whereas experts' average experience was 5.1 years (range 6 months – 10 years). 10 (47.6%) employees and 17 (81.0%) experts had at least 3 years of offshore experience. Almost one third (28.6%) of the employees were technicians. 11 (52.4%) experts worked as health and safety managers and 4 (19.0%) as occupational physicians. 11 (52.4%) employees were aged between 31 and 40 years. 18 (85.7%) employees were in a relationship.

Table 1 Interview topic list

Introduction	study information, confidentiality, informed consent
Socio-demographics	offshore occupation, offshore experience in years
	employees: age, relationship status
Working conditions	job demands *(example question: "When you think about your offshore work, what are particular [physical / psychological] demands of your work?")*
	job resources *(example question: "When you think about your offshore work, what do you particularly like about your work?")*
	employees: needs for improvement *(example question: "In general, what needs for improvement do you see regarding your working conditions offshore?")*

Table 2 Participant characteristics (*n* = 42)

Variable	Employees (*n* = 21)		Experts (*n* = 21)	
	n	%	*n*	%
Gender				
male	19	90.5	17	81.0
female	2	9.5	4	19.0
Offshore experience				
< 1 years	2	9.5	3	14.3
1 – 2 years	9	42.9	1	4.8
3 – 4 years	5	23.8	7	33.3
> 4 years	5	23.8	10	47.6
	Mean: 3.4 years Range: 7 months – 8 years		Mean: 5.1 years Range: 6 months – 10 years	
Occupation				
technician	6	28.6	–	–
quality and maintenance	5	23.8	–	–
paramedic	3	14.3	–	–
health and safety	3	14.3	11	52.4
management offshore	4	19.0	3	14.3
occupational physician	–	–	4	19.0
managing director of offshore service providers	–	–	3	14.3
Age				
20 – 30 years	5	23.8	n.a.	n.a.
31– 40 years	11	52.4	n.a.	n.a.
41– 50 years	4	19.0	n.a.	n.a.
> 50 years	1	4.8	n.a.	n.a.
Relationship status				
relationship	18	85.7	n.a.	n.a.
single	3	14.3	n.a.	n.a.

Offshore employees' working conditions

The job demands and resources that emerged from the interviews can be summarized into the five main categories depicted in Fig. 1.

In addition to the main categories, we identified various associated sub-categories. All main categories and their

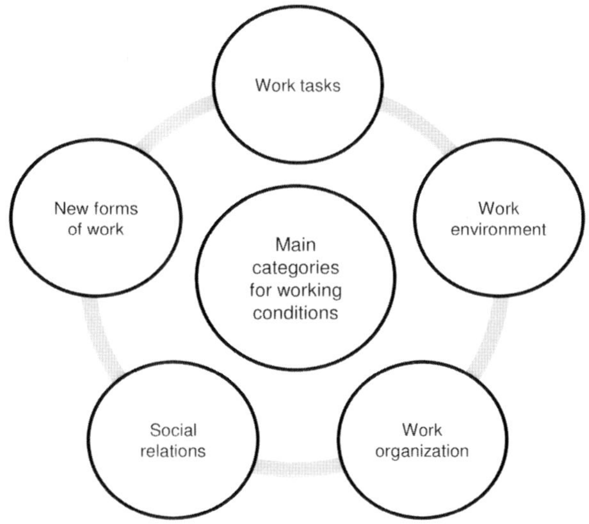

Fig. 1 Main categories for offshore employees' working conditions

related sub-categories are depicted in tables and elaborated below. In particular, central aspects are further expanded upon in the next paragraphs. A table with all main and sub-categories can be found in the Additional file 1.

Category 1: Work tasks

All job demands and resources named in terms of the category 'work tasks' are depicted in Table 3.

Table 3 Job demands and resources in terms of the work tasks

Main category: Work tasks	
Job demands	
physical work	hard physical work
transfer and access to installations	physically and psychologically challenging
accident risks	e.g. danger of falling or slipping
workloads	intermittent periods of high workloads
demanding work tasks	demanding work tasks that require high concentration
work equipment	heavy work tools and personal protective equipment
Job resources	
meaning of work	associations: adventure, freedom, fulfilment, pioneer spirit
perception of safety	high perception of safety, strict safety procedures
motivation and satisfaction	high work motivation and satisfaction
challenging work tasks	positively challenging work tasks
skills and competencies	work requires high skills and competencies
versatility of work	great versatility of the work
scope of action	wide scope of action at work

Job demands

Physical work

The physical work was considered demanding by all workers and experts:

> *"Generally, the work is very physically taxing." [employee, ID #17, age 31–40 years, offshore experience 1–2 years].*

According to the interviewees, climbing the installations was challenging, in particular when wearing survival suits and carrying heavy materials. Moreover, tasks involving the climbing of ladders, working at heights, or in forced postures on and inside the installations were regarded as physically demanding by both workers and experts:

> *"There is a huge physical component [that comes with the job], with climbing and working in awkward positions and at heights, etc." [expert, ID #4, offshore experience > 4 years].*

Transfer and access to installations

Transfer and access to the offshore installations were considered particularly demanding by the interviewees. Accessing the installations was perceived to be physically challenging:

> *"Skipping up a ladder in a survival suit is certainly not everyone's cup of tea." [expert, ID #3, offshore experience > 4 years].*

Beyond that, it was also seen as a psychological challenge, since unstable weather conditions could increase accident risks during the transfer and lead to mental stress and tenseness:

> *"In that kind of situation there is a definite feeling of tenseness." [employee, ID #2, age 31–40 years, offshore experience 3–4 years].*

Furthermore, some workers reported to feel a certain form of social pressure to access the installations despite situations of marginal weather conditions, as they reported that they didn't want to be regarded as the only ones expressing reservations to access the installations. Notably, the level of stress seemed to correspond with the workers' previous experiences working under such circumstances, the less-seasoned workers experiencing more difficulties. Besides, interviewees reported that rough weather during transfer to the installations could cause seasickness among the workers, thereby further complicating the task:

"The problem of seasickness became apparent. It's a very real problem, affecting many people." [expert, ID #14, offshore experience > 4 years].

Job resources

Meaning of work

For many offshore employees and experts, the job was reported to be of very high personal meaning. For instance, to many of the interviewees, working offshore meant adventure, challenge, and freedom:

"For me personally it's still a great adventure." [employee, ID #2, age 31–40 years, offshore experience 3–4 years].

In particular, the large-scale idea behind the offshore wind industry – the green energy revolution – contributed substantially to the sensation of performing meaningful work. Many of the interviewees further perceived offshore work as being something new and special. The pioneer spirit of the growing offshore branch was often emphasized:

"You're not just an electrician in a small company that does routine house calls, rather you're a pioneer – there are not many people who do this type of work." [expert, ID #8, offshore experience > 4 years].

Perception of safety

Employees and experts felt that safety had the highest priority for their work offshore. Most of the workers claimed to generally feel safe due to strict safety procedures and well-organized work processes. Employees reported feeling well prepared for emergencies and described the medical care offshore as being readily accessible. Furthermore, some of the workers highlighted that colleagues always kept an eye on each other:

"You are not only responsible for yourself, but also for your colleagues. And that is true in everything you do." [employee, ID #4, age 41–50 years, offshore experience > 4 years].

Motivation and satisfaction

Both work motivation and job satisfaction were reported as being high among the interviewees:

"They love their job out there. When they go to work and are assigned an exciting task, you can see the smiles light up their faces, they are really fired up for it." [employee, ID #8, age 31–40 years, offshore experience 1–2 years].

Category 2: Work organization

All job demands and resources named in terms of the category 'work organization' are depicted in Table 4.

Job demands

Work time

In general, offshore workers and experts described the daily 12-h shifts as lengthy and tedious. Interviewees stated that it was common to work a lot offshore:

"I am here [offshore] anyway, what else is there to do? I may as well work." [expert, ID #9, offshore experience 3–4 years].

Some workers described a certain loss of sense of time, stating that the hours spent offshore sometimes seemed to fade into the background; it was *"just normal that you always work" [employee, ID #7, age 20–30 years, offshore experience 1–2 years].* Working night shifts and on call was perceived as being strenuous. Some employees noted difficulties in completing their tasks within the 12-h shifts, e.g. due to work time being invested in daily

Table 4 Job demands and resources in terms of the work organization

Main category: Work organization	
Job demands	
work time	lengthy and tedious, overtime
time pressure	prevalent in specific work situations
waiting times, weather days	occurrence of waiting times, e.g. due to bad weather
workflow	occurrence of delays and modifications
cost pressure	high costs involved in offshore projects
work schedule	14 days offshore perceived as long
personnel	too few offshore personnel
communication on –/offshore	difficulties in the communication and information flow between colleagues onshore and offshore
experts only: emergency medical care	knowledge of limited treatment options and lengthy emergency routes
Job resources	
work time	still manageable in length
payment	attractive remuneration
waiting times, weather days	occasionally helpful for relaxation
workflow	well-structured and coordinated
work schedule	allows much free time onshore, suitable regularity
experts only: emergency medical care	readily accessible
experts only: medical check-ups	suitable regularity, important in its function

preparation, follow-up, or documentation. Working overtime was also described as demanding, being particularly prevalent among workers with planning and management responsibilities:

> *"I was told from the very beginning that, 'yes, having to work overtime is fairly common here' [at management level]." [employee, ID #12, age 20–30 years, offshore experience 1–2 years].*

Time pressure

Some of the interviewees mentioned time pressure as a job demand that especially appeared to arise during sudden weather changes or in emergency situations:

> *"When you start work and then get the message from the client that, 'bad weather is coming, we have to hurry, hurry, hurry' – that's a form of psychological stress." [employee, ID #18, age 31–40 years, offshore experience > 4 years].*

The feeling of time pressure seemed to depend on the project stage, being more pronounced in the construction phase of the wind parks, where a strict time schedule was specified.

Waiting times, weather days

Both employees and experts described waiting times offshore as burdensome. Although it was recognized that waiting times served the offshore workers' own safety, many of the employees perceived their occurrence as paternalistic. Waiting times in the form of so-called 'weather days' (days when work was impeded by bad weather) were described as particularly strenuous. Such days were accompanied by increased feelings of discontentment among the workers, even resulting in sensations of cabin fever:

> *"They want to work, not just hang around. It is almost unbearable! After a week stuck on a ship, you start to feel like a rat in a cage." [employee, ID #4, age 41–50 years, offshore experience > 4 years].*

Job resources

Work schedule

Although the 14/14-work schedule was regarded as demanding, it was also considered a substantial job resource. Employees expressed their satisfaction with being able to spend much free time onshore and in regular intervals throughout the year. To many of the employees, this fixed work schedule represented one of the main benefits of offshore work:

> *"That's an important factor for me, if not the most important factor. That I have a regular schedule and can say: OK, at that time, I'll be away, but afterwards, I'll be 100% at home." [employee, ID #15, age 41–50 years, offshore experience 1–2 years].*

Payment

Payment and related surcharges were described as main job resources and motives for working offshore:

> *"Financially, offshore work is always a good decision. If I'm being honest, I would have to say that that is the main reason why I do it." [employee, ID #5, age 31–40 years, offshore experience 1–2 years].*

Category 3: Work environment

All job demands and resources named in terms of the category 'work environment' are depicted in Table 5.

Job demands

Weather conditions

Both employees and experts highlighted the dependency on weather conditions as a relevant stressor of the offshore workplace. Seasonal complications (e.g. in the summer when temperatures were high, or in the winter when cold and rainy weather prevailed) were perceived as burdensome:

> *"The weather conditions out there are relatively extreme. When the sun is shining, it shines intensely; when the wind is blowing, it blows very hard." [expert, ID #16, offshore experience 3–4 years].*

According to the interviewees, unfavourable weather could result in work interruptions and delays of crew transfer, which could lead to negative feelings among the workers.

Table 5 Job demands and resources in terms of the work environment

Main category: Work environment	
Job demands	
weather conditions	dependency on the weather, bad weather causes work interruptions, delays and waiting times
workplace design	confined spaces on platforms and installations
physicochemical factors	e.g. noise, vibrations, conditioned air, artificial light, chlorinated water
Job resources	
weather conditions	good weather offshore

Job resources

Weather conditions

On a positive note, good weather was regarded as a job resource. Employees reported to appreciate being able to enjoy good conditions during their lunch breaks and free time offshore. They particularly highlighted the *"fresh air and magnificent sunrises and sunsets" [employee, ID #16, age 31–40 years, offshore experience > 4 years].*

Category 4: Social relations

All job demands and resources named in terms of the category 'social relations' are depicted in Table 6.

Job demands

Job demands regarding social relations were rarely described by the interviewees. For example, employees mentioned discussions with colleagues regarding work methods or differences in remuneration:

> *"There are disputes about the fact that people receive varying compensation for the same jobs. I mean, it's loudly discussed why someone else earns more money than I do for the same type of work." [employee, ID #16, age 31–40 years, offshore experience > 4 years].*

Job resources

Social support

Both offshore employees and experts described the social support from colleagues and executives as one of the greatest resources of offshore work. In particular, employees reported strong ties as well as a sense of comradeship within the group, and highlighted the fact that new friendships developed quickly when working offshore:

> *"It's a really great thing that, after 14 days, you have 55 good friends here, with whom you enjoy spending your time." [employee, ID #7, age 20–30 years, offshore experience 1–2 years].*

Table 6 Job demands and resources in terms of social relations

Main category: Social relations	
Job demands	
conflicts with colleagues	e.g. regarding work methods or differences in remuneration
international work environment	language barriers
Job resources	
social support	good comradeship and strong support from the team
international work environment	possibilities to improve language skills

Some of the interviewees pointed out that the offshore business in Germany was still a manageable, relatively small market. Thus, there is a good chance that offshore colleagues will meet again over time in different projects, which was regarded positively:

> *"We all keep saying, offshore is like a small village." [employee, ID #4, age 41–50 years, offshore experience > 4 years].*

International work environment

Some of the employees described meeting international colleagues and improving their language skills as positive side effects of working offshore:

> *"You meet so many new, interesting people from different countries." [employee, ID #5, age 31–40 years, offshore experience 1–2 years].*

Category 5: New forms of work

All job demands and resources named in terms of the category 'new forms of work' are depicted in Table 7.

Job demands

Absence from home

Most of the workers considered the intermittent absences from home as one of the main challenges of their job, and feelings of homesickness were expressed by some workers. Such feelings seemed to increase when communication with the families and partners onshore was limited:

Table 7 Job demands and resources in terms of new forms of work

Main category: New forms of work	
Job demands	
absence from home	absence from home, family, and friends
catering	too rich in calories, hearty, unhealthy
accommodation	confined spaces, cramped cabins, double cabins
opportunities for leisure activities and retreat	limited possibilities for sports, leisure activities, and retreat
means of communication	often location dependent or only partially available
Job resources	
free time at home	intensive time at home during free time onshore
catering	healthy food offers available
accommodation	sufficient in size
opportunities for leisure activities and retreat	various opportunities: exercising, watching movies, playing games, reading books, participating in social activities

"Generally, the men here are 'tough guys'. But when the telephone for calling home doesn't work, they are suddenly 12 years old again, get really homesick, and then they are useless." [employee, ID #8, age 31–40 years, offshore experience 1–2 years].

Offshore workers described that they found it particularly hard not being able to help their partners at home in their daily tasks. Missing pivotal moments in their children's development and missing out of events onshore was also described as being difficult. The struggle of dealing with *"two different everyday lives" [expert, ID #8, offshore experience > 4 years]* – one onshore and one offshore – was highlighted. The level of burden experienced appeared to depend on the workers' personality and their personal situations. Fathers, for example, reported to suffer more from the absences from home in comparison to non-fathers in a relationship and singles:

"It also depends on whether you're married or single. All these younger, single people have no problem working four weeks straight. Those of us who are married, however, wish they could have some more family time." [employee, ID #4, age 41–50 years, offshore experience > 4 years].

Catering

Catering offshore was regarded as extremely important by the interviewees for their well-being and work performance. However, some workers complained about certain aspects of the catering, e.g. that it was too rich in calories, too hearty, or consisted of too much meat:

"There is meat, and then meat, and then even more meat." [employee, ID #5, age 31–40 years, offshore experience 1–2 years].

Accommodation

Depending on the specific type of accommodation, some interviewees described to sleep in cramped, uncomfortable cabins, causing a feeling of discomfort. Especially those required to share a double cabin reported to experience a lack of privacy. Furthermore, a few employees stated that the boundary between work and leisure time sometimes seemed to blur due to the shared or overlapping spaces of their offshore workplaces and living accommodations. However, other workers reported to have eventually been able to adjust to the particularity of working and living at the same place:

"It's just how it is; where you work is where you live." [employee, ID #3, age > 50 years, offshore experience 3–4 years].

Opportunities for leisure activities and retreat

In general, employees and experts perceived the limited opportunities for retreat and leisure activities as demanding:

"You actually just sit there for 14 days in this form of prison; you sit there in your cell and are very limited in your free-time activities." [expert, ID #7, offshore experience 3–4 years].

Employees particularly complained about the limited possibilities for sports and exercise. For instance, gyms (when available) were described as being too small and insufficiently equipped.

Job resources

Free time at home

Employees reported positive effects of offshore work on their private and family life. They highlighted the fact that they were able to spend intensive time with their families and to actively engage in childcare during their free time periods onshore:

"My son is now 7 months old. When we go to baby swimming lessons I am the only dad there, because all of the other dads are at work." [employee, ID #6, age 20–30 years, offshore experience < 1 year].

Catering

Even though some employees complained about unhealthy food, the majority of the interviewees expressed their satisfaction with the catering. The experts were in particular of the opinion that offshore workers were provided with a great variety of high-quality food offers:

"The food is healthy. It's like when you're staying in a good hotel." [expert, ID #12, offshore experience 3–4 years].

Employees' needs for improvement

In the interviews, we asked offshore employees about their needs for improvement regarding their working conditions. Few of the employees reported being satisfied with their current job situation and provided no recommendation for change. The majority of workers, however, suggested various needs for improvement. These are related to the work categories and depicted in Table 8.

Table 8 Employees' needs for improvement

Category 1: Work tasks	
transfer and access to installations	promotion of greater awareness among the workers when accessing installations definition of maximum waiting times when accessing installations
Category 2: Work organization	
communication off–/onshore	promotion of a better mutual understanding and flow of information between colleagues offshore and onshore
personnel	increase in offshore personnel
workflow	definition of clear work processes
work time	changes in work tasks to avoid overtime work reduction of working hours (e.g. from 12 to 10 h) definition of break and leave regulations
work schedule	changes in work schedule (e.g. from 14 to 10 days offshore)
payment	increase in payment
medical care & check-ups	establishment of uniform international standards for check-ups
Category 3: Work environment	
workplace design	assurance of ergonomic workplace design
physicochemical factors	provision of room humidifiers in cabins to avoid dry air
Category 4: Social relations	
	–
Category 5: New forms of work	
private and family life	assurance of stable telephone and internet connections
accommodation	provision of single cabins of reasonable size
catering	arrangements with catering to improve healthy diet
opportunities for leisure activities and retreat	improvement of sports and leisure opportunities

Most of the suggestions made by the employees fell under the categories of work organization and new forms of work. With regard to work organization, employees expressed a particular need for changes in the working hours:

> *"I think it would make sense to reduce the 12-hour shifts. Maybe make them 10 hours... something along those lines." [employee, ID #18, age 31–40 years, offshore experience > 4 years].*

Regarding new forms of work, they stressed the importance of stable telephone and internet connections, the improvement of leisure possibilities, and the provision of single cabins:

> *"In order to ensure that everything runs smoothly, every employee who works out here should have access to a single cabin." [employee, ID #7, age 20–30 years, offshore experience 1–2 years].*

For the category of social relations, there was no perceived need for improvement.

Discussion

The aim of our study was to investigate the working conditions of employees in the German offshore wind industry and to identify areas in need of improvement. By conducting our interview study, we were able to gain important insights into these topics.

Offshore employees' working conditions

By drawing on the JD-R model [23, 25], we were able to classify a broad range of demands and resources of offshore work. In summary, employees and experts perceived most of the job demands to be under the categories of work organization and new forms of work, whereas the fewest demands where expressed for the category of social relations. In contrast, most of the job resources were found in the category of work tasks. Consistent with the JD-R model's assumptions, we found that employees perceived job demands as hindering factors, whereas job resources were regarded as facilitating offshore work.

Interestingly, we found that some aspects were considered to be both a potential job demand *and* job resource, depending on the specific context (e.g. weather conditions: good weather was seen as a resource, and harsh weather was regarded as a demand). In the literature, offshore employees' working conditions have been exclusively described unilaterally, either as a job demand *or* as a resource. In our study, we were able to achieve a further differentiation.

With respect to the work tasks, the hard physical work and challenging transfer and access to the installations were identified as job demands. This is consistent with certain considerations made for workers in the German [7–10] and international offshore wind industry [27], as well as in the offshore oil and gas industry [13, 17, 28]. Findings from the offshore wind industry indicate the most frequent incidents offshore to occur during the transport of people and material, including accessing wind farms and installations [27]. Despite this, the topic hasn't received particularly much attention as a job demand for workers in the German offshore wind industry. Our result reinforces the relevance of this demand, being made further important by the fact that offshore workers may transfer to and from the installations several times per shift.

An important finding from our study is that the workers reported to feel safe at their place of work. Because the offshore workplace presents specific hazards, particular importance has been placed on safety concepts in the offshore wind industry [7] and other high-risk industries [29, 30]. Since it was found that risk perceptions present a stressor for offshore workers [17, 31] with potential negative impacts on their health [32], the strong perception of safety among our interviewees can be considered an important resource.

Demands associated with the work organization consisted, in part, of long working hours and shift work. This agrees with theoretical assumptions and empirical findings for employees in the German [7, 9, 10] and international offshore wind industry [14] as well as in the offshore oil and gas sector [13, 29, 33]. A relevant finding of our study is that waiting times and weather days represented a substantial job demand for the interviewees. There has been discussion concerning waiting times and the burden they represent in the form of work delays [9, 34]; however, waiting times haven't been described as a burden in of themselves. This might be due to the fact that, until now, primary focus has been placed on demands regarding employees' work situation, and not on the demand of *not* being able to work.

We found that the 14/14-work schedule, on the one hand, represented a particularly positive factor of offshore work for many interviewees. In studies from the offshore oil and gas sector, the work schedule has also been described as a potential benefit of offshore work, allowing the employees long periods of time off work [12, 29, 33]. However, preferences concerning work schedules have generally been found to vary across different age groups [35], such that our finding should be interpreted with caution. Our interviewees were relatively young, and older offshore workers might be less satisfied and able to cope with the 14/14-work schedule. Research indicates, for example, that aging workers cannot tolerate shift-work as well as their younger colleagues [36, 37], and that they have a higher need for recovery after work [38]. On the other hand, the work schedule was also perceived as demanding. In particular, our findings reinforce that being away from home represents a job demand for workers in the German offshore wind industry [7, 9]. Work-family-interface has also been described as a stressor for offshore oil and gas workers [13, 17, 31] and seafarers [20]; these workers tend to spend even longer periods of time away from home. Our findings show that some workers felt difficulties reconciling work and family life, supporting the notion that intermittent absences from home can contribute to work-family-conflicts for offshore wind industry workers [39]. In addition, we found workers to experience difficulty switching between their two social environments (offshore and onshore), an aspect that has also been revealed for offshore oil and gas workers [40, 41].

Job demands concerning the work environment were found to be in line with existing considerations for workers in the offshore wind industry, underlining unfavourable weather conditions and confined spaces at the workplace as demanding [7, 10, 27]. Such demands have similarly been discussed for offshore oil and gas workers [13, 17, 29] and seafarers [18].

In our study, conflicts with colleagues and language barriers were rarely described by either workers or experts. This finding is somewhat contradictory with theoretical considerations for workers in the German and international offshore wind industry, in which the limited social contact, conflicts with colleagues, and language barriers have been described [7, 9, 14, 27]. Likewise, in studies from the oil and gas sector and seafaring branch, a lack of social support [13, 18] and loneliness on board [20] have been reported. It should be noted that our finding only reflects the views of workers fluent in the German language; non-German speakers might encounter more difficulties in social interactions with German colleagues. However, results from other studies also support our finding of good social relations between offshore colleagues. For example, many workers in the offshore oil and gas industry were found to describe their colleagues as their second family [29], and social support was identified as a job resource with positive effects on offshore oil and gas workers' health [15, 16, 32, 42, 43].

Remarkably, interviewees put special emphasis on job demands concerning new forms of work. Identified demands regarding the offshore accommodations (e.g. confined cabins, lack of privacy) and limited opportunities for leisure activities are in line with findings and theoretical considerations for workers in the offshore wind [7, 9] and oil and gas industry [17, 31]. Furthermore, our result that suitable catering was particularly important to the workers in our study agrees with findings from the offshore oil and gas industry [43–45].

Interestingly, we were able to identify additional job demands which have not been previously described in the literature, such as a perceived cost pressure at work. Employees felt that the perception of cost pressure was associated with time pressure (in the way that economic losses were anticipated when employees weren't able to finish their work in time). Despite there being little discussion concerning cost pressure, the related aspect of time pressure has been described as a job demand in the offshore wind industry [9, 14, 27]. Another previously unknown demand revealed in our study was the limited access to means of communication. As limited chances for communication were described to provoke dissatisfaction among the workers, adequate means of communication seem to be essential for their well-being.

Influencing factors regarding employees' working conditions

We found that interviewees' working conditions varied considerably, e.g. in terms of their specific work tasks, work contracts and salaries, as well as work and living environment (e.g. type of accommodation, catering, and opportunities for leisure activities). Moreover, the working conditions appeared to differ according to project phase (e.g. time pressure was reported to be more prevalent in the construction stage of the wind parks). These results are in line with findings from the offshore oil and gas industry, showing that, for example, sources of stress were specific to certain groups of offshore personnel with different work tasks and workplaces [31, 42, 46, 47]. In addition, employees perceived the level of burden of the job demands to varying extents, depending on their previous experiences in the offshore work environment or related industries. There was a tendency towards the perception of less job demands, the more experienced workers were. Furthermore, the workers' personality and attitude seemed to play a role in their perceptions of job demands. Similarly, personality was found to be relevant for offshore oil and gas workers' well-being, high extraversion and low neuroticism being associated with adaptability [46].

Comparison of employees' and experts' perceptions

The views of offshore employees and experts mostly coincided with regards to job demands and resources. Observed differences mainly involved the emphasis they put on specific aspects. Experts, for example, spoke more often of demands related to heavy work equipment, the workplace design, or the emergency medical care. This finding should be interpreted in the context of offshore experts' professions, since demands concerning the work equipment and workplace directly relate to experts' occupational fields (e.g. health and safety). The fact that demands regarding emergency medical care were stressed by the experts is also reasonable, as they are directly involved in the design of offshore rescue concepts. In contrast, offshore workers emphasized demands associated with new forms of work, e.g. inconvenient accommodations and limited means of communication. Naturally, the living conditions offshore should be of greater importance to the workers in comparison to the experts who spend less time offshore. Regarding job resources, experts emphasized the medical care and medical check-ups, and spoke more positively about the living conditions offshore. In contrast, the scope of action, well-structured workflow, and international work environment were more in the forefront for the workers.

Strengths and limitations

An important strength of our study is the fact that we conducted interviews with offshore workers *and* offshore experts. Therefore, we were able to incorporate different points of view and to contrast interviewees' perspectives with each other. Workers and experts differed in their ages and years of experience in the offshore branch, which allowed us to incorporate a wider range of subjective perceptions. Moreover, we utilized rich descriptions of the results and direct quotes from the interviewees, which contributes to the trustworthiness of qualitative research results [48]. Another strength of our study stems from the fact that, during the data analysis process, the results were discussed thoroughly within the group of researchers involved in the study, which strengthened the transparency of the research process. In addition, the findings were compared with an appropriate theoretical framework (JDR-model), and empirical references [49]. Over time, the various job demands and resources were repetitively described by the interviewees, eventually reaching a point at which no new information were collected. Hence, it can be assumed that the 42 interviews we conducted were sufficient to achieve data saturation [50]. However, further quantitative studies are needed to generalize the results. Since our results are solely based on the views of persons directly related to the industry, it would be interesting to focus on external evaluations of the working conditions by involving independent authorities. Future studies should also investigate offshore workers' health and study the impact of the working conditions on health-related outcomes. To date, many German offshore workers are relatively young. As the workers age, special focus should be placed on the question of whether or not the offshore workplace can be considered ageing-appropriate.

A restriction of our study is the fact that we conducted telephone interviews instead of face-to-face-interviews. Telephone interviews have generally been found to provide detailed, high quality data [51]; however, the asynchronous communication of place by telephone and subsequent reduction of certain social cues might have influenced the results [51, 52]. Moreover, the potential influence of the interviewer on interviewees' responses as well as answer tendencies due to social desirability must be borne in mind. Some of the workers and experts were interviewed during their offshore assignments, while others were interviewed during their free-time periods onshore. The diverse geographical settings (work sector versus leisure sector) might also have influenced interviewees' perceptions. Furthermore, interviewees were rather young in age and had relatively few years of offshore work experience. It might be assumed that our study could have revealed different results for older workers with more years of offshore experience. We only interviewed employees fluent in German and mostly spoke with male workers, so we could not account for the views of non-German speakers nor include gender perspectives in our findings. However, the male-dominated sample accurately reflects the predominance of male workers in the German offshore wind industry. Due to the qualitative nature of our study and the fact that we didn't apply a statistical method to select interviewees, our sample cannot be considered as representative of the entire German offshore working population.

Conclusions

To our knowledge, this is the first study to systematically analyse the working conditions and self-perceived needs of employees in the German offshore wind industry. Overall, our results can provide a basis for further quantitative research in order to generalize the findings. Moreover, the results can be utilized to develop needs-based interventions to improve the working conditions offshore. Since most of the needs for improvement expressed were in regard to the work organization and living conditions offshore, we highly recommend that these aspects be accounted for in the design of suitable interventions.

Acknowledgements
We gratefully acknowledge all offshore employees and experts who participated in the study. Moreover, we wish to thank Iris Richrath, Nora Colli and Maria Kirchhöfer for their help in data preparation as well as Rosalie McDonough for language editing.

Funding
This research was supported by a grant from the German Federal Ministry of Education and Research (grant number: 01FA15029; URL: https://www.bmbf.de/). The funder had no role in the study design, data collection, data analysis and interpretation, preparation of the manuscript and decision to submit the paper for publication.

Authors' contributions
JM, MVG, VH, AP and SM planned the study and participated in the study design. JM carried out the qualitative study and analysed the data. JM, MVG, AP and SM interpreted the data. JM drafted the manuscript and all co-authors contributed substantially to its revision. All authors read and approved the final version of the manuscript.

Authors' information
Not applicable.

Competing interests
JM, MVG, VH, AP and SM declare that they have no competing interests.

References

1. van der Slot A, Hader, M, de Vries, M, van den Berg, W: Think act. Offshore wind power - Takeaways from the Borssele wind farm. Munich: Roland Berger GmbH; 2016.
2. Lüers S, Wallasch A-K, Vogelsang K. Status des Offshore-Windenergieausbaus in Deutschland. 1. Halbjahr 2017. Varel: Deutsche Windguard GmbH; 2017.
3. Lehr U, Ulrich P. Beschäftigung in Deutschland durch Windenergie - Bundesländerergebnisse. 2017. http://www.offshore-stiftung.de/sites/offshorelink.de/files/documents/Besch%C3%A4ftigung%20Windenergie.pdf. Accessed 25 Apr 2017.
4. Schwieters N, Ull T, Meyer R: Volle Kraft aus Hochseewind. Bremerhaven, Bremen: PricewaterhouseCoopers AG Wirtschaftsprüfungsgesellschaft (PwC); 2012.
5. Institut für Innovation und Technik, dsn: Bericht Plattform Zukunftsberufe Offshore-Windenergie. Hamburg, Berlin: Behörde für Wirtschaft, Verkehr und Innovation; 2012.
6. Velasco Garrido M, Mette J, Mache S, Harth V, Preisser AM. Belastungen und Gefährdungen der Beschäftigten in der Offshore-Windindustrie. Arbeitsmed Sozialmed Umweltmed. 2017;52:138–41.
7. Puskeppeleit M: Medizin im Offshore-Bereich. In Maritime Medizin: Praxiswissen für Schiffsärzte und Ärzte im Offshore-Bereich. Edited by Ottoman C, Seidenstücker KH. Berlin, Heidelberg: Springer; 2015: 35-47.
8. Preisser AM, Töpel M, Harth V. Arbeitsmedizinische Eignungsuntersuchung für Mitarbeiter auf Offshoreinstallationen – Von der DGMM-Empfehlung zur AWMF-Leitlinie. Flug u Reisemed. 2016;23:14–8.
9. Hennings S: Psychische Belastungen bei Offshore-Arbeiten. 2015. https://www.bghm.de/fileadmin/user_upload/Seminare/Veranstaltungen/Werftentagung/Hennings_Psychische_Belastungen_bei_Offshore-Arbeiten_20150630.pdf. Accessed 2 Apr 2017.
10. Landesamt für Gesundheit und Soziales Mecklenburg-Vorpommern: Staatlicher Arbeitsschutz im Offshorebereich. 2012. http://service.mvnet.de/_php/download.php?datei_id=68240. Accessed 15 Apr 2017.
11. Mette J, Velasco Garrido M, Preisser AM, Harth V, Mache S. Psychische Belastung von Beschäftigten in der deutschen Offshore-Windindustrie. Zbl Arbeitsmed. 2016;66:307–11.
12. Parkes KR. Psychosocial aspects of stress, health and safety on North Sea installations. Scand J Work Environ Health. 1998;24:321–33.
13. Chen WQ, Wong TW, Yu TS. Mental health issues in Chinese offshore oil workers. Occup Med. 2009;59:545–9.
14. Brun E, Suarez A. European Agency for Safety and Health at Work: Occupational safety and health in the wind energy sector. Luxembourg: European Agency for Safety and Health at Work; 2013.
15. Berthelsen M, Pallesen S, Bjorvatn B, Knardahl S. Shift schedules, work factors, and mental health among onshore and offshore workers in the Norwegian petroleum industry. Ind Health. 2015;53:280–92.
16. Ljosa CH, Tyssen R, Lau B. Mental distress among shift workers in Norwegian offshore petroleum industry - relative influence of individual and psychosocial work factors. Scand J Work Environ Health. 2011;37:551–5.
17. Parkes KR. Psychosocial aspects of work and health in the North Sea oil and gas industry. Research report 002. Sudbury: University of Oxford for the Health and Safety Executive; 2002.
18. Wadsworth EJK, Allen PH, McNamara RL, Smith AP. Fatigue and health in a seafaring population. Occup Med. 2008;58:198–204.
19. Chen WQ, Wong TW, Yu TS. Reliability and validity of the occupational stress scale for Chinese off-shore oil installation workers. Stress Health. 2001;17:175–83.
20. Carotenuto A, Molino I, Fasanaro AM, Amenta F. Psychological stress in seafarers: a review. Int Marit Health. 2012;63:188–94.
21. Gardner R. Overview and characteristics of some occupational exposures and health risks on offshore oil and gas installations. Ann Occup Hyg. 2003;47:201–10.
22. Niven K, McLeod R. Offshore industry: management of health hazards in the upstream petroleum industry. Occup Med. 2009;59:304–9.
23. Demerouti E, Bakker AB, Nachreiner F, Schaufeli WB. The job demands-resources model of burnout. J Appl Psychol. 2001;86:499–512.
24. Bakker AB, Demerouti E. The job demands-resources model: state of the art. J Manag Psychol. 2007;22:309–28.
25. Karasek RA. Job demands, job decision latitude, and mental strain: implications for job redesign. Adm Sci Q. 1979;24:285–308.
26. Siegrist J. Adverse health effects of high-effort/low-reward conditions. J Occup Health Psychol. 1996;1:27–41.

27. Tveiten CK, Albrechtsen E, Heggset J, Hofmann M, Jersin E, Leira B, Norddal PK. HSE challenges related to offshore renewable energy. Report no. A18107. Trondhelm: SINTEF Technology and Society; 2011.
28. Sneddon A, Mearns K, Flin R. Stress, fatigue, situation awareness and safety in offshore drilling crews. Saf Sci. 2013;56:80–8.
29. Ulven AJ. Medical and psychological challenges in the offshore petroleum industry. Int Marit Health. 2009;60:40–2.
30. Bjerkan AM. Health, environment, safety culture and climate – analysing the relationships to occupational accidents. J Risk Res. 2010;13:445–77.
31. Sutherland VJ, Cooper CL. Stress in the offshore oil and gas exploration and production industries: an organizational approach to stress control. Stress Med. 1996;12:27–34.
32. Ulleberg P, Rundmo T. Job stress, social support, job satisfaction and absenteeism among offshore oil personnel. Work Stress. 1997;11:215–28.
33. Ross JK. Offshore industry shift work – health and social considerations. Occup Med. 2009;59:310–5.
34. Sutherland VJ, Cooper CL. Stress prevention in the offshore oil and gas exploration and production industry. Geneva: International Labour Office; 1996.
35. Eurofond. Working time and work-life balance in a life course perspective. Dublin: Eurofond; 2012.
36. Harrington JM. Health effects of shift work and extended hours of work. Occup Environ Med. 2001;58:68–72.
37. Costa G. Shift work and occupational medicine: an overview. Occup Med. 2003;53:83–8.
38. Kiss P, De Meester M, Braeckman L. Differences between younger and older workers in the need for recovery after work. Int Arch Occup Environ Health. 2008;81:311–20.
39. Kirchhoefer M, Mache, S, Harth, V, Mette, J: Vereinbarkeit von Berufs- und Familienleben bei Offshore-Beschäftigten – eine Übersicht. *Zbl Arbeitsmed* 2017. doi:10.1007/s40664-017-0189-x.
40. Rodrigues VF, Fischer FM, Brito MJ. Shift work at a modern offshore drilling rig. J Hum Ergol (Tokyo). 2001;30:167–72.
41. Solheim J. Coming home to work. In: Lewis J, Porter M, Shrimpton M, editors. Women, work and family in the British, Canadian and Norwegian offshore oilfields. London: Palgrave Macmillan UK; 1988. p. 140–62.
42. Håvold JI. Stress on the bridge of offshore vessels: examples from the North Sea. Saf Sci. 2015;71:160–6.
43. Riethmeister V, Brouwer S, van der Klink J, Bültmann U. Work, eat and sleep: towards a healthy ageing at work program offshore. BMC Public Health. 2016;16:134.
44. Parkes KR. Demographic and lifestyle predictors of body mass index among offshore oil industry workers: cross-sectional and longitudinal findings. Occup Med. 2003;53:213–21.
45. Horsley H, MacKenzie I. Lifestyle survey amongst North Sea oil workers. In Proceedings of the Occupational Health Offshore Conference. Edited by Gardner R. HSE Books: Sudbury; 1997. pp. 161–79.
46. Parkes KR, Farmer E, Carnell S: Psychosocial aspects of work and health in the North Sea oil and gas industry: A survey of FPSO installations and comparison with platforms and drilling rigs. Sudbury: Health & Safety Executive; 2004.
47. Bjerkan AM. Work and health: a comparison between Norwegian onshore and offshore employees. Work. 2011;40:125–42.
48. van Nes F, Abma T, Jonsson H, Deeg D. Language differences in qualitative research: is meaning lost in translation? Eur J Ageing. 2010;7:313–6.
49. Malterud K. Qualitative research: standards, challenges, and guidelines. Lancet. 2001;358:483–8.
50. Guest G, Bunce A, Johnson L. How many interviews are enough?: an experiment with data saturation and variability. Field Methods. 2006;18:59–82.
51. Novick G. Is there a bias against telephone interviews in qualitative research? Res Nurs Health. 2008;31:391–8.
52. Opdenakker RJG. Advantages and disadvantages of four interview techniques in qualitative research. Forum Qual Soc Res. 2006;7(4):11. http://nbn-resolving.de/urn:nbn:de:0114-fqs0604118.

13

A case-case study on sinonasal cancer prevention: effect from dust reduction in woodworking and risk of mastic/solvents in shoemaking

Enzo Emanuelli[1], Enrico Alexandre[1*], Diego Cazzador[1], Vera Comiati[2], Tiziana Volo[1], Alessia Zanon[1], Maria Luisa Scapellato[2], Mariella Carrieri[2], Alessandro Martini[1] and Giuseppe Mastrangelo[2]

Abstract

Background and aims: Sinonasal cancers (SNCs) are rare neoplasms, accounting for about 3 % of head and neck cancers, with squamous cell carcinoma (SCC) and adenocarcinoma (ADC) as the most common subtypes. ADCs present strong associations with occupational wood dust exposure. Preventive measures have progressively reduced wood dust concentrations in workplaces but no study has evaluated the effectiveness of such interventions. Few studies indicate associations between ADC and exposure to solvents, which is common in the shoe industry, but this hypothesis still needs confirmation.

Methods: In a case-case study, we contrasted 32 ADCs against 21 Non-Adenocarcinoma Epithelial Tumors (NAETs) – all recruited from the same clinical setting (Padua's University Hospital; period 2004–2015) – using questionnaires and clinical records to collect information on potential predictors. Non-occupational factors were age, sex, smoking, allergy and chronic sinusitis. Occupational factors were intensity and frequency of wood dust exposure, protection from wood dust, type of wood (in woodworking); frequency of exposure to leather dust or mastic/solvent (in shoemaking). Odds-ratio (OR), 95 % confidence interval (95 % CI) and two-tail p-values were obtained through stepwise backward logistic regression for each industry, always using as reference patients never employed in either trade and adjusting for non-occupational risk factors.

Results: Adjusted OR was 22.5 (95 % CI = 3.50–144; $p = 0.001$) and 9.37 (95 % CI = 1.29–67.6; $p = 0.026$), respectively, in patients with low or high degree of protection against wood dust. In the shoe industry, adjusted OR was 1 and 18.8 (95 % CI = 1.29–174; $p = 0.030$), respectively, in patients with low or high exposure to only mastic/solvent; and 1 and 22.5 (95 % CI = 2.07–244; $p = 0.011$), respectively, in patients with low or high exposure to only leather dust.

Discussion and conclusions: The questionnaire used was able to estimate with simple algorithms past exposures in wood and footwear industries. The case-case design considerably increased the validity of this small study. Results in this study were always consistent with the extant literature; this could support reliability of novel findings. In woodworking, respiratory protective equipment and local exhaust ventilation reduced the risk of occupational SNC; in footwear manufacture, where preventive interventions were seldom adopted, SNC risk was significantly greater for high exposure from mastic/solvent and leather dust.

Keywords: Wood dust, Wood industry, Leather dust, Mastic solvent, Shoe industry, Sinonasal cancer, Occupational risk, Case-case study

* Correspondence: alexandre.enrico@gmail.com
[1]Department of Otolaryngology and Endoscopic Surgery of the Upper Airways, University Hospital of Padua, Via Giustiniani 2, 35100 Padua, Italy
Full list of author information is available at the end of the article

Background

Sinonasal cancers (SNCs) are rare neoplasms that account for about 3 % of all cancers of the head and neck. The majority (59 %) of SNCs diagnosed in the USA between 2004 and 2008 were epithelial neoplasms, with squamous cell carcinoma (SCC) and adenocarcinoma (ADC) being the most common subtypes, accounting for 38 % and 10 % of all sinonasal cancers, respectively [1].

SNCs have been associated with various occupational risk factors. In Monograph 100, the International Agency for Research on Cancer (IARC) classified wood dust, leather dust, nickel compounds, isopropyl alcohol production, radium 226 and 228 and their relative decay products as Group 1 carcinogens for sinonasal mucosa. The numerous epidemiological studies on occupational exposure and sinonasal cancer risk have been recently reviewed [2–4]. In a meta-analysis, exposure to wood dust as well as to leather dust showed associations with SNC, the strongest relative risk (RR) association being with ADC ($RR_{pooled} = 29.43$; 95 % CI = 16.46, 52.61 for wood dust; and $RR_{pooled} = 35.26$; 95 % CI = 20.62, 60.28 for leather dust) [4].

Preventive measures to reduce wood dust concentration have been progressively introduced. For example, in the furniture industry of Viborg County, Denmark, two cross-sectional studies investigated wood dust exposure six years apart (winter 1997/1998, study 1; and winter 2003/2004, study 2), using 2627 personal dust exposure measures carried out in 1907 persons. The geometric mean (geometric standard deviation) of inhalable wood dust concentration decreased from 0.95 mg/m^3 (2.05) in study 1 to 0.60 mg/m^3 (1.63) in study 2, representing a 7 % annual decrease in dust concentration [5]. Likewise, occupational exposure in the wood processing industry in Estonia improved considerably over the years 1990–2000 [6]. The better work conditions in wood industry were generally gained with effective ventilation and consistent cleaning of the work areas [5, 6].

In data from the 1989–2009 nation-wide Netherlands Cancer Registry, the incidence of both SCC and ADC decreased gradually in males, while in females the incidence of SCC increased. The incidence of adenocarcinoma remained stable for both sexes [7]. Since ADC in males is likely related to occupational exposures, the decrease could be attributed to the implementation of measures preventing exposure or to the decreasing number of workers in the furniture and leather industry or the building industry. To the best of our knowledge, no study has yet addressed this issue.

A significant association and a dose–response relationship between exposure to organic solvents and sinonasal ADC has been observed in one study [8]. This finding, which supports the hypothesis of a causal relationship between solvents and ADC, still needs confirmation.

Exposure to mastic/solvents is common in the shoe industry; both woodworking and shoe industry are well represented in the Veneto region. We therefore aimed to investigate in these industrial sectors the SNC risk resulting from the two new aspects of occupational experience: 1) use of personal protective equipment/presence of local exhaust ventilation in wood industry and 2) exposure to glues/organic solvents in shoe industry.

Methods

Patient selection

The source of patients was the database of the Departments of Otolaryngology and Endoscopic Surgery of Airways of Padua's University Hospital. Out of 92 patients with SNCs observed between 2004 and 2015, 26 were excluded because of histology (mesenchymal cancers or epithelial cancers not of sinonasal mucosa, i.e. melanoma). The remaining 66 patients (affected by sinonasal ADC, SCC, undifferentiated carcinoma, mucoepidermoid carcinoma and adenoid cystic carcinoma) were invited by phone to participate in the study; 53 patients (40 males and 13 females) agreed to participate. Written informed consent was obtained before examination. The sample included eight (15 %) decedents; for dead or elderly/disable patients, a letter with the informed consent was sent to the patient's home, together with a return addressed envelope. For dead patients, closest next of kin signed the informed consent and answered the questionnaire telephonically. Elderly/disabled patients, who were not able to be interviewed face-to-face at the hospital, completed the questionnaire telephonically.

Study design

As already reported, ADC is largely associated with woodworking and leather working, while other Non-Adenocarcinoma Epithelial Tumors (NAETs) can be viewed as a background risk. We therefore used a case-case study design contrasting two groups of patients: 32 ADCs and 21 NAETs (the latter including SCC and a few cases of adenoid cystic carcinoma, undifferentiated carcinoma and mucoepidermoid carcinoma) for their occupational exposure. Since the two groups were recruited from the same clinical setting, they are likely to be similar in terms of geographical background, social class and symptoms that lead the patients to seek clinical attention. Moreover, since NAET and ADC share non-occupational risk factors (smoking, age, others), the two samples were well matched for such risk factors, reducing background noise and increasing both the validity and specificity of the association [9].

Variables

The site of onset of both ADCs and NAETs and the histologic subtypes of ADCs were obtained from clinical records. The site of onset was coded as: 0 = ethmoid; 1 = maxillary; 2 = nasal septum. ADC subtypes were coded as: 0 = Intestinal-Type Adenocarcinoma (ITAC); 1 = Non Intestinal-Type Adenocarcinoma (non-ITAC).

All other variables used in the analysis were collected through interview-based questionnaires (Additional file 1). Non-occupational risk factors were:

- age at diagnosis (continuous variable) and gender (1 = male; 0 = female);
- clinical history for allergies, chronic polypoid sinusitis and chronic non-polypoid sinusitis (1 = present; 0 = absent);
- smoking: pack-years (= cigarettes per day/20 × years of smoking) and a variable that was 0 for never smokers; 0.5 for ex-smokers quitting >15 years from interview; 1 for current smokers and former smokers quitting < 15 years.

Using the same questionnaire, we collected the following circumstances of past occupational exposures.

Wood industry

- Intensity. We considered calendar year of first exposure as a surrogate of intensity of wood dust exposure because, depending on technological advancements, it has been reduced over time. Four classes were coded: 0 (subjects never exposed to wood or leather dusts); 1 (year of first exposure ≥1971); 2 (1956 to 1970); 3 (≤1955).
- Frequency. We presumed that the jobs involving high exposure to wood dust were cutting, sanding, planing and use of compressed air; each job was scored as a dichotomous variable (0 = No; 1 = Yes). Then, we collected the workshift frequency (hours per shift/8) of each high exposure job. Finally, we multiplied (job × frequency) summing up as many products as were necessary to take into account the overall work experience of each patient. The latter index ranged from 0 to 1. The frequency of high exposure was then coded: 0 (for subjects never exposed to wood dusts nor leather dusts); 1 (frequency ≤0.5); 2 (frequency >0.5).
- Protection. The original variables were: frequency of high exposure (as above); personal protective equipment (PPE) such as masks (codes = 0/1); and presence of local exhaust ventilation (LEV) (codes = 0/1). The level of protection against wood dust was calculated as: ((PPE + (2 × LEV)) × frequency), summing up all the exposed tasks. The index ranged from 0 to 3.75, increasing with increasing level of protection. The variable was recoded as: 0 (subjects never exposed to wood dusts nor leather dusts); 1 (≥2.6, most protected subjects); 2 (0.1–2.5, least protected subjects).
- Wood type. Coded as 0 for subjects never exposed to wood nor leather dusts; 1 (softwood or mixed wood types); 2 (only hardwoods).
- Duration. Coded as 0 for subjects never exposed to wood nor to leather dusts; 1 and 2 for those with <15 and ≥15 years of exposure to wood dust, using as threshold the value suggested by Binazzi et al. [4].

Shoe industry

- Frequency (leather dust). The jobs presuming to involve a high exposure to leather dust (cutting, polishing and sole preparation) were converted in 0/1 variables and multiplied by the corresponding frequencies (hours per workshift/8). The products were summed up into an index ranging from 0.05 to 1. Three classes of increasing exposure were coded: 0 (subjects never employed into wood industry nor leather industry); 1 (frequency ≤0.05, least exposed workers); 2 (frequency >0.05, most exposed workers).
- Frequency (mastic solvents). The jobs presuming to involve a high exposure to mastic and/or solvents (shoe-assembling and gluing) were converted in 0/1 variables that were multiplied with the corresponding frequency (hours per workshift/8). The products were summed up into an index ranging from 0.05 to 1. Three classes of increasing exposure were coded: 0 (subjects never employed into wood industry nor leather industry); 1 (frequency ≤0.5, least exposed workers); 2 (frequency >0.5, most exposed workers).

Statistical analysis

Analyses were performed within each specific industrial sector (woodworking or shoe industry). The reference group for all analyses consisted of patients never exposed to wood and leather dust. Seven logistic regression models were built in which the dependent variable was dichotomous (1 = ADC; 0 = NAET) and the primary variables were: exposure (model 1); frequency (model 2); protection (model 3); type of wood (model 4); and duration of exposure in wood industry (model 5); frequency of leather dust exposure in shoe industry (model 6); and frequency of mastic solvent exposure in shoe industry (model 7). Some employees less exposed to mastic solvent were mainly involved in tasks that had higher exposures to leather dust, and vice versa. Therefore, the analysis according to models 6 and 7 were repeated excluding those with simultaneous high exposure to the other factor. The non-occupational risk factors (smoking, gender, age at diagnosis, allergies, chronic sinusitis) entered every model. Backward stepwise selection was used to exclude non-statistically significant variables and determine the best-fit model. The statistical procedure provided the odds-ratio (OR) together with 95 % confidence interval (95 % CI) and two-tail p-value. Statistical significance was set at $p < 0.05$; all analyses were performed with STATA 13.0 software.

Results

Table 1 shows the main characteristics of ADC and NAET patients. It can be seen that industrial sector was highly related with the development of ADC, while all non-occupational risk factors were not. The site of onset for ADCs was the ethmoid sinus (100 %); for NAETs the most frequent site was the maxillary sinuses (38 %), followed by nasal septum (33 %), and ethmoid (29 %). ADC cases were mostly ITAC (94 %).

Table 2 shows the distribution of patients (ADC or NAET) as well as the OR with 95 % CI and p-value of developing ADC in wood industry. In model 1, the highest ORs were observed for the remotest years of first exposure to wood dust. In model 2, ORs increased with increasing frequency of high exposure to wood dust. In model 3, ORs tended to decrease with increasing level of protection from wood dust. In model 4, exposure to hardwood and (to a lesser extent) softwood significantly increased the risk of ADC. In model 5, ORs tended to increase with increasing duration of exposure to wood dust (OR being 1 in the subgroup with <15 years of exposure because there were no ADC cases). Non-occupational risk factors did not enter in any model.

Table 3 shows the distribution of patients (ADC or NAET) as well as the OR with 95%CI and p-value of developing ADC in the shoe industry. ORs were found to increase with increasing frequency of estimated exposure to both leather dust (model 6) and mastic/solvent (model 7) although, in the latter model, the relationship was not monotonic probably because employees lesser exposed to mastic solvent had higher exposure to leather dust. Non-occupational risk factors did not enter any of these models.

Discussion and Conclusions

We contrasted two groups of patients (ADC against NAET) for circumstances of exposure in wood and shoe industry. The role of traditional risk factors was always confirmed; regarding the two new hypotheses, we found that use of PPE and/or presence of LEV reduced the risk of occupational SNC in wood industry, while exposure

Table 1 Main characteristics of patients with adenocarcinoma (ADC), non-adenocarcinoma epithelial tumor (NAET) and in the whole sample

Patients' characteristics		ADC Number (%)	NAET Number (%)	Whole sample Number (%)	Chi square (*p*-value)
Industrial sector	*Wood*	16 (50)	5 (24)	21 (40)	14.60 (0.001)
	Leather	11 (34)	2 (10)	13 (25)	
	Other	5 (16)	14 (67)	19 (36)	
Age (years)	≤59	8 (25)	10 (48)	18 (34)	4.17 (0.125)
	60–74	8 (25)	6 (29)	14 (26)	
	>74	16 (50)	5 (23)	21 (40)	
Smoking (pack-years)	*0*	17 (53)	14 (67)	31 (58)	2.67 (0.263)
	≤*18*	6 (19)	5 (24)	11 (21)	
	>*18*	9 (29)	2 (9)	11 (21)	
Sex	*M*	26 (81)	14 (67)	40 (75)	1.46 (0.227)
	W	6 (19)	7 (33)	13 (25)	
Chronic Sinusitis	*Yes*	6 (19)	4 (19)	10 (19)	0.001 (0.978)
	No	26 (81)	17 (81)	43 (81)	
Allergies	*Yes*	4 (13)	2 (10)	6 (11)	0.11 (0.738)
	No	28 (87)	19 (90)	47 (89)	
Site of onset	*Ethmoid*	32 (100)	6 (29)	38 (72)	
	Maxillary	0	8 (38)	8 (15)	
	Septum	0	7 (33)	7 (13)	
ADC subtype	*ITAC*[a]	30 (94)	-	-	
	Non-ITAC	2 (6)	-	-	

[a]Intestinal-Type Adenocarcinoma

Table 2 Distribution of patients and results of five models of logistic regressions (wood industry only)

Terms	ADC	NAET	OR	95 % CI	p-value
Model 1. First exposure to wood dust					
Reference	4	15	1	-	-
1970-today	5	2	9.37	1.29–67.6	0.026
1956–1970	6	1	22.5	2.06–245.	0.011
Pre-1956	6	1	22.5	2.06–245.	0.011
Model 2. Frequency of exposure to wood dust					
Reference	4	15	1	-	-
Low	7	2	13.1	1.92–89.5	0.009
High	10	2	18.8	2.87–122.	0.002
Model 3. Protection from wood dust					
Reference	4	15	1	-	-
Low	12	2	22.5	3.50–144.	0.001
High	5	2	9.37	1.29–67.6	0.026
Model 4. Wood used					
Reference	4	15	1	-	-
Other woods	8	3	10.0	1.78–56.1	0.009
Hardwood	9	1	33.8	3.22–351.	0.003
Model 5. Duration of exposure to wood dust					
Reference	4	15	1	-	-
<15 years	4	0	1.0	-	.
≥15 years	13	4	12.2	2.52–58.7	0.002

ADC adenocarcinoma, *NAET* non-adenocarcinoma epithelial tumor, *OR* odds-ratio, 95%CI 95 % confidence interval

Table 3 Distribution of patients and results of two models of logistic regressions (shoe industry only)

Terms	ADC	NAET	OR	95 % CI	p-value
Model 6. Frequency of exposure to leather dust					
Reference	4	15	1	-	-
Low	5	1	18.75	1.67–209.	0.017
High	6	1	22.5	2.06–244.	0.011
Model 6. Frequency of exposure to leather dust (no exposure to mastic/solvent)					
Reference	4	15	1	-	-
Low	1	0	1	-	-
High	6	1	22.5	2.06–244.	0.011
Model 7. Frequency of exposure to mastic/solvent					
Reference	4	15	1	-	-
Low	7	1	26.25	2.45–280.	0.007
High	4	1	15.00	1.29–174.	0.030
Model 7. Exposure to mastic/solvent (no exposure to leather dust)					
Reference	4	15	1	-	-
Low	1	0	1	-	-
High	4	1	15.00	1.29–174.	0.030

ADC adenocarcinoma, *NAET* non-adenocarcinoma epithelial tumor, *OR* odds-ratio, 95%CI 95 % confidence interval

to mastic/solvents increased such risk in the shoe industry.

Internal validity

A weakness of the present study is the limited size. However, according to Curtis [9], the choice of a case-case study rather than the classic case-control study could lower the background noise because two similar diseases share most of non-occupational risk factors. In fact, as shown in Table 1, there were no differences between ADC and NAET groups for gender, age at diagnosis, clinical history of allergies, chronic polypoid or non-polypoid sinusitis, and smoking habits. Thus, despite the low number of our subjects, the case-case design has considerably increased the validity of the study, overcoming the several difficulties that often affect investigations on these rare diseases.

The proportion of NAET patients exposed to risks was about 20 % in our study group in contrast to 8 % in a clinical series reported by Bonzini et al. [10]. Since the corresponding percentage was about 2.2 % in the general population of the Veneto region in 1996 (about 100.000 workers in 4.500.000 inhabitants); using NAETs as references probably has underestimated the true risk of developing ADC.

Besides SCC, we included in the reference group cases with different histologies (adenoid cystic carcinoma, undifferentiated carcinoma and mucoepidermoid carcinoma). Although this could represent a major limit to the study, given the low number of patients and the scarce evidence of association between these histologies and exposure to wood and leather dust [10], it is unlikely that such inclusion could have severely biased our results.

A questionnaire was specifically designed for this study. In agreement with Hernberg [11], we assumed that calendar year of first exposure could be a reliable surrogate of intensity of exposure, because occupational hygiene in general has improved in many countries and work methods have changed substantially over the years. In agreement with Schluenssen [5], we considered sanding, cutting, sanding and cutting, mixed task, and use of compressed air work as tasks involving high level of exposure to wood dust – moreover we also collected the frequency (hours per workshift/8) spent in each high exposure task. In the same study [5], manual assembling/packing, sanding with adequate exhaust ventilation, adequate exhaust ventilation, vacuum cleaning of machines and special cleaning staff were found to decrease wood dust concentration. Accordingly, we built an algorithm to characterize protection against wood dust exposure, using the presence of LEV and use of PPE. Building an algorithm of protection in shoe sector was not feasible because PPE and respiratory protective equipment were seldom used by our subjects and in literature [12]. In short, using literature data we created a questionnaire that was able to estimate with relatively simple algorithms past exposures to occupational pollutants in wood and leather industry.

Collecting occupational history from next-of-kin should could lower the quality of information because relatives tend to over- or under-estimate such exposure [11]. The latter fact increases the non-differential misclassification that underestimates the true OR. Despite this fact, our findings resulted statistically significant.

Interpretation of findings

As clearly reported in Table 1, ITAC arisen from ethmoid sinus was the commonest subtype of ADC in our study, in agreement with extant literature [10, 13–15]. Notwithstanding, SNCs that originate from other sinonasal sites can be associated with occupational exposure [4, 16]. For woodworking, moreover, we were able to confirm the increasing trend of SNC with duration of exposure to wood dust (model 5) [4]. Our results were coherent with extant literature [2–4], and this could support the reliability of the new findings reported in this study in spite of the low number of cases and the wide confidence intervals of risk estimates.

The novel finding was the evidence that PPE and/or LEV could be effective in preventing occupational SNCs. It could be noted, however, that OR was still as high as 9 in the group with maximal protection (model 3). This finding, which also suggests that further improvements need to be done, could be the residual effect of high wood dust exposures prior to 1981 – year in which woodworking was first classified by IARC as class I carcinogen – that became manifest after the typical long latency of these tumors. Likely, in fact, woodworking industries started providing their employees with PPEs or installing exhaust systems or more technically advanced protective machines only starting in 1981. In our subjects, moreover, when intensity or duration of exposure, frequency of exposure and protection from exposure were forced with the non-occupational risk factors in a same model of stepwise logistic regression, protection was the only significant predictor (same results of model 3). Therefore, the ultimate risk for sinonasal cancer in woodworking was the lack of primary prevention. A review of the literature shows no other reports on this topic. In Italy, in the sector of wood and cabinet making, the number of employees increased progressively from the year 1951 to 1981 to then decrease to levels of 1961 in the year 2001 (seriestoriche.istat.it). The corresponding values are not available for the Veneto region. Presuming that values were similar in the Veneto region and given the long latency period of the disease, the decreasing number of employees is too recent to explain the decrease of SNC risk.

In the shoe industry, the novel finding was the association between exposure to mastic/solvent and risk of developing ADC. An overestimation of such risk was unlikely because neither patients nor interviewers had any prior knowledge of organic solvents as a suspected occupational risk factor for SNC. There are in fact few reports on this issue. In a case-control study carried out in Piedmont (Italy) in 113 incident cases and 336 hospital controls, d'Errico [8] reported a significant association and a dose–response relationship between occupational exposure to organic solvents and sinonasal ADC, after controlling for age, sex, smoking and co-exposure to wood dust. Exposure to solvents was evaluated based on the information provided in the questionnaires in conjunction with two job-exposure matrices by economic sector and job title [8]. In a population-based case-control study undertaken in Southern Germany, involving 427 cases (cancers of the paranasal sinuses, cancers of the nasal cavity, nasopharyngeal cancer) and 2401 controls, Greiser [17] found a significant excess of nasal cancer in smokers after exposure to organic solvents but not a dose-response relationship. Exposure to organic solvents was determined at the time of the interview with questions about exposure during any occupation as well as by a detailed questionnaire module about specific tasks in metalwork [17]. The majority of our subjects reported exposure to solvents in absence of personal protective equipment, task barriers and mechanical ventilation. Likewise, in a study conducted in Hebron City, 81 % of the shoe factory workers had never used respiratory protective equipment and 92 % had never used work clothes; while 97 % of the workers in the shoe workshops had never used respiratory protective equipment, 94 % had never worn gloves, and 90 % had never used work clothes [12]. Other studies found that workers in footwear manufacture are routinely exposed to complex mixtures of solvents, including acetone, n-hexane, methylethylketone, and large amounts of toluene [18, 19]. None of these solvents is considered genotoxic or carcinogenic [20–22]. The results observed in this study could possibly be explained by the presence of some elastomer in adhesives such as chloroprene, which is used mainly in the footwear industry and is ranked as 2B carcinogen by IARC [23].

The duration of exposure in this industry was not analyzed because of the few cases with specific exposure to either of the substances studied. However, in a recent meta-analysis, no relationship was reported between duration of exposure and SNC risk in the shoe industry [4].

Acknowledgements
We thank Professor G.B. Bartolucci for allowing us to use the materials and spaces to perform the interviews in the setting of this study.

Funding
Ministero dell'Istruzione, dell'Università e della Ricerca (Fondi quota ex60% 2015); recipient: Professor G. Mastrangelo.

Authors' contributions
GM conceived of the study, participated in the design of the study and its coordination and helped to draft the manuscript. EA drafted and revised this manuscript and helped in performing the interviews. AM and EE provided all of the cases together with DC and TV who also helped in coordinating the study. VC performed the interviews and developed the questionnaire. MLS and MC helped to develop the questionnaire. All authors critically read/revised and approved the final version of the manuscript.

Competing interests
The authors declare that they have no competing interests.

Author details
[1]Department of Otolaryngology and Endoscopic Surgery of the Upper Airways, University Hospital of Padua, Via Giustiniani 2, 35100 Padua, Italy. [2]Department of Occupational Medicine, University Hospital of Padua, Via Giustiniani 2, 35100 Padua, Italy.

References
1. Youlden DR, Cramb SM, Peters S, Porceddu SV, Møller H, Fritschi L, et al. International comparisons of the incidence and mortality of sinonasal cancer. Cancer Epidemiol. 2013;37(6):770–9.
2. Husgafvel-Pursiainen K, Carton M, Luce D, Wolff CHJ, Holmila R, Schlünssen V et al. Sinonasal cancers. Occupational Cancers. 2014. 139-168. http://link.springer.com/chapter/10.1007%2F978-1-4471-2825-0_7.
3. Alonso-Sardón M, Chamorro AJ, Hernández-García I, Iglesias-de-Sena H, Martín-Rodero H, Herrera C, et al. Association between occupational exposure to wood dust and cancer: a systematic review and meta-analysis. PLoS One. 2015;10(7):e0133024.
4. Binazzi A, Ferrante P, Marinaccio A. Occupational exposure and sinonasal cancer: a systematic review and meta-analysis. BMC Cancer. 2015;15(1):1.
5. Schlünssen V, Jacobsen G, Erlandsen M, Mikkelsen AB, Schaumburg I, Sigsgaard T. Determinants of wood dust exposure in the Danish furniture industry—results from two cross-sectional studies 6 years apart. Ann Occup Hyg. 2008;52(4):227–38.
6. Traumann A, Reinhold K, Tint P. The model for assessment of health risks of dust connected with wood manufacturing in Estonia. Agron Res. 2013; 11(2):471–8.
7. Kuijpens J, Hans LP, Louwman MWJ, Peters R, Janssens GORJ, Burdorf AL, et al. Trends in sinonasal cancer in The Netherlands: More squamous cell cancer, less adenocarcinoma: A population-based study 1973–2009. Eur J Cancer. 2012;48(15):2369–74.
8. d'Errico A, Pasian S, Baratti A, et al. A case-control study on occupational risk factors for sino-nasal cancer. Occup Environ Med. 2009;66:448–55.
9. Curtis D, Vine AE, McQuillin A, Bass NJ, Pereira A, Kandaswamy R. Case-case genome wide association analysis reveals markers differentially associated with schizophrenia and bipolar disorder and implicates calcium channel genes. Psychiatr Genet. 2011;21(1):1.
10. Bonzini M, Battaglia P, Parassoni D, Casa M, Facchinetti N, Turri-Zanoni M, et al. Prevalence of occupational hazards in patients with different types of epithelial sinonasal cancers. Rhinology. 2013;51(1):31–6. https://www.researchgate.net/profile/Mario_Turri_Zanoni/publication/235730863_Prevalence_of_occupational_hazards_in_patients_with_different_types_of_epithelial_sinonasal_cancers/links/00b7d526d35d5a908d000000.
11. Hernberg S. Introduction to occupational epidemiology. CRC Press; 1992.
12. Nijem K, Kristensen P, Thorud S, Al-Khatib A, Takrori F, Bjertness E. Solvent exposures at shoe factories and workshops in Hebron City, West Bank. Int J Occup Environ Health. 2001;7(3):182–8.
13. Bimbi G, Saraceno MS, Riccio S, Gatta G, Licitra L, Cantù G. Adenocarcinoma of ethmoid sinus: an occupational disease. Acta Otorhinolaryngol Ital. 2004; 24(4):199–203.
14. Khademi B, Moradi A, Hoseini S, Mohammadianpanah M. Malingant neoplasms of the sinonasal tract: report of 71 patients and literature review and analysis. Oral Max Fac Surgery. 2009;13(4):191–9.
15. Bossi P, Saba NF, Vermorken JB, Strojan P, Pala L, de Bree R, Takes RP. The role of systemic therapy in the management of sinonasal cancer: A critical review. Cancer Treat Rev. 2015;41(10):836–43.
16. Mensi C, Consonni D, Sieno C, De Matteis S, Riboldi L, Bertazzi PA. Sinonasal cancer and occupational exposure in a population-based registry. Int J Otolaryngology. 2013;2013:672621.
17. Greiser EM, Greiser KH, Ahrens W, Hagen R, Lazszig R, Maier H, et al. Risk factors for nasal malignancies in German men: the South-German Nasal cancer study. BMC Cancer. 2012;12(1):1.
18. Uuksulainen SO, Heikkilä PR, Olkinuora PS, Kiilunen M. Self-reported occupational health hazards and measured exposures to airborne impurities and noise in shoe repair work. Int J Occup Environ Health. 2002;8(4):320–7.
19. Pitarque M, Vaglenov A, Nosko M, Hirvonen A, Norppa H, Creus A, et al. Evaluation of DNA damage by Comet assay in shoe-workers exposed to toluene and other organic solvents. Mutat Res. 1999;441(1):115–27.
20. ASTDR (Agency for Toxic Substances and Disease Registry)-ToxFAQs, Toxicological Profile for: 2-butanone (1995). Nhexane (1999). Toluene (2001). Acetone (2002).http://www.atsdr.cdc.gov/substances/index.asp. Accessed 19 Jan 2016
21. WHO (World Health Organization). Air quality Guidelines, second edition, Chapter 5.14. Toluene. Regional Office for Europe, Copenhagen, Denmark. http://www.who.int/. 2000. Accessed 19 Jan 2016
22. EPA (Environmental Protection Agency). In Support of Summary Information on the Integrated Risk Information (IRIS). Toxicological Review ofMethyl Ethyl Ketone. http://epa.gov/iris. 2003. Accessed 16 Jan 2016
23. International Agency for Research on Cancer (IARC). IARC Monographs on the evaluation of carcinogenic risks to humans. Re-evaluation of some organic chemicals, hydrazine and hydrogen peroxide. Lyon: IARC, 71. 1999.

14

Utilization of personal protective equipment and associated factors among textile factory workers

Sebsibe Tadesse[1*], Temesgen Kelaye[2] and Yalemzewod Assefa[1]

Abstract

Background: Use of personal protective equipment is one of the important measures to safeguard workers from exposure to occupational hazards, especially in developing countries. However, there is a dearth of studies describing personal protective equipment utilization in Ethiopia. The present study has determined the magnitude of personal protective equipment utilization and identified associated factors among textile factory workers at Hawassa Town, southern Ethiopia.

Methods: An institution-based cross-sectional study was conducted among textile factory workers at Hawassa Town, southern Ethiopia from January to March 2014. Stratified sampling followed by simple random sampling techniques was used to select the total of 660 study participants. A pre-tested and structured questionnaire was used to collect data. Multivariate analyses were employed to see the effect of explanatory variables on dependent variable.

Results: The magnitude of personal protective equipment utilization was 82.4 %. Service duration of >10 years [AOR: 0.23, 95 % CI: (0.09, 0.58)], availability of personal protective equipments [AOR: 21.73, 95 % CI: (8.62, 54.79)], shift work [AOR: 2.28, 95 % CI: (1.12, 4.66)], alcohol drinking [AOR: 0.26, 95 % CI: (0.10, 0.66)], and cigarette smoking [AOR: 0.20, 95 % CI: (0.05, 0.78)] were factors significantly associated with use of personal protective equipment.

Conclusion: In this study a relatively higher personal protective equipment utilization rate was reported compared to other studies in developing countries. However, this does not mean that there will be no need for further strengthening the safety programs as there are significant proportion of the workers still does not use all the necessary personal protective equipment during work. Interventions to promote use personal protective equipment should focus on areas, such as service duration, availability of protective equipment, presence of shift work, and control of substance abuse.

Keywords: Hazard control, Personal protective equipment, Safety, Textile factory, Workers

Background

The International Labour Organization has estimated that over 2 million people die every year from work-related accidents and diseases, and over 300 million non-fatal accidents are recorded each year [1]. This translates into more than 6000 deaths and over 800,000 non-fatal accidents every day. As a result of these, there is an estimated economic loss of more than $1.25 trillion each year, which is equivalent to 4.0 % of the world's Gross Domestic Product. This loss is 4 times higher for developing countries than that of industrialized countries [2, 3]. In many low and middle income countries, such as Ethiopia statistics on occupational accidents and injuries are limited. In cases where such information is available it is largely impaired by

* Correspondence: sbsbtadesse90@gmail.com
[1]Institute of Public Health, The University of Gondar, Gondar, Ethiopia
Full list of author information is available at the end of the article

underreporting. Considering the differences between countries, it is reasonable to agree that occupational deaths and injuries take a heavy toll among the poor and least protected.

Textile industry is one of labor intensive production and most technologically complex of all industries, and is a place of work where workers are exposed to different safety hazards, like cotton dust, excessive noise, accidents and diseases [4–7]. As result of this, workers, employers and government lost direct and indirect costs related to workplace injuries and illnesses [8]. The direct costs for employers include compensation and treatment costs that has to be paid to the disabled workers, and while the indirect costs include production disturbance costs, lost time of injured worker, time lost by supervisors or executive to follow the injured worker, training costs for new workers. The direct costs for workers include pain and suffering from the injury or illness, loss of income, loss of a job and health-care costs, and while the indirect costs include time lost by family members to care the disabled worker and utmost economic shock and social chaos [9, 10].

Use of personal protective equipment (PPE) is one of the important measures to safeguard workers from exposure to occupational hazards, especially in developing countries where conventional occupational safety control principles remain a challenge to implement [11–13]. Workers use of PPE is affected by socio-demographic, behavioral and work environment factors [14]. In textile factory they use different protective devices at different production sections. For example, they need to wear respirator, gloves, goggle, boot shoes, overall, ear plugs and mask at spinning section, and while reflector and helmet are worn in addition at engineering section.

Policies or measures for delivering health and safety services to factory workers are limited in Ethiopia. This not only limits their access to information and training opportunities but also places the workers at a greater risk to occupational injuries and diseases. Furthermore, literatures show that factory workers lack the knowledge on proper use of protective measures and are least aware of health effects emanating from the activities and materials in their work environments [13, 15, 16].

There is a dearth of studies describing PPE utilization among textile factory workers in most of Subsaharan African countries, like Ethiopia. This paper presents the findings of a study which investigated PPE utilization and associated factors among textile factory workers in southern Ethiopia, a low-income country in East Africa. This study addresses a critical gap in understanding PPE utilization in Ethiopia and contributes to the growing workplace safety research in low-income countries. Such studies may also help in developing evidence-based intervention strategies targeted at promoting workers safety and health.

Methods

Study design, area and period, and source population

An institution-based cross-sectional study was conducted to assess the magnitude of PPE utilization and associated factors among textile factory workers at Hawassa Town, southern Ethiopia, from January to March 2014. The town is located at 275 km South of Addis Ababa, the capital city of Ethiopia. During the investigation, there are about 1370 workers in the factory. Of whom, 65.0 % are permanent, 32.3 % temporary, and 2.7 % daily workers [17].

Participants and data collection

All textile factory workers who directly involved in the process of production at spinning, weaving, finishing, engineering, and garmenting departments were included in the study until the required sample size was obtained. Workers who were absent from work due to reasons other than work-related injuries during the time of data collection were excluded from the study. A pre-tested and structured interview questionnaire was used to collect the data. The questionnaire contained detail information on socio-demographic, behavioral and environmental factors, and utilization of PPE. Except age, all the factors were measured using a categorical scale of measurement.

Sample size calculation

Epi info version 7 was used to determine the sample size required for this study by taking 1370 total population, 49.3 % expected proportion of sickness absenteeism, 3 % confidence limit, and 95 % confidence level. By adding 10 % non-response rate, the total sample size was 660.

Sampling procedure

Stratified sampling followed by simple random sampling techniques was used to select the study participants. That is, the manufacturing units were stratified into five departments: spinning, weaving, finishing, engineering, and garment department. Then, the total of 660 samples was proportionally allocated to each department. The participants were drawn from the factory's list of workers using simple random sampling.

Data analyses

The training of data collectors and supervisors emphasized issues such as data collection instrument, field methods, inclusion–exclusion criteria, and record keeping. The principal investigator and supervisors coordinated the interview process, spot-checked and reviewed the completed questionnaire on a daily basis to ensure the completeness and consistency of the data collected. The interview questionnaire was pre-tested on 20 workers who work in a factory nearly similar to Hawassa Textile Factory in order to identify potential problem areas, unanticipated interpretations, and cultural objections to any of the questions. Based on the pre-test results the questionnaire was adjusted contextually.

Data entered and cleaned using Epi info version 7 statistical software were analyzed on SPSS version 16. Frequency distribution, mean, standard deviation, and percentage, were used for descriptive analyses. All independent variables were fitted separately into bivariate logistic regression model to evaluate the degree of association with utilization of PPE. Then, variables with a p-value < 0.20 were exported to multivariate logistic regression model to control confounders. The odds ratio (OR) with a 95 % confidence interval (CI) was used to test the statistical significance of variables. The crude OR was used to present the bivariate model outputs while the adjusted OR to the multivariate outputs.

Operational definitions

Utilization of PPE

Use of all the necessary worker-specialized clothing or equipment by workers for protection against health and safety hazards in the workplace [18]. Workers were classified as *those who used PPE* when they were observed wearing of all the PPE that were necessary to be worn during work in a particular working section. The necessarily worn PPE were: 1) a respirator, gloves, eye protector, boot shoes, overall, ear plugs and mask at spinning section, 2) respirator, gloves, eye protector, boot shoes, ear plugs and overall at weaving section, 3) respirator, gloves, mask, ear plugs, boot shoes and overall at finishing section, 4) respirator, gloves, boot shoes, eye protector, overall, reflector, mask and helmet at engineering section, and 5) gloves, boot shoes, mask and overall at garmenting section.

Worker

A person who is directly involved in the process of production and has an employment relationship with an employer [19].

Marital status

Workers are classified as married and single based on their risk difference to unsafe acts.

Ethical considerations

The study protocol was reviewed and approved by the Institutional Review Board of the University of Gondar via the Institute of Public Health. Permission was obtained from Hawassa Textile Factory Administrative Office prior to data collection. Study participants were interviewed after informed written consent was obtained. They were also informed that their participation was voluntary and that they could withdraw from the interview at any time without consequences. The participants were assured that their responses would be treated confidentially through the use of strict coding measures. Finally, safety education was given to workers who reported not utilizing the necessary PPE.

Results

Socio-demographic characteristics

A total of 660 workers who directly involved in the process of production participated in the study which makes the response rate 100 %. Of whom 80.8 % were males and 19.2 % females. The mean age with a standard deviation of the workers was 32.9 ± 9.3. More than two-thirds, 68.8 %, of them belonged to the age group of 18-39 years. The majority, 60.5 %, attended secondary and above education. About half, 47.0 %, served for more than 10 years in the factory. The majority, 58.0 %, of the workers were married. Nearly two-thirds, 63.3 %, had a monthly income of less than or equal to Birr 1500 (Table 1).

Table 1 Socio-demographic characteristics of textile factory workers at Hawassa Town, southern Ethiopia, 2014

Variables	Number	Percent
Sex		
Male	533	80.8
Female	127	19.2
Age (in years)		
18–25	200	30.3
26–39	254	38.5
> 39	206	31.2
Educational status		
Illiterate	17	2.5
Primary	244	37.0
Secondary	203	30.8
Above secondary	196	29.7
Service duration (in years)		
1–10	350	53.0
> 10	310	47.0
Marital status		
Married	383	58.0
Single	277	42.0
Monthly income (in Birr)		
1–1000	243	36.8
1001–1500	241	36.5
> 1500	176	26.7

Behavioral characteristics and environmental conditions

The majority, 80.3, 84.1 and 85.9 %, of the workers reported that they did not drink alcohol, chew khat and smoke cigarette, respectively. Three-fourths, 74.5 %, stated that they were satisfied with their job. The majority, 98.6, 93.6 and 62.9 %, informed that they used work guidelines, received safety orientation and attended safety training, respectively. Nearly two-thirds, 61.5 %, complained that there was no safety supervision during their work. Eighty five percent of the workers reported that there was a work shift in the factory. Nearly half, 47.0 %, stated that there was no work rotation. Poor conditions of ventilation and light in the working rooms were testified by 72.3 and 48.9 % of the workers, respectively (Table 2).

Magnitude of PPE utilization

Out of 660 workers 82.4 % were observed wearing of all the necessary PPE during work at the time of interview. Of whom 82.0 % were males and 18.0 % females. The majority, 68.6 %, of them belonged to the age group of 18 to 39 years. Fifty eight percent were married.

The magnitude of PPE utilization was 73.0 % spinning section, 76.0 % weaving section, 87.6 % finishing section, 87.3 % engineering section, and 88.2 % garmenting section (Table 3).

More than 17.0 % of the workers reported that they did not use all the necessary PPE during work. The reasons for not using PPE were for 43.0 % lack of PPE, for 20.0 % lack of practice, for 20 % uncomfortable to use, and for 17.0 % lack of safety education.

Factors associated with PPE utilization

Table 4 presents factors which remained statistically significant in the bivariate and multivariate logistic regression analyses. In this study, the independent predictors of PPE utilization on the multivariate analysis include service duration of >10 years [AOR: 0.23, 95 % CI: (0.09, 0.58)], availability of PPE [AOR: 21.73, 95 % CI: (8.62, 54.79)], shift work [AOR: 2.28, 95 % CI: (1.12, 4.66)], alcohol drinking [AOR: 0.26, 95 % CI: (0.10, 0.66)], and cigarette smoking [AOR: 0.20, 95 % CI: (0.05, 0.78)], (Table 4).

Table 2 Behavioral characteristics and environmental conditions of workers at Hawassa Textile Factory, southern Ethiopia, 2014

Variables	Number	Percent
Drink alcohol		
Yes	130	19.7
No	530	80.3
Chew khat		
Yes	105	15.9
No	555	84.1
Smoke cigarette		
Yes	93	14.1
No	567	85.9
Satisfied with job		
Yes	492	74.5
No	168	25.5
Used work guideline		
Yes	651	98.6
No	9	1.4
Attended safety training		
Yes	415	62.9
No	245	37.1
Orientation given		
Yes	618	93.6
No	42	6.4
Safety supervision		
Yes	254	38.5
No	406	61.5
Work shift		
Yes	562	85.2
No	98	14.8
Work rotation		
Yes	350	53.0
No	310	47.0
Ventilation		
Good	183	27.7
Poor	477	72.3
Light		
Good	337	51.1
Poor	323	48.9

Discussion

In this study, the magnitude of PPE utilization among textile factory workers was 82.4 %. This finding is by far higher than that of studies from Asia (12.0–49.4 %) [14, 20] and Africa (16.7–75.3 %) [12, 13, 15, 18, 21]. The difference could be due to methodological differences, like study population and methods of data collection, and workplace conditions, like employees' level of awareness on hazard control and disease prevention and accessibility to safety services. However, this does not mean that there will be no need for further strengthening the safety programs as there are significant proportion of the workers still does not use all the necessary PPE during work. The interventions should consider designing and provision of PPE, and regular safety education.

One important finding of this study was the identification of independent predictors influencing PPE utilization.

Table 3 Magnitude of PPE utilization by working section among textile factory workers in Hawassa Town, southern Ethiopia, 2014

Working section	Number	Percent
Spinning section		
Used	199	73.0
Not used	73	27.0
Weaving section		
Used	109	76.0
Not used	34	24.0
Finishing section		
Used	65	87.6
Not used	9	12.4
Engineering section		
Used	57	87.3
Not used	8	12.7
Garment section		
Used	94	88.2
Not used	12	11.8

It was found that the odds of PPE utilization among workers who served for greater than 10 years were 0.77 times less when compared to those who served for less than or equal to 10 years. The possible explanation for this may be that those who served for longer period could be accustomed to the work environment and developed false consciousness of safety which might drive them not to comply with safety precautions including proper use of PPE. Thus, giving attention for this segment of workers may contribute for safety improvement.

Table 4 Factors associated with associated with PPE utilization among textile factory workers in Hawassa Town, southern Ethiopia, 2014

Variables	Utilized PPE		Crude OR (95 % CI)	Adjusted OR (95 % CI)
	Yes	No		
Service duration (in year)				
1–10	272	78	1.0	1.0
> 10	272	38	2.05 (1.35, 3.13)	0.23 (0.09, 0.58)
PPE available				
Yes	531	62	0.03 (0.02, 0.05)	21.73 (8.62, 54.79)
No	13	54	1.0	1.0
Shift work				
Yes	475	87	0.44 (0.27, 0.71)	2.28 (1.12, 4.66)
No	69	29	1.0	1.0
Drink alcohol				
Yes	106	24	1.08 (0.66, 1.77)	0.26(0.10, 0.66)
No	438	92	1.0	1.0
Smoke cigarette				
Yes	86	7	0.34 (0.15, 0.76)	0.20 (0.05, 0.78)
No	458	109	1.0	1.0

Like in previous studies [16, 18], availability of PPE was found to be strong independent predictor of PPE utilization in this study. Cognizant of this fact, safety administration programs should consider availing of all the necessary PPE on regular bases to promote health and safety in the workplace.

In this study the odds of PPE utilization among workers who worked in shift were about two times high when compared to those who did not. The reason behind this could be that shift work encourages workers towards PPE utilization by providing adequate time to think for and communicate about their safety. This signifies that there is a need for revising of work schedule to promote use of PPE in the factory.

Cigarette smoking and alcohol drinking also showed significance association with PPE utilization. The odds of PPE utilization among cigarette smokers and alcoholists were 0.80 and 0.74 times less, respectively when compared to their counter parts. This might be due to the fact that smoking and drinking are proxy indicators of a certain degree of risk tolerance. A high blood level of such substances during work will endanger both safety and efficiency, and be the cause of increased likelihood of mistakes, poor decision making, and errors in judgment. As the result of this fact, the factory's safety policy should consider control of substance abuse at workplace.

Social desirability bias is a potential limitation in self–reported studies like this one, in that workers might report socially acceptable responses than their actual day to day practice. As this is a cross–sectional study, the limitations that come with this type of design need to be taken into consideration when interpreting the findings.

Conclusion

In this study a relatively higher PPE utilization rate was observed compared to other studies in developing countries. However, this does not mean that there will be no need for further strengthening the safety programs as there are significant proportion of the workers still does not use all the necessary PPE during work. Interventions to promote PPE utilization should focus on areas, such as service duration, availability of PPE, presence of shift work, and control of substance abuse.

Competing interests
The authors declare that they have no competing interest.

Authors' contribution
Author 1. ST: Involved in write up of the research proposal, the data analyses, and wrote the manuscript, Author 2. TK: Involved in write up of the research proposal, the data analyses, and wrote the manuscript, Author 3. YA: Involved in write up of the research proposal. All authors read and approved the final manuscript.

Acknowledgments
The authors wish to thank the Southern Nations Nationalities and Peoples Regional State Bureau of Labor and Social Affairs for logistic and administrative support, and data collectors for their support in making this study possible. They also extend their deepest gratitude to the study participants.

Author details
[1]Institute of Public Health, The University of Gondar, Gondar, Ethiopia.
[2]Southern Nations Nationalities and People's Regional State Health Bureau, Hawassa, Ethiopia.

References

1. International Labour Organization. Safety and Health at Work; 2015. [Accessed at: 25/09/2015]. [Available from: http://ilo.org/global/topics/safety-and-health-at-work/lang–en/index.htm.]
2. International Labor Organization.Workplace health promotion;2014. [Accessed at: 1/15/2014].
3. International Labor Organization. World Day for Safety and Health at Work; 2013. [Accessed at: 1/15/2014].
4. Conn R, Barclay L. Health education in the workplace. AAOHN J. 2008;2(28):407–12.
5. Gawenda D. Occupational Health Nursing Care Guidelines. Springer Publishing Company, Boston 2008; 2(2):17-30.
6. Danton S. Prevention of Injury and Disease in occupational Health Nursing Practice, Harris CJ 2009; second edition, 48-75.
7. Sewefy A. Health hazard and safety. J Egypt Med Assoc. 2009;51(3):757.
8. Health and Safety Executive. Costs to Britain of workplace fatalities and self reported injuries and ill health; 2010/2011: 5-36.
9. Aghera N. Occupational health and safety with special reference to textile industry research scholar. Singhania university, Acheri Bari-Jhunjhunu 2013;2(3):2277-8160.
10. Hildegunn K. The global textile and clothing industry post the agreement on textiles and clothing. World Trade Organization Geneva, Switzerland 2007; 2(3):6.
11. Malik N, Mean AA, Pasha TS, Akhtar S, Ali T. Role of hazard control measures in occupational health and safety in the textile industry of Pakistan. Pak J Agri Sci. 2010;47(1):72–6.
12. Kamal A, Sayed M, Massoud A. Usage of personal protective devices among Egyptian industrial workers. Am J Ind Med. 2007;13(6):706–16.
13. Akintayo WL. Knowledge, attitude and practice on the use of personal protective equipment by traditional resist Fabrics workers in Abeokuta, Nigeria. Kuwait Rev Chapter Arabian J Bus Manag Rev. 2013;2(7):31–3.
14. Jaiswal A. Case Control study among carpet thread factory workers in Uttar Pradesh, India: Occupational injury and its deteriorating factors. Global J Human Soc Sci History and Anthr 2012;12:22-30.
15. Motbainor A, Kumie A, Melkamu Y. Assessment of knowledge and practice on safety information among factory workers Addis Ababa, Ethiopia. Addis Ababa University; 2007.
16. Ahmad I, Qadir S, Muhammad, Yasir M, Irfanullah M, Khan MA, Aslam, SZ, Alam J, Iqbal J, Sikandar I, Waqas M. Knowledge, attitude and practice related to occupational health and safety among textile mills workers in Dera Ismail Khan. Gomal J Med Sci 2012;10 222-226.
17. Southern Nations Nationalities and Peoples Regional State. Hawassa textile factory manpower summary data. Hawassa: Hawassa Textile Factory; 2013.
18. Zungu L, Gabe SG. A survey of work, health and safety conditions in small-scale garment enterprises in Gaborone, Botswana. Occup Health Southern Africa 2011;17:13-19.
19. Ministry of Labor and Social Affairs. Labor proclamation No. 377/2003. Addis Ababa: Labor and Social Affairs; 2004.
20. Parimalam P, Kamalamma N, Kumar A. Knowledge, attitude and practices related to occupational health problems among garment workers in Tamil Nadu, India. J Occup Health. 2007;49(6):528–34.
21. Aderaw Z, Engedaw D, Tadesse T. Determinants of occupational injury: a case control study among textile factory workers in Amhara Regional State, Ethiopia. J Trop Med. 2011;2011:1–8.

15

Assessment of long-term cultivated human precision-cut lung slices as an ex vivo system for evaluation of chronic cytotoxicity and functionality

Vanessa Neuhaus[1], Dirk Schaudien[1], Tatiana Golovina[2], Ulla-Angela Temann[2], Carolann Thompson[2], Torsten Lippmann[3], Claus Bersch[4], Olaf Pfennig[4], Danny Jonigk[3], Peter Braubach[3], Hans-Gerd Fieguth[5], Gregor Warnecke[6], Vidadi Yusibov[2], Katherina Sewald[1*†] and Armin Braun[1,7†]

Abstract

Background: Investigation of basic chronic inflammatory mechanisms and development of new therapeutics targeting the respiratory tract requires appropriate testing systems, including those to monitor long- persistence. Human precision-cut lung slices (PCLS) have been demonstrated to mimic the human respiratory tract and have potential of an alternative, ex-vivo system to replace or augment in-vitro testing and animal models. So far, most research on PCLS has been conducted for short cultivation periods (≤72 h), while analyses of slowly metabolized therapeutics require long-term survival of PCLS in culture. In the present study, we evaluated viability, physiology and structural integrity of PCLS cultured for up to 15 days.

Methods: PCLS were cultured for 15 days and various parameters were assessed at different time points.

Results: Structural integrity and viability of cultured PCLS remained constant for 15 days. Moreover, bronchoconstriction was inducible over the whole period of cultivation, though with decreased sensitivity (EC_{50}1d = 4×10^{-8} M vs. EC_{50}15d = 4×10^{-6} M) and reduced maximum of initial airway area (1d = 0.5% vs. 15d = 18.7%). In contrast, even though still clearly inducible compared to medium control, LPS-induced TNF-α secretion decreased significantly from day 1 to day 15 of culture.

Conclusions: Overall, though long-term cultivation of PCLS need further investigation for cytokine secretion, possibly on a cellular level, PCLS are feasible for bronchoconstriction studies and toxicity assays.

Keywords: Precision-cut lung slices, PCLS, Long-term cultivation, Bronchoconstriction, Human, Cytokines, Cytotoxicity

Background

Respiratory diseases, both chronic and acute, account for millions of deaths every year. In 2012 about 68% of global deaths were caused by noncommunicable diseases (NCD), with chronic lung disease being one of the four main reasons [1]. The very fact that of the approximately 38 million annual deaths attributed to NCD about 10.5% are accounted for by chronic respiratory diseases (CRD) [2], emphasizes the urgent need for improved respiratory therapies.

In this context of understanding physiological lung behavior *in-vitro,* it is essential to develop new therapeutic substances. In recent years, the technique of precision-cut lung slices (PCLS) has expanded the tools available for respiratory research with a link between human based in-vitro models and complex cellular anatomy [3]. PCLS, as a 3D organotypic tissue model, reflects the natural and relevant microanatomy of the respiratory tract, as well as its functional responses to specific stimuli [4–7]. Especially with regard to the three Rs principle, PCLS represents an

* Correspondence: katherina.sewald@item.fraunhofer.de
†Equal contributors
[1]Fraunhofer Institute for Toxicology and Experimental Medicine, Hannover, Germany, Biomedical Research in Endstage and Obstructive Lung Disease Hannover (BREATH), Member of the German Centre for Lung Research (DZL), Member of the REBIRTH Cluster of Excellence, Hanover, Germany
Full list of author information is available at the end of the article

alternative to *in-vivo* models and can help to reduce the number of animal studies [3].

Since the description of human agarose-filled lung slices in 1994 [8], optimizations have been made to reproducibly prepare very thin tissue slices of defined thickness. These improvements have led to the wide application of the PCLS technique [7, 9–11]. Ever since, PCLS from different species have been used for the assessment of pharmacological and toxicological compounds [7, 9, 10], as well as to model airway constriction [6]. Additionally, the use of PCLS as a model has expanded into the fields of nanotechnology [12, 13] and virology [14]. However, most of these studies using PCLS were conducted under short-term culturing conditions (≤72 h) [9, 13, 15], which limits their value to certain questions investigating rapid and acute effects. Accordingly, slowly metabolized therapeutics or chemicals, as well as repeated applications, which might be important to investigate basic mechanisms and treatments of CRD, have not been addressed with cultured PCLS. Even though some effort has been made prior to 2000 to establish long-term cultivation of agarose-embedded tracheal and lung tissue [16–18], these studies only focused on limited endpoints to evaluate the feasibility of long-term cultivation of lung tissue.

The maintenance of structural and cellular integrity of long-term cultivated murine or porcine lungs has primarily been evaluated microscopically [16, 17]. Recently a manuscript has been published that uses different endpoints for long-term cultivation of human PCLS, focusing on PCLS as a "high-throughput, *ex vivo* system for evaluating the safety, and potentially immunogenicity, of vaccines and pharmaceuticals" [19]. However, to our knowledge there is no study investigating multiple structural and functional endpoints after long-term cultivation of human lung tissue slices.

In the context of CRD research models, PCLS have been used as a supportive tool after disease establishment *in-vivo* [20]. This approach limits pre-clinical CRD research to either animal in-vivo studies or the use of human material from patients with the desired but very advanced disease qualifying them for lung resection.

In order to extend the research applications that PCLS can be used for, the current study evaluated long-term cultivated human PCLS with regard to their feasibility as a model for CRD research in terms of viability, physiology and structure. The intention of the study was not to introduce PCLS as a new technique, but to combine established methods and investigate the value of PCLS at a functional level as a long term cultivation model, which in our opinion has been lacking so far. The results of the present study extend the published work on long-term organ cultures and demonstrate the feasibility of using human PCLS as a long-term model for bronchoconstriction and cytotoxicity studies.

Methods

Culture media and reagents

Bicinchoninic acid (BCA) total protein kit, Earle's Balanced Salt Solution (EBSS) and Dulbecco's Modified Eagle's Medium Nutrient Mixture F-12 Ham (DMEM, pH 7.2–7.4, without phenol red) with L-glutamine and 15 mM HEPES were obtained from GIBCO (Thermo Fisher Scientific, Rockford, IL, USA). DMEM was supplemented with 100 U/mL penicillin and 100 μg/mL streptomycin. Phosphate buffered solution (PBS, pH 7.4) and lyophilized lipopolysaccharide (LPS) of *Escherichia coli*, serotype 0111:B4 were purchased from Lonza (Verviers, Belgium). WST-1 assay kit was obtained from Roche (Mannheim, Germany). Low-gelling agarose and protease inhibitor cocktail P1860 were obtained from Sigma Aldrich (Munich, Germany).

Human donors and ethics statement

Providing written informed consent for PCLS experiments from all patients, lung lobes were obtained immediately after surgical resection at Hannover Medical School or KRH Klinikum Oststadt-Heidehaus. For lung tumor patients, only tumor-free tissue was used. Experiments were in accordance with *The Code of Ethics of the World Medical Association* and approved by the Ethics Committee of the Hannover Medical School.

Lung donors for this study were diverse regarding age, gender, medical history and cause of resection. The average age of donors was 64 years (Additional file 1: Table S1). The number of patients is indicated in each figure.

Preparation of PCLS

Human PCLS were prepared as previously described [7]. Briefly, lungs were gently inflated with warm 1.5% agarose-DMEM mix. Afterwards, lung explants were macroscopically assessed by an experienced pulmopathologist to identify regions of interest and exclude previously unknown medical conditions (e.g. neoplasias or infections). Sections (∅ 8 mm) were sliced in cold EBSS using a Krumdieck tissue slicer (Alabama Research and Development, Munford, AL, USA) into approx. 250–300 μm thin slices. PCLS were washed thoroughly before cultivation in DMEM (2 slice per 500 μl) under normal immersion culture conditions (37 °C, 5% CO_2, and 100% air humidity) for up to 15 days. PCLS treated for 1 h with 1% Triton X-100 served as a dead reference.

WST-1 assay

Viability of PCLS was assessed by metabolic activity using the WST-1 assay according to the manufacturer's instructions and as described before [7]. PCLS were incubated with 0.125 mL/slice of diluted WST-1 solution (1:10, according to manufacture's instructions) for 1 h at

37 °C. Optical density (OD) was measured at 420–480 nm with a reference wavelength of 690 nm.

Calcein AM/ethidium homodimer-1 ("LIVE/DEAD®") staining and quantitative image analysis

For microscopic assessment of viability, PCLS were incubated with 2 µM Calcein AM and 5 µM Ethidium homodimer-I (EthD-1) for 45 min at room temperature in the dark on an orbital shaker (150 rpm) using the Live/Dead® Viability/Cytotoxicity kit from Life Technologies (Darmstadt, Germany), as previously described [7]. After washing, the slices were imaged on a confocal laser scanning microscope Meta 510 (LSM, Zeiss, Jena, Germany) using a 10× objective. From each PCLS, triplicates of 30 µm thick 3D stacks were recorded randomly and analyzed using IMARIS 7.4.0 software (Bitplane Scientific Software, Zurich, Switzerland), as described previously [7]. The ratio of counted dead cell nuclei (ex/em 517 nm/617 nm; red fluorescence) to total volume of cytoplasm of living cells (ex/em 494 nm/517 nm; green fluorescent) was calculated (dead cell nuclei/10^6 μm^3 cytoplasm volume).

Measurement of cytokine secretion by enzyme-linked immunosorbent assay (ELISA)

PCLS culture supernatants were collected, supplemented with 0.2% P1860, and stored at −80 °C. Human Tumor necrosis factor-alpha (TNF-α) was measured using the human TNF-α DuoSet from R&D Systems (Wiesbaden-Nordenstadt, Germany) according to the manufacturer's specifications and as described elsewhere [7]. OD was determined at 450 nm (reference wavelength 540 nm) using the Tecan reader Infinite 200 PRO (Crailsheim, Germany). Cytokine concentration refers to 2 slices per time point and donor, measured in duplicate.

Methacholine-induced bronchoconstriction

Bronchoconstriction was measured according to the protocol by Seehase et al. [21]. One slice was transferred into a 6-well plate with 2 mL DMEM (supplemented with 25 mM HEPES) per measurement and fixed with a slice anchor (Warner Instruments, Hamden, CT, USA). Methacholine (Mch) was added stepwise. After addition of each concentration of Mch (10^{-9} to 10^{-3} M), pictures were recorded in 5 s intervals for 3 min with a stereo microscope (Discovery V8; Zeiss, Jena, Germany) controlled by the Axio Vision 4.8.2. software program (Zeiss, Jena, Germany). Images were analyzed with the ImageJ analysis program (National Institute of Health).

Histopathology analysis

PCLS were fixed in 10% neutral buffered formalin, embedded in paraffin, and sliced into 4–5 µm thin slices. The paraffin slices were stained with hematoxylin and eosin (H&E) using standard histological procedures and mounted for light microscopy. Magnification and scale bars are indicated in the figure.

Statistical analysis

Mann-Whitney tests were performed for statistical analyses using GraphPad 4.03 (GraphPad, San Diego, CA). Data were expressed as Box and Whiskers or mean ± standard error of the mean (SEM). Differences between different time points were considered statistically significant at the level of $p < 0.05$.

Results

Human PCLS showed persistent viability during 15-day long-term cultivation

In order to determine the viability of freshly prepared human lung tissue slices in immersion culture, PCLS were cultivated for 15 days and analyzed using different assays. Within this time frame no significant decrease of metabolic activity was detected by the WST-1 assay, indicating no long-term loss in viability after several days in culture. In contrast, a 1-h treatment with Triton X-100, a commonly used detergent, abrogated metabolic activity completely (Fig. 1).

Additionally, Calcein AM staining of the tissue showed an overall presence of living tissue with visible alveolar structures, which were maintained for the entire period of cultivation. Quantitative analysis of Live/Dead® staining showed no significant differences over time. The dead cell control with Triton X-100 showed only nuclei of dead cells and no vital tissue (Fig. 2).

Human PCLS sustained the ability for bronchoconstriction

In order to determine the physiology of long-term cultured human PCLS, Mch -induced bronchoconstriction was measured. Slices were treated with different concentrations of Mch and constriction of the airways was imaged via stereo microscopy (Fig. 3a). The ability of the PCLS to constrict upon Mch stimulus was sustained over the 15-day cultivation time (Fig. 3b). The reactivity of the airway, however, decreased during cultivation (Table 1). The capability to fully constrict upon treatment with the highest concentration of Mch, which was observed on the first day, decreased until day 15, with a maximal constriction of 81% (equals 19% initial airway area [IAA] remaining; Table 1). Additionally, the sensitivity of the airways decreased, as shown by increased EC_{50} values (Table 1). For the first 24 h after preparation,

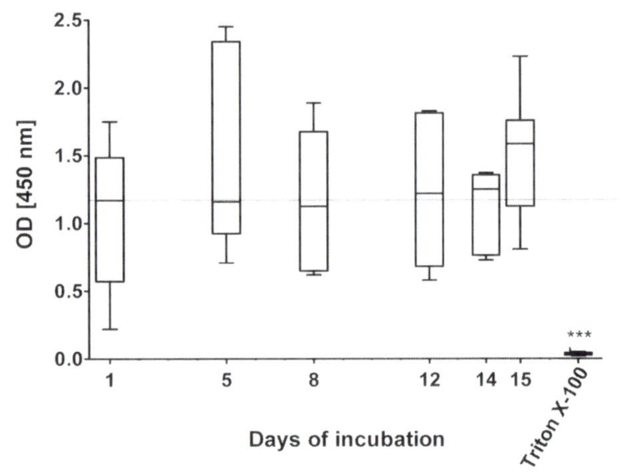

Fig. 1 Metabolic activity of long-term cultured human PCLS. Metabolic activity in human PCLS was determined by the WST-1 assay. The negative control Triton X-100, a commonly used detergent, decreased metabolic activity in human PCLS to an OD corresponding to background (~0.04). Data are presented as *Box* and *Whiskers*, Mann-Whitney test (WST-1: $n = 8_{(\text{day 1, 8, 15, Triton})}$, $n = 5_{(\text{day 5})}$, $n = 6_{(\text{day 12, 14})}$). The dotted line marks the mean measured OD on day 1. PCLS = precision cut lung slices

a dose of 0.37 nM Mch was sufficient to induce a 50% reduction of the IAA. In contrast, 15 days after preparation a 100-fold higher dose (38 nM Mch) was needed to achieve this same IAA reduction. A high variability between different donors, however, needs to be pointed out. Slices from different donors do not constrict equally at the same day, though the trend towards a steady decrease in reactivity and sensitivity were observed for each donor individually.

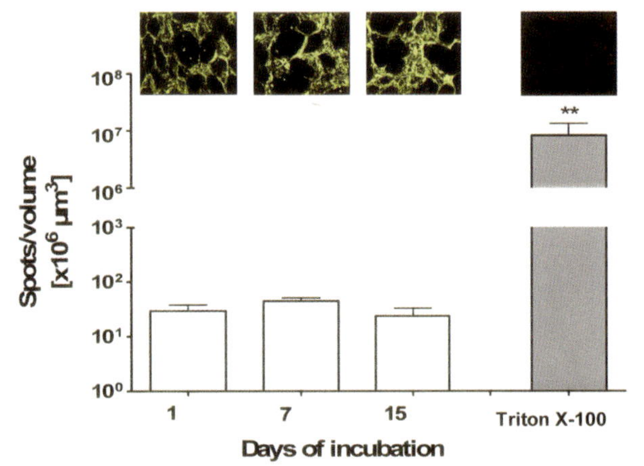

Fig. 2 Three dimensional detection and quantitative image analysis of viability staining of long-term cultured human PCLS. Human lung slices were stained with Calcein AM (yellow) and Ethidium homodimer 1 (EthD-1; red). Three stacks per slice of 30 µm thickness were taken randomly at days 1, 7 and 15. One representative images for each time point is shown. The stacks were analysed using IMARIS 5.5.3. software and were quantitatively evaluated as the number of *red* nuclei of dead cells (*spots*) per 10^6 μm^3 volume of *yellow vital tissue* Triton X-100 served as a dead cell control. Data are presented as *Box* and *Whiskers*, $^{**}p < 0.01$ compared to day 1, Mann-Whitney test ($n = 6_{(\text{day 1, 7, Triton})}$, $n = 4_{(\text{day15})}$)

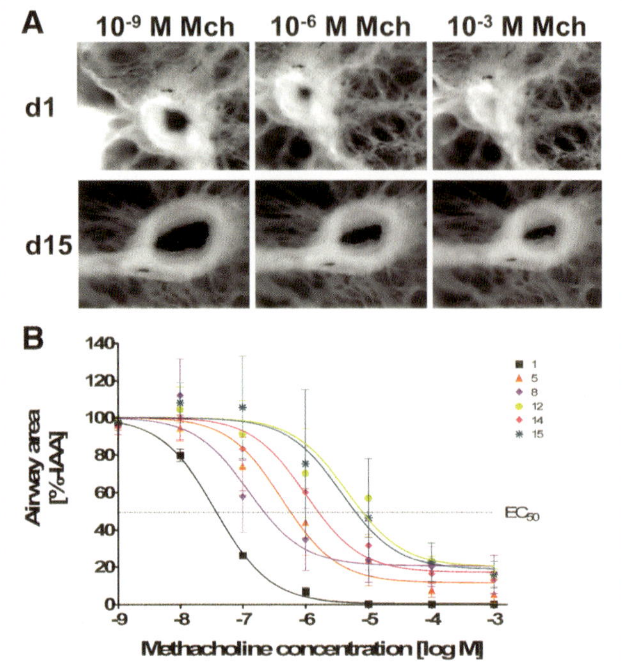

Fig. 3 Methacholine-induced bronchoconstriction in long-term cultured human PCLS. PCLS with intact airways and surrounding epithelium were used to measure methacholine-induced bronchoconstriction at different time points. Different concentrations of methacholine (10^{-9} to 10^{-3} M) were added to the slice and slice constriction was recorded by a stereo microscope (**a**). Images were analyzed by the ImageJ analysis program. The first control picture of the non-constricted airway was set to 100%. The methacholine-induced reduction of the airway area was related to the 100% airway area of the initial airway (**b**). Measurements were conducted in at least duplicate. Data are presented as mean ± SEM, $n = 3$. Mch = methacholine, %-IAA = percentage of initial airway area, EC_{50} = half maximal effective concentration

LPS-induced release of TNF-α was declining during 15-day long-term cultivation

The ability of PCLS to release the pro-inflammatory cytokine TNF-α upon LPS stimulation was evaluated at different time points during culture (Fig. 4). Human PCLS were stimulated once with 100 ng/mL LPS for 20 h before the released TNF-α was measured. Media-treated slices served as controls. The level of LPS-induced and secreted TNF-α was shown to continuously decrease over time, from 1168 ± 223 pg/mL at the first day post preparation to 93 ± 54 pg/mL at day 15.

Table 1 Maximal airway constriction and EC_{50} concentrations of methacholine at different days of cultured human PCLS

Days of incubation	1	5	8	12	14	15
Maximal constriction [% IAA]	0.426	11	20	20	17	19
EC50 [$\times 10^{-9}$ M]	0.37	4	1	47	10	38

However, the level of basal TNF- α measured in the untreated medium-controls also diminished drastically from 238 ± 122 pg/mL (day 1) to 13 ± 5 pg/mL (day 5) and further to 7 ± 3 pg/mL (day 15). Therefore, after 15-day cultivation, LPS-induced TNF-α secretion is still 13 times higher than the baseline level measured in the control medium (93 ± 54 pg/mL vs. 7 ± 3 pg/mL).

The overall structural integrity of human PCLS maintained over a 15-day cultivation period

In order to visualize pathological changes in lung tissue, PCLS were stained and imaged for histopathological analyses (Fig. 5a-i). The H&E staining revealed intact maintenance of the extracellular matrix of the lung, such as collagen and alveolar septal structure, although the slight beginning of separation of the connective tissue fibers was observed on day 7. The best preservation was observed for the bronchiolar epithelium, followed by the bronchiolar wall, the vasculature and the connective tissue. A high number of intact macrophages were observed within the tissue over time from day 1 until day 15 (Arrows Fig. 5b, e & h). The number of pneumocytes, on the other hand, seemed to be reduced during long-term cultivation. The smooth muscles remained intact for the entire period of cultivation (Arrows Fig. 5c, f & i). Also of note, there was no overgrowth of fibroblasts observable at any time point.

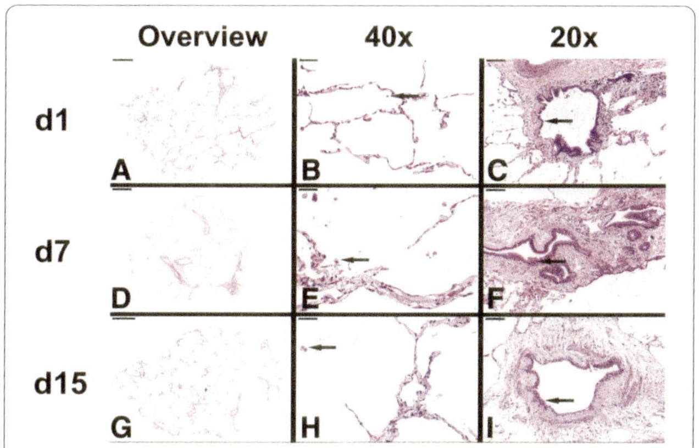

Fig. 5 Histopathological staining of long-term cultured human PCLS. Representative pictures of human PCLS stained at days 1, 7 and 15 post preparation. The pictures show an overview of PCLS at different time points (**a**, **d** & **g**; left row), close-up pictures of alveolar regions with alveolar macrophages (**b**, **e** & **h**; arrow; middle row, 40× magnification) and close-up pictures of larger airways with bronchiolar epithelium (**c**, **f** & **i**; arrows; right row, 20× magnification)

Discussion

The aim of the current study was to evaluate long-term maintenance of human PCLS as a tool for CRD research, as defined by a range of viability and physiology markers. Our study completes the data set of long-term cultivation of human PCLS presented by the work of Temann et al. [19] by several important structural and functional (e.g. bronchoconstriction) assays. Overall, the present study demonstrates that human PCLS can be kept in culture for up to 15 days without the loss of structural integrity, which is consistent with earlier studies focusing only on the structure of murine tissue slices [17, 18]. Further, the here presented histology data shows no overgrowth of fibroblasts during the serum-free cultivation of human PCLS, which is in agreement with the work of Siminski et al. on mouse lungs [17]. The presented study investigates on the one hand different vitality markers, completing the recently published work of Temann et al., and on the other hand functionality markers of long-term cultivated human PCLS, which to our knowledge have not been described before. Thus, this manuscript adds useful data to evaluate the overall quality of human PCLS as a long-term tool for CRD research. For the present study, a standard slice thickness range of 250–300 μm was used in an immersion culture. In contrast, some other groups investigating long-term cultivation of lung tissue have used several millimeter thick slices and cultured them as air-liquid interface (ALI) cultures, for example either on a foam matrix or in a rotating fashion (e.g. in Leighton tubes) [16, 18]. ALI culture mimics the natural *in-vivo* air contact of the epithelial cells in-vitro [22], with one side of the tissue being exposed to about 21% oxygen. Oxygen supply is an important factor for maintaining tissue culture and the well-being of lung cells. Several years ago, an influence of tissue slice thickness and oxygen penetration was evaluated, demonstrating that

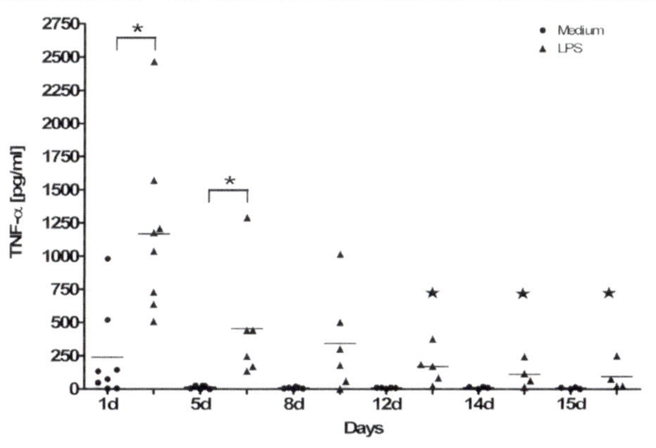

Fig. 4 Extracellular LPS-induced release of TNF-α in long-term cultured human PCLS. Human PCLS were treated once at indicated time points without (control) or with 100 ng/mL LPS and incubated for 20 h. The cytokine levels of TNF-α in PCLS culture supernatants were determined by ELISA. TNF-α levels are depicted as mg/mL. Data are presented as mean ± SEM, *$p < 0.05$ compared to TNF-α secreted by untreated PCLS, ★$p < 0.05$ compared LPS-induced TNF-α at day 1, Mann-Whitney test ($n = 8_{(day\ 1)}$, $n = 6_{(day5,\ 8,\ 12)}$, $n = 4_{(day\ 14,\ 15)}$). TNF-α = Tumor necrosis factor alpha, LPS = Lipopolysaccharide, ELISA = Enzyme Linked Immunosorbent Assay

increased slice thickness decreased the oxygen supply due to reduced diffusion, which subsequently leads to a decreased viability of cells in the center of the slices [23]. Although these observations were made for non-agarose filled organs different from the lung, they are conforming to the observations we made here. In line with an earlier report on long-term cultivated PCLS [19], the slice viability in the presented study was evaluated by several different assays, demonstrating a constant number of vital cells with metabolic activity over the duration of cultivation. A decreased cell vitality in the middle of the slices can mostly be excluded by microscopically Live/Dead® staining (max. Penetration depth ~ 150 μm). Application of a second assay (WST-1 in this case), however, supports the microscopic data that the tissue remains vital over the described culturing period. Additionally, microscopically observed cilia movement, as well as the ability of the airways to constrict upon Mch stimulation, both observed for the complete duration of cultivation, indicated the presence of intact, functional and vital smooth muscle and epithelial cells. This suggests a sufficient oxygen supply to PCLS, even in the immersion tissue culture.

Despite the constant viability measurements, the results of the present study also demonstrate that changes in the cellular composition and/or the functionality of certain cells may have occurred. The sensitivity of the airways to Mch stimulation decreased time-dependently (EC_{50}day1 = 0.37 nM Mch vs. EC_{50}day15 = 38 nM Mch). Likewise, the reactivity to Mch decreased from day 1 to day 8, as seen by the altered maximal bronchoconstriction values (IAA_{day1} = 0% vs. IAA_{day8} = 20%). However, it seems that the reactivity reached a plateau and does not further decrease after 1 week of cultivation (IAA_{day8} = 20% vs. IAA_{day15} = 19%). Therefore, a clear Mch-induced bronchoconstriction was detectable for the complete duration of the long-term cultivation.

Another alteration at the cellular level within the PCLS, which has also been described before [19], is indicated by the decreased ability to secrete the pro-inflammatory cytokine TNF-α upon LPS stimulation. Even though cells still secreted 13-times more TNF-α upon LPS stimulation at day 15 compared to the baseline level measured in the untreated controls, secretion of TNF-α decreased significantly from day 1 to day 15 (1168 ± 222.8 pg/mL vs. 93 ± 54 pg/mL). One explanation might be the serum-free or Granulocyte macrophage-colony stimulating factor (GM-CSF)-free culturing conditions used for PCLS, as TNF-α is mostly secreted by macrophages, but also by natural killer cells, B and T cells and epithelial cells [24, 25]. Macrophages in single cell culture, however, seemed to depend on the presence of GM-CSF or serum for better cell survival and TNF-α secretion upon activation [26, 27]. These macrophages secreted about twice as much TNF-α upon stimulation compared with control [26]. Noteworthy, monocytes at day 1 secreted about 4-times as much TNF-α as GM-CSF-cultivated macrophages at day 3, indicating that differentiated macrophages in culture lose TNF-α-secreting ability over time, even in the presence of GM-CSF [26]. The observations made in single cell culture systems that upon stimulation TNF-α secretion by macrophages decreases per se over time, with or without medium supplements, indicate that altered TNF-α secretion in long-term PCLS culture may be a problem of cultivation in general rather than specifically of PCLS. Further, we also observed a decline in TNF-α secretion, even for the untreated media control PCLS, from day 1 to day 5 and further until day 15 (238 ± 122 pg/mL vs. 7 ± 3 pg/mL) as has been described before [19]. This suggests that some basal TNF-α secretion occurs at the initiation of culture (day 1), either due to PCLS preparation or because of the origin of the tissue. The slicing process induces some stress for the cells, especially for those located at the cutting edge. Moreover, the complete preparation process of the human lungs (surgery, agarose filling, transport to the laboratory, cutting) takes several hours, where the lungs, though kept on ice and in media, are exposed to several stress factors. However, experience has demonstrated that after a resting phase (in medium at 37 °C) the induction of immediate early responses (e.g. genes & cytokines) are not affected [3]. In order to minimize the effect of the PCLS preparation process, the slices were thoroughly washed with medium and left for several hours under cell culture conditions before experiments were started. Yet, the influence of the cutting process, though minimized, cannot be fully excluded. It is important to note, however, that the level of this non-induced basal TNF-α release is significantly lower than what was observed after LPS treatment. In the context of a general decrease in TNF-α secretion in cell culture, it might be plausible that without the addition of essential supplements to the culture, cells responsible for TNF-α secretion may rapidly die. Yet, in the present study, macrophages appeared to survive 15-day long-term PCLS cultivation, as demonstrated by complementary histopathological analysis. However, macrophages and monocytes are not the only source of TNF-α, and other cells in PCLS may also undergo cell death in serum-free long-term culture. To elucidate this question, further studies need to look in more detail into the cellular composition of PCLS after long-term cultivation.

Working with human samples includes another important factor that needs to be considered: high inter-individual variation. Wouters et al. investigated inter- and intra-individual variations of LPS-induced cytokine (e.g. TNF-α) responses in a human whole blood assay

[28]. In the present study, high inter-individual variation can be observed, especially at the first day of culture. This inter-individual variation declined during cultivation, at least for the medium control. The variations in response to LPS stimulation observed here may have been caused by the different medical background of the donors (diseases and/or different treatments, such as chemotherapy). The inter-individual variations may also play a key role in the scattering observed for the Mch-induced bronchoconstriction. Yet, regardless of the inter-individual variations, inducible bronchoconstriction and cytokine responses were observed, even after a 15-day long-term cultivation.

Conclusions

Overall, the here presented data complement the work of Temann and colleagues [19], that long-term cultivation of PCLS for chronic exposure experiments are feasible with regard to their viability. Additionally, and new to this field is that this assumption is also supported by the maintenance of some physiological features such as bronchoconstriction. However, other questions still need to be further elucidated and protocols further adapted, to determine the exact cellular composition of lung tissue after long-term cultivation and chronic exposure. Yet, the presented data show convincingly that the extended culturing time frame of vital and functional human tissue, in regard to long-term cultivation, might increase the application of the ex-vivo technique of PCLS. PCLS have mainly been used to investigate local respiratory irritation and immunotoxicity of potential sensitizers or anti-cancer drugs [9, 29]. On the other hand, PCLS were established as disease models, reflecting features of inflammation, infection or early allergic responses mimicked by passive sensitization [14, 30–33]. Disease models involving cellular remodeling have hardly been established in PCLS. Kasper et al. established an early fibrosis model in rat PCLS using a 3-day protocol monitoring early pathohistological changes, such as extracellular matrix accumulation and myofibroblast transdifferentiation and activation of microvascular endothelial cells [34]. In line with this, Lin and colleagues also established a lung fibrosis model using 1–2 mm thick rat slices in an ALI culture, observing the fibrosis with typically increased alveolar septa thickness [35]. However, these protocols were used in rodent tissue and either did not require cultivation for longer than 3 days or did not monitor viability or functionality.

Corresponding to these earlier PCLS models of slowly progressive pulmonary diseases (e.g. interstitial lung diseases), our data might contribute to the development of further subacute or even CRD ex-vivo disease models and new therapeutic substances for these, particularly including slowly metabolized therapeutics.

Acknowledgments

The authors would like to thank Susanne Romberg, Christopher Fromm, Emma Spies and Olga Danov for their technical assistance. Furthermore, the authors would like to thank Natasha Kushnir and Stephen J. Streatfield for critical reading of the manuscript, as well as Dr. R. Kellner for statistical advice.

Funding

The work was part of a funded study by the Defense Threat Reduction Agency (DTRA; HDTRA-12-C-092). DTRA was not involved in the design of the study or collection, analysis, or interpretation of the data or in writing the manuscript.

Authors' contributions

Conception or design of the work or acquisition: VN, KS, TG, U-AT, CT, TL, CB, OP, DJ, PB, H-GF, GW, VY, AB. Analysis and interpretation: VN, KS, DS, TG, U-AT, CT, VY, AB. Drafting the manuscript: VN. Revising it critically for important intellectual content: VN, KS, DS, TG, U-AT, CT, TL, CB, OP, DJ, PB, H-GF, GW, VY, AB. Final approval of the version to be published: VN, KS, DS, TG, U-AT, CT, TL, CB, OP, DJ, PB, H-GF, GW, VY, AB. All authors read and approved the final manuscript.

Competing interests

Fraunhofer ITEM is an independent public non-profit research organization for applied research performing contract research with many companies in biotechnology, and pharmaceutical, chemical and cosmetic industries. Fraunhofer USA is also a non-profit research organization. The authors declare that they have no competing interests.

Author details

[1]Fraunhofer Institute for Toxicology and Experimental Medicine, Hannover, Germany, Biomedical Research in Endstage and Obstructive Lung Disease Hannover (BREATH), Member of the German Centre for Lung Research (DZL), Member of the REBIRTH Cluster of Excellence, Hanover, Germany. [2]Fraunhofer USA Center for Molecular Biotechnology, Newark, DE, USA. [3]Institute for Pathology, Hannover Medical School, Hanover, Germany, Biomedical Research in Endstage and Obstructive Lung Disease Hannover (BREATH), Member of the German Centre for Lung Research (DZL), Hanover, Germany. [4]Klinikum Region Hannover (KRH), Institute of Pathology, Hanover, Germany. [5]Klinikum Region Hannover (KRH), Division of Thoracic and Vascular surgery, Hanover, Germany. [6]Division of Cardiac, Thoracic, Transplantation, and Vascular Surgery, Hannover Medical School, Hanover, Germany, Biomedical Research in Endstage and Obstructive Lung Disease Hannover (BREATH), Member of the German Centre for Lung Research (DZL), Hanover, Germany. [7]Institute of Immunology, Hannover Medical School, Hanover, Germany.

References

1. World Health Organization (WHO). The top 10 causes of death. Fact Sheet. Available at: http://www.who.int/mediacentre/factsheets/fs310/en/index2.html. [Accessed 8-1-2016].
2. World Health Organization (WHO). Noncommunicable diseases. Fact Sheet. Available at: http://www.who.int/mediacentre/factsheets/fs355/en/. [Accessed 8-1-2016].
3. Sewald K, Braun A. Assessment of immunotoxicity using precision-cut tissue slices. Xenobiotica. 2013;43(1):84–97. doi:10.3109/00498254.2012.731543.
4. Brown SM, Koarai A, Sturton RG, Nicholson AG, Barnes PJ, Donnelly LE. A role for M(2) and M(3) muscarinic receptors in the contraction of rat and human small airways. Eur J Pharmacol. 2013;702(1–3):109–15. doi:10.1016/j.ejphar.2013.01.054.
5. Henjakovic M, Sewald K, Switalla S, Kaiser D, Muller M, Veres TZ, et al. Ex vivo testing of immune responses in precision-cut lung slices. Toxicol Appl Pharmacol. 2008;231(1):68–76. doi:10.1016/j.taap.2008.04.003.
6. Schleputz M, Rieg AD, Seehase S, Spillner J, Perez-Bouza A, Braunschweig T, et al. Neurally mediated airway constriction in human and other species: a comparative study using precision-cut lung slices (PCLS). PLoS One. 2012;7(10):e47344. doi:10.1371/journal.pone.0047344. PONE-D-12-11366 [pii]
7. Switalla S, Lauenstein L, Prenzler F, Knothe S, Forster C, Fieguth HG, et al. Natural innate cytokine response to immunomodulators and adjuvants in human precision-cut lung slices. Toxicol Appl Pharmacol 2010;246(3):107-115;10.1016/j.taap.2010.04.010.
8. Fisher RL, Smith MS, Hasal SJ, Hasal KS, Gandolfi AJ, Brendel K. The use of human lung slices in toxicology. Hum Exp Toxicol. 1994;13(7):466–71.
9. Lauenstein L, Switalla S, Prenzler F, Seehase S, Pfennig O, Forster C, et al. Assessment of immunotoxicity induced by chemicals in human precision-cut lung slices (PCLS). Toxicol in Vitro. 2014;28(4):588–99. doi:10.1016/j.tiv.2013.12.016.
10. Ressmeyer AR, Larsson AK, Vollmer E, Dahlen SE, Uhlig S, Martin C. Characterisation of guinea pig precision-cut lung slices: comparison with human tissues. Eur Respir J. 2006;28(3):603–11. doi:10.1183/09031936.06.00004206.
11. Rieg AD, Suleiman S, Perez-Bouza A, Braunschweig T, Spillner JW, Schroder T, et al. Milrinone relaxes pulmonary veins in Guinea pigs and humans. PLoS One. 2014;9(1):e87685. doi:10.1371/journal.pone.0087685.
12. Nassimi M, Schleh C, Lauenstein HD, Hussein R, Hoymann HG, Koch W, et al. A toxicological evaluation of inhaled solid lipid nanoparticles used as a potential drug delivery system for the lung. Eur J Pharm Biopharm. 2010;75(2):107–16. doi:10.1016/j.ejpb.2010.02.014.
13. Sauer UG, Vogel S, Aumann A, Hess A, Kolle SN, Ma-Hock L, et al. Applicability of rat precision-cut lung slices in evaluating nanomaterial cytotoxicity, apoptosis, oxidative stress, and inflammation. Toxicol Appl Pharmacol. 2014;276(1):1–20. doi:10.1016/j.taap.2013.12.017.
14. Dobrescu I, Levast B, Lai K, Delgado-Ortega M, Walker S, Banman S, et al. In vitro and ex vivo analyses of co-infections with swine influenza and porcine reproductive and respiratory syndrome viruses. Vet Microbiol. 2014;169(1–2):18–32. doi:10.1016/j.vetmic.2013.11.037.
15. Umachandran M, Howarth J, Ioannides C. Metabolic and structural viability of precision-cut rat lung slices in culture. Xenobiotica. 2004;34(8):771–80. doi:10.1080/00498250400000816.
16. Williams PP, Gallagher JE. Preparation and long-term cultivation of porcine tracheal and lung organ cultures by alternate exposure to gaseous and liquid medium phases. In Vitro. 1978;14(8):686–96.
17. Siminski JT, Kavanagh TJ, Chi E, Raghu G. Long-term maintenance of mature pulmonary parenchyma cultured in serum-free conditions. Am J Phys. 1992;262(1 Pt 1):L105–10.
18. Shapiro P, Absher PM, Casty F, Evans J. Maintaining intact mature lung tissue in culture using low melt agarose. Methods Cell Sci. 1995;17(4):245–9. http://dx.doi.org/10.1007/BF00986229
19. Temann A, Golovina T, Neuhaus V, Thompson C, Chichester JA, Braun A, et al. Evaluation of inflammatory and immune responses in long-term cultured human precision-cut lung slices. Hum Vaccin Immunother. 2017;13(2), S.):351–8.
20. Hansen NU, Karsdal MA, Brockbank S, Cruwys S, Ronnow S, Leeming DJ. Tissue turnover of collagen type I, III and elastin is elevated in the PCLS model of IPF and can be restored back to vehicle levels using a phosphodiesterase inhibitor. Respir Res. 2016;17(1):76. doi:10.1186/s12931-016-0394-8. 10.1186/s12931-016-0394-8 [pii]
21. Seehase S, Schleputz M, Switalla S, Matz-Rensing K, Kaup FJ, Zoller M, et al. Bronchoconstriction in nonhuman primates: a species comparison. J Appl Physiol (1985). 2011;111(3):791–8. doi:10.1152/japplphysiol.00162.2011.
22. Switalla S, Knebel J, Ritter D, Krug N, Braun A, Sewald K. Effects of acute in vitro exposure of murine precision-cut lung slices to gaseous nitrogen dioxide and ozone in an air-liquid interface (ALI) culture. Toxicol Lett. 2010;196(2):117–24. doi:10.1016/j.toxlet.2010.04.004.
23. Berndt WO. Use of the tissue slice technique for evaluation of renal transport processes. Environ Health Perspect. 1976;15:73–88.
24. Rahman MM, McFadden G. Modulation of tumor necrosis factor by microbial pathogens. PLoS Pathog. 2006;2(2):e4. doi:10.1371/journal.ppat.0020004.
25. Sekine-Okano M, Lucas R, Rungger D, De KT, Grau GE, Leuenberger PM, et al. Expression and release of tumor necrosis factor-alpha by explants of mouse cornea. Invest Ophthalmol Vis Sci. 1996;37(7):1302–10.
26. Eischen A, Vincent F, Bergerat JP, Louis B, Faradji A, Bohbot A, et al. Long term cultures of human monocytes in vitro. Impact of GM-CSF on survival and differentiation. J Immunol Methods. 1991;143(2):209–21.
27. Kreutz M, Krause SW, Hennemann B, Rehm A, Andreesen R. Macrophage heterogeneity and differentiation: defined serum-free culture conditions induce different types of macrophages in vitro. Res Immunol. 1992;143(1):107–15.
28. Wouters IM, Douwes J, Thorne PS, Heederik D, Doekes G. Inter- and intraindividual variation of endotoxin- and beta(1 -> 3)-glucan-induced cytokine responses in a whole blood assay. Toxicol Ind Health. 2002;18(1):15–27.
29. Behrsing HP, Furniss MJ, Davis M, Tomaszewski JE, Parchment RE. In vitro exposure of precision-cut lung slices to 2-(4-amino-3-methylphenyl)-5-fluorobenzothiazole lysylamide dihydrochloride (NSC 710305, Phortress) increases inflammatory cytokine content and tissue damage. Toxicol Sci. 2013;131(2):470–9. doi:10.1093/toxsci/kfs319.
30. Cooper PR, Zhang J, Damera G, Hoshi T, Zopf DA, Panettieri RA Jr. C-027 inhibits IgE-mediated passive sensitization bronchoconstriction and acts as a histamine and serotonin antagonist in human airways. Allergy Asthma Proc. 2011;(5):359–65. doi:10.2500/aap.2011.32.3460.
31. Delgado-Ortega M, Melo S, Punyadarsaniya D, Rame C, Olivier M, Soubieux D, et al. Innate immune response to a H3N2 subtype swine influenza virus in newborn porcine trachea cells, alveolar macrophages, and precision-cut lung slices. Vet Res. 2014;45:42.1297-9716-45-42 [pii]. doi:10.1186/1297-9716-45-42.
32. Lambermont VA, Schleputz M, Dassow C, Konig P, Zimmermann LJ, Uhlig S, et al. Comparison of Airway Responses in Sheep of Different Age in Precision-Cut Lung Slices (PCLS). PLoS One. 2014;9(9) e97610.10.1371/journal.pone.0097610
33. Seehase S, Lauenstein HD, Schlumbohm C, Switalla S, Neuhaus V, Forster C, et al. LPS-induced lung inflammation in marmoset monkeys - an acute model for anti-inflammatory drug testing. PLoS One. 2012;7(8):e43709. doi:10.1371/journal.pone.0043709. PONE-D-12-00746 [pii]
34. Kasper M, Seidel D, Knels L, Morishima N, Neisser A, Bramke S, et al. Early signs of lung fibrosis after in vitro treatment of rat lung slices with CdCl2 and TGF-beta1. Histochem Cell Biol. 2004;121(2):131–40. doi:10.1007/s00418-003-0612-6.
35. Lin CJ, Yang PC, Hsu MT, Yew FH, Liu TY, Shun CT, et al. Induction of pulmonary fibrosis in organ-cultured rat lung by cadmium chloride and transforming growth factor-beta1. Toxicology. 1998;127(1–3):157–66.

16

Use of an audience response system to maximise response rates and expedite a modified Delphi process for consensus on occupational health

Tar-Ching Aw[1,2*], Tom Loney[1], Anza Elias[1], Soha Ali[1] and Balázs Ádám[1,3]

Abstract

Background: Different methods have attempted to obtain consensus on occupational health issues. The objective of this paper is to describe a modified three-stage Delphi process that uses a wireless audience response system to enable consensus to be attained in a single day and to maximise response rates. The modified Delphi approach required: a) agreeing the topic/s of interest for which consensus is sought, b) identifying key stakeholders whose opinions are required; c) assembling the stakeholders for a one-day event. Participants' opinions were recorded primarily through use of a system of individual wireless audience response devices ('clickers') linked to a computer. Providing immediate feedback enabled the audience to consider the group's views before proceeding to the next stage. From an initial round of responses, participants were asked to narrow their choices to any five preferred options. A third round was conducted, using the 'clickers' to rank 5 of the most popular group options. Through this iterative exercise, stakeholder consensus was achieved after three decision rounds.

Results: The use of the modifications and the wireless audience response system described enabled stakeholders to provide a group view on specific occupational health issues e.g. priorities or barriers or resources needed. Completing the three-stage iterative exercise in a day maximised the response rate with advantages for both the participants and the researchers. Careful design of the protocol is essential, with a team familiar with information technology to ensure smooth execution of the various stages.

Conclusions: Modification of the Delphi method with the use of a wireless audience participation system facilitates rapid consensus.

Keywords: Audience response system, Consensus, Delphi technique, Occupational health

Background

The Delphi method was originally developed by the US Rand Corporation as a method for decision making and forecasting [1–3]. The technique used an iterative approach for obtaining consensus. It appeared to be especially useful in the absence or non-availability of definitive data, and when expert opinion is therefore sought as a possible alternative to decisions based on published evidence. The subject area in which it was first used was defence, but the technique was then adopted by other disciplines, such as business, social science and medicine for research, education and training purposes [4–10]. The Delphi approach allowed agreement to be reached, even in areas as potentially contentious as determination of priorities, provision of services and barriers to delivery. The technique has also been used for occupational health in several countries, including Malaysia, the United Arab Emirates and the United Kingdom [11–15].

One of the limitations of the multi-stage iterative process is the low response rate, especially during the subsequent rounds of iteration, as it has been experienced in

* Correspondence: tcaw11@gmail.com
[1]Institute of Public Health, College of Medicine and Health Sciences, United Arab Emirates University, PO Box 17666 Al Ain, United Arab Emirates
[2]PAPRSB Institute of Health Sciences, Universiti Brunei Darussalam, Japan Tungku Link, Gadong BE1410, Brunei Darussalam
Full list of author information is available at the end of the article

various settings [16, 17]. This has led to considerations as to whether there is a possibility of completing the exercise in a shorter period of time to reduce poor participation from the first round through to completion. Single-round, almost real-time methods and use of online systems have been proposed [18, 19], and researchers have attempted to modify the method to improve participation rates and shorten the process time. We have trialled the use of a computerised audience-response system for determining key issues and barriers to effective provision of occupational health in the United Arab Emirates (UAE) [20]. The method was refined and used in 2014 to determine consensus on health and safety issues and obstacles to successful implementation of health and safety programmes for a large utilities company in Abu Dhabi.

Methods

The Delphi approach was modified to obtain results in a short time, requiring only one day of direct contact with stakeholders. This is possible with the use of a back-up computer team, and through the use of an automated audience response system to obtain almost instantaneous feedback. The modified process involves several stages:

a. Identification of the topic of interest
   Two occupational health projects using the modified Delphi method were conducted in Abu Dhabi (in 2009 and 2014). The two organisations involved were a government health authority (2009), and a large utilities company (2014). In 2009, the purpose was to obtain a consensus view on three key areas of occupational health and safety in the United Arab Emirates. These were i) specific priority issues, ii) data gaps and iii) resources needed. In 2014, the aim was to determine within the company i) priorities, and ii) barriers to success, in developing and implementing provisions for occupational health and safety.
b. Selection of participants
   Stakeholders were identified by the organisations involved to participate in the Delphi exercise. The main requirement was that they should represent a spectrum of those involved or with a major interest in occupational health and safety. The 2009 project included 64 stakeholders with a balanced representation from employers and employees, government officials, representatives of industry, academics and other health and safety practitioners in the United Arab Emirates. In the 2014 exercise the participants consisted of 80 managers, safety representatives and members of the workforce at different seniority levels and from different geographical regions served by the organisation (i.e. Eastern, Western and Central region of the Emirate of Abu Dhabi).
c. Listing of options
   The initial step in our modified Delphi method involved the selected participants listing as many options as possible in regards to the topic of interest. In 2009, this was completed on a single blank sheet of paper that was then collected for immediate analysis and tabulation of all the responses. Thirty-two specific priority issues and ten items each as data gaps and resources required were listed. In 2014, a list of 20 priorities and 20 barriers for occupational health was available for the organisation from a recent questionnaire survey of approximately 750 employees. The items were entered into a computer program linked to the automated audience response system.
d. Use of the audience response system
   The 2009 study used a three-stage iterative process. Some adjustments to the procedure were made in 2014, based on the experience and feedback from the 2009 exercise. Due to substantial overlap, only the methodological details of the improved three-stage process used in the 2014 study are discussed below.

On the day of the exercise, the stakeholders were instructed on the necessity to provide their own views without involving any discussion with their colleagues. The importance of obtaining a personal individual opinion was stressed. Each participant was provided with a 'clicker' (Keepad Interactive, NSW, Australia; see illustration, Fig. 1) and received oral instructions and practice sessions on how to use the device.

The personal wireless 'clicker' allowed individuals to make a choice from several options, with their choices logged directly onto a computer.

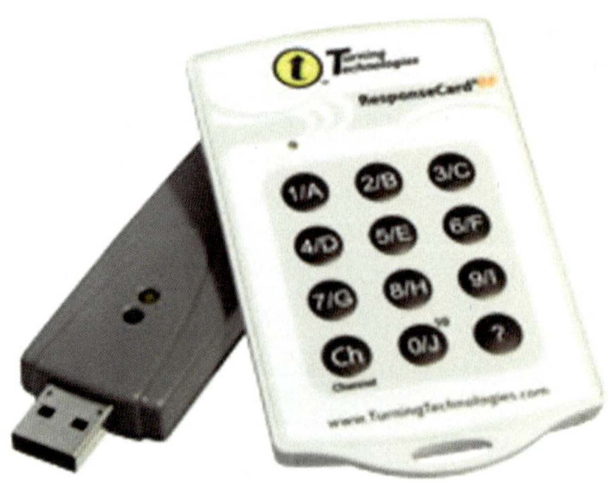

Fig. 1 Photo of a 'clicker' as part of the audience response system hardware

Round 1: Indicating the relevance of the pre-identified items

The participants were asked to indicate on a pre-printed color-coded single-sheet form whether they felt that each of the 20 items (separately for priorities, and then for barriers in the case of the 2014 project) were very relevant, somewhat relevant or of minor relevance. The participants were then required to use the information that they had provided on the forms to indicate their choice by use of the 'clicker', so that the group's views are summarised automatically through the computer, thereby providing quick analysis for the research team and feedback to the audience on the views of the group at the appropriate stage of the modified Delphi process.The data from stage 1 were analysed to exclude approximately one third (33 %) of the listed priorities and barriers from further consideration. About one third of the items, those with the highest number of participants indicating that they were of 'minor relevance', were discarded.

Round 2: Choosing the five most preferred items

Following exclusion of a third of the initial options, a shorter list of items was printed on a single sheet of color-coded paper and distributed to the audience. Next, the participants from the utilities company were instructed to select only five of their most preferred choices from each list (13 residual priorities items and 12 barriers). The selections were again transferred to the computer through use of the audience response system and the five items indicated by the highest number of participants as their preferred choice were determined. The selections of the audience were displayed on screen through the computer to provide feedback on the views of the group before the next stage.

Round 3: Ranking the five items most favoured by the group

The five most preferred items by the whole group for both priorities and barriers were distributed on color-coded paper and participants were asked to rank these five items. The audience response system was then used to determine the rank of each item on a scale from 1 to 5 with 1 indicating the most important. The final rank of the top five occupational health issues for priorities and the top five barriers was determined by the average rank of the items voted by the participants.

The study was approved by the Social Sciences Research Ethics Committee of the United Arab Emirates University.

Results

Study participants

In 2009, the 64 participants consisted of 23 (38 %) individuals from government agencies, 17 (28 %) from industry, and 20 (33 %) from other groups (including academia, health and safety practitioners and employee interest groups). In 2014, the 80 participants were all employees of the utilities company. Fifty-five (69 %) were mainly office-based staff and the remaining 25 (31 %) were either only field-based or largely field-based with some office-based duties. They represented different levels of seniority (the majority, 50 %, working in middle management) and worked in several different geographical regions (i.e. Eastern, Western and Central region of the Emirate of Abu Dhabi). Thirty-eight (48 %) of the participants worked in the power supply division of the company, whilst fourteen (18 %) were in the water supply division, and twenty-seven (34 %) in customer services and other smaller sections.

Response rate

In 2009, the participation rate was 94 % in our three-stage Delphi project. There were slight changes in the number of respondents during the three stages of the 2014 Delphi exercise. Altogether 80 employees participated in the study with 14 leaving during the process and a two arriving after it had been started. There were 78 (98 % of the total) and 79 (99 %) responses in the first stage of indicating relevance of priorities and barriers, respectively (Fig. 2). A small drop in the response rate was experienced in the second stage to 89 and 91 %, respectively (Fig. 2). The decrease continued in the last stage; 84 % completed ranking of the top five priorities and 83 % for the top five barriers (Fig. 2).

Final ranks

The 2009 Delphi exercise identified the top five priority areas, data gaps and resource needs for the UAE in occupational health and safety (Table 1).

The top five priorities and barriers of occupational health and safety determined by the 2014 Delphi study for the utilities company are shown in Table 2.

There was an expected difference in consensus regarding priorities for health and safety for the country, versus priorities and barriers for health and safety within a company.

Discussion

The two exercises in Abu Dhabi showed that the modified Delphi method using an automated audience response system had many advantages in obtaining a consensus view from stakeholders on pre-determined issues in occupational health, most importantly the exercise could be completed in a short period of time with a very high response rate in the consecutive rounds. The use of a combination of written responses and the computerised audience response system proved effective in enabling a multi-round iterative exercise to be conducted over a day, thereby reducing dropouts from participation. The majority of previous

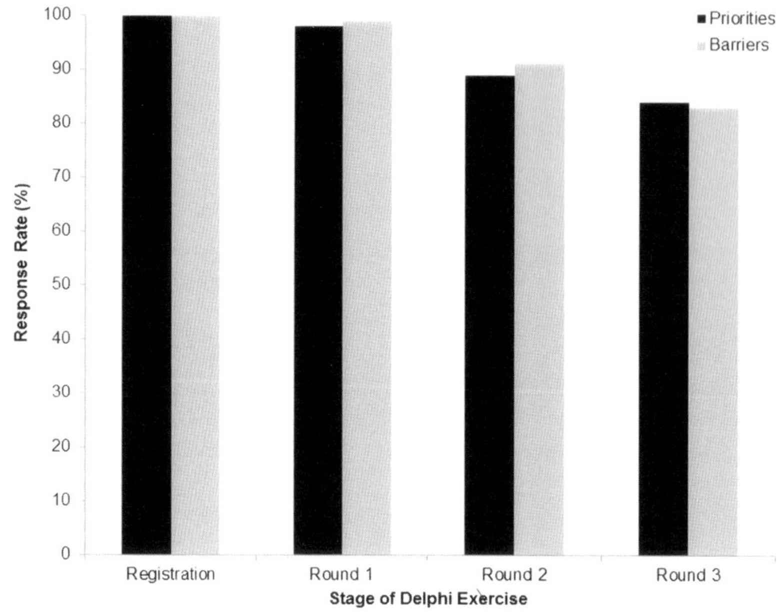

Fig. 2 Response rate (%) for three-round Delphi study conducted in 2014

Delphi projects have taken several weeks or months [5, 14]. This was because several iterations were required, and a postal or online system was used to gather information, with time allocated between iterations in order for responses to be received.

The computer-aided audience response system also enabled almost immediate feedback to the group about their responses at specific stages of the modified Delphi study. Stages 2 and 3 of the iterative process could then proceed after participants had received feedback from the preceding stages, allowing them for comments and questions. At the end, the final results of the exercise were shared with the participants so that everybody could express their final opinion. Informal feedback through initial provision of the findings to the company suggests that there was general agreement with the priorities and barriers identified through the Delphi exercise.

Completion of all stages in a day reduced the dropout rate. The final participation rate for multi-stage Delphi exercise is often low and would be affected by the number of rounds involved, and the time given between stages. A recent study employed a two-round online Delphi study to develop consensus on remote healthcare practitioners' competency for oil and gas operations and the valid response rate for round one and two was 27 and 24 %, respectively [17]. Study authors reported that technical issues with the recruitment, sampling and data collection techniques accounted for 59 % of the non-response across the two rounds: out-of-office replies (26 %), incorrect email addresses (19 %), and burst rate limit exceeded (14 %) [17]. In the two-stage postal exercise on priorities for occupational health research involving 53 senior occupational physicians, Harrington obtained an 86 % response to round 1, and 91 % for round 2 [12]. When the exercise was repeated as a postal questionnaire to personnel

Table 1 Top five priorities, data gaps and resource needs for the United Arab Emirates in occupational health and safety, Delphi exercise, 2009

Priorities	Data gaps	Resource needs
1. Adequate occupational health and safety legislation	1. Absence of workplace injury reporting system	1. Government support and commitment for occupational health and safety
2. Availability of guidelines on health and safety	2. Lack of accurate health and safety statistics	2. National guidelines on industry-specific health and safety standards
3. A central government authority for developing occupational health strategy	3. Data on the extent and results of occupational health screening	3. Education and training for different groups of health and safety practitioners
4. Competency of occupational health professionals	4. Data on occupational diseases	4. A central health and safety resource
5. Prevention of work-related illness and injury	5. Information on occupational exposure assessment	5. A system for collecting occupational health and safety statistics

Table 2 Top five priorities and barriers of occupational health and safety for a utilities company in the United Arab Emirates, Delphi exercise, 2014

Priorities	Barriers
1. Personal protective equipment	1. Lack of management commitment
2. Training	2. Production taking priority over safety considerations
3. Quality of work equipment	3. Workload
4. Regular safety inspections	4. Poor communication regarding health and safety
5. First aid facilities and training	5. A 'blame' culture

managers, the response rate was 24 % despite two reminders and a second mailing to non-responders. For our three-stage Delphi project in 2009, the participation rate was 94 %, and in 2014, 83 % of registered participants completed all three stages of the exercise. With a postal questionnaire the participation rate often decreases after each round. Follow up of non-responders is difficult if there are concerns about preservation of the confidentiality of responses. With our modified system, all participants were requested to remain until all stages were completed. Despite the whole process taking only one day, a 17 % drop-out rate was still experienced, with a few individuals leaving before completing either stage three or stages two and three. This may be partly due to inadequate communication or commitment by the participants regarding the importance to remain till the end of the exercise.

Although neither the Delphi process nor the computerised audience response system was familiar for the participants, the majority could understand and complete the expected tasks. The modified approach enabled individual views to be expressed, with equal weighting given to each person's opinion, regardless of position or rank within the organisation, or professional or managerial background or experience. The likelihood of opinions being influenced by the views of senior or more vocal colleagues was reduced by providing an individual 'clicker' for each participant. Individual participant choices could then be transmitted to the computer with preservation of anonymity. Participants were reminded to provide their own opinions without group discussion, and that the projects were designed to obtain individual opinion and not necessarily company policy or views of the group. Therefore, there was a strong likelihood that the views of individuals were obtained. With postal or even online questionnaires there is no certainty as to whether the views expressed or the choices made were completed as a group exercise or completed by persons other than the identified respondent.

A major limitation of the modified approach is the requirement for stakeholders to be physically present to participate for a day. This requires time away from work, and the costs of accommodating a large number of individuals including finding a suitable venue and providing meals and refreshments. This was feasible in the two projects in Abu Dhabi as there was commitment and support from the employers for the process. There is also a need for a small team of experienced support staff to facilitate the distribution and collection of questionnaires and 'clickers', and to analyse data captured by the audience response system in a limited time between the stages. The availability of a set of 100 clickers (to include spare devices) that had to be checked and tested ahead of the exercise was essential. The process required a smooth transition from one stage of the Delphi procedure to the next, without unnecessary delay that could well reduce the likelihood of participants remaining for subsequent stages. Good audio-visual facilities were essential, and a preliminary explanation as to the purpose of the process, and the importance of full participation was key to the success of the modified Delphi study.

The selection of participants was not random therefore it did not assure that opinions were representative for the views of the organisations they represented. Nevertheless, random selection is not the main purpose of selecting participants for a Delphi exercise; rather, purposeful sampling was used to recruit knowledgeable and experienced participants on the topic of interest [10]. This concept was obtained by inviting acknowledged professionals from the field of occupational health and safety available in the United Arab Emirates in the 2009 study. In 2014, the organisers of the initial survey within the company were entrusted to recruit employees related to occupational health and safety issues from various sectors of the company in a number that is manageable in a one-day exercise. The choice of participants with different levels of seniority, representing different professional groups or working in different geographical areas allowed views to be gathered from a wide area of representation.

Conclusions

The presented modified Delphi technique with the use of a wireless audience participation system enables rapid consensus that proves especially advantageous in effectively identifying priorities and barriers of occupational health and safety in countries and workplace settings where such knowledge is particularly needed.

Competing interests

The authors declare that they have no competing interests.

Authors' contributions

TCA and TL initiated the study, formulated the concept and outlined the manuscript. BA elaborated the detailed study design. TCA, TL, BA AE and SA completed the final protocol and implemented the study. All authors contributed to manuscript preparation, read and approved the final manuscript.

Authors' information

TCA has had extensive experience with applying the Delphi technique to obtain consensus on occupational health issues in the United Kingdom,

Malaysia and recently in the United Arab Emirates. All authors have special interest in identifying priority issues of occupational health in the United Arab Emirates and in the WHO Eastern Mediterranean Region.

Acknowledgements
We thank Carpenter S, Cooling RF and Barlis J (Parsons Brinckerhoff Middle East Limited, Dubai, United Arab Emirates) for their assistance with the project.

Author details
[1]Institute of Public Health, College of Medicine and Health Sciences, United Arab Emirates University, PO Box 17666 Al Ain, United Arab Emirates. [2]PAPRSB Institute of Health Sciences, Universiti Brunei Darussalam, Japan Tungku Link, Gadong BE1410, Brunei Darussalam. [3]Department of Preventive Medicine, Faculty of Public Health, University of Debrecen, PO Box 9, Debrecen H-4012, Hungary.

References

1. Dalkey N, Helmer O. An experimental application of the Delphi method to the use of experts. Manag Sci. 1963;9(3):458–67.
2. Gupta UG, Clarke RE. Theory and applications of the Delphi technique: a bibliography (1975–1994). Technol Forecast Soc Chang. 1996;53:185–211.
3. Linstone HA, Turoff M. Delphi: A brief look forward and backward. Technol Forecast Soc Chang. 2011;78:1712–9.
4. MacDonald E, Ritchie K, Murray K, Gilmour W. Requirements for occupational medicine training in Europe: a Delphi study. Occup Environ Med. 2000;57(2):98–105.
5. van der Beek AJ, Frings-Dresen MH, van Djik FJ, Houtman IL. Priorities in occupational health research: a Delphi study in the Netherlands. Occup Environ Med. 1997;54(7):504–10.
6. Van Djik JAGM. Delphi method as a learning instrument. Technol Forecast Soc Chang. 1990;37:399–407.
7. Landeta J. Current validity of the Delphi method in social sciences. Technol Forecast Soc Chang. 2006;73:467–82.
8. Powell C. The Delphi technique: myths and realities. J Adv Nurs. 2002;42(4): 376–82.
9. Graham B, Regehr G, Wright JG. Delphi as a method to establish consensus for diagnostic criteria. J Clin Epi. 2003;56:1150–6.
10. Okoli C, Pawlowski SD. The Delphi method as a research tool: an example, design considerations and applications. Inform Manag. 2004;42:15–29.
11. Agius RM. Priorities for managing occupational allergy – a Delphi consensus. Clin Exp Allergy. 1993;23:634–7.
12. Harrington JM. Research priorities in occupational medicine: a survey of United Kingdom medical opinion by the Delphi technique. Occup Environ Med. 1994;51:289–94.
13. Harrington JM, Calvert IA. Research priorities in occupational medicine: a survey of United Kingdom personnel managers. Occup Environ Med. 1996;53:642–4.
14. Sadhra S, Beach JR, Aw TC, Sheikh-Ahmed K. Occupational health priorities in Malaysia: a Delphi study. Occup Environ Med. 2001;58:426–31.
15. Loney T, Aw TC. Development of occupational health in the Gulf Cooperation council countries: The UAE experience. J Inst Remote Hlth Care. 2014;5(1):18–24.
16. Reetoo KN, Harrington JM, Macdonald EB. Required competencies of occupational physicians: a Delphi survey of UK customers. Occup Environ Med. 2005;62:406–13.
17. Klein S, Mohamed H. Developing consensus on remote healthcare practitioners' competency for oil and gas operations: A Delphi study: Institute of Remote Healthcare: conference proceedings, October 07–08, 2014. London: Olympia London; 2014.
18. Gordon T, Pease A. RT Delphi: An efficient, "round-less" almost real time Delphi method. Technol Forecast Soc Chang. 2006;73:321–33.
19. Steinert M. A dissensus based online Delphi approach: An explorative research tool. Technol Forecast Soc Chang. 2009;76:291–300.
20. Aw TC. Occupational health and safety priorities for the UAE. Internal report for the Health Authority of Abu Dhabi. Al-Ain: UAE University report; 2010.

17

Application of the ICF based Norwegian function assessment scale to employees

Sylvia Jankowiak*, Uwe Rose and Norbert Kersten

Abstract

Background: At the interface of the occupational setting and rehabilitation, normative values for functional ability are desirable and worthwhile. The Norwegian Function Assessment Scale (NFAS) is a 39 item self-report instrument based on the International Classification of Functioning, Disability and Health (ICF). As the questionnaire was not used in a working population, we aimed to obtain functional levels of employees in Germany as measured through the NFAS.

Methods: The NFAS was included in the Study on Mental Health at Work (S-MGA) 2011/12, a representative German survey of employees aged 31 to 60 years. For descriptive analyses, 95% confidence intervals were applied through bootstrap estimation to the skewed data of the NFAS (range from 1 = 'no difficulty' to 5 = 'could not do it'). The data were analysed by age decades, professional qualification, and by disabilities, congenital diseases and accidents, stratified by sex. Linear regression analyses were conducted to estimate adjusted effects of age, professional qualification, and health limitations.

Results: The NFAS total score was 1.17 (95% CI = 1.15–1.17). Thirty-five percent of the employees' (1378 out of 3937 participants) reported the best possible functional ability (NFAS total score of 1.00). Managing and walking/standing were the NFAS' most affected domains with a score of 1.26 (95% CI = 1.23–1.27), respectively. The regression analysis confirmed more functional difficulties for elder employees, females, employees with low professional qualification, and for employees suffering from disability and accidents.

Conclusions: The study presents normative values of functional ability for the workforce. The results are useful for score interpretation in rehabilitation and return-to-work processes.

Keywords: Occupational health, Employee health, International classification of functioning, disability and health, Surveys and questionnaires

Background

Functional ability is the actual or potential capacity of an individual to perform the activities and tasks that are common in daily life [1]. Functional ability is a key factor in determining an individual's quality of life, and an important asset for both employees and the society [2]. National and international reports based on assessments by the respective social insurance systems revealed that a considerable proportion of the population suffers from reduced capacities for workforce participation [3, 4]. The social security systems are ultimately required to make the decision on disability pension applications. In Norway, in 2012, the percentage of disability pensioners in the population age group of 18–66 years was 9.5% [5]. In Germany, at the same time, the percentage of disability pensioners in the same age group was only 5.1% [6], and the Norwegian share also exceeds that of most other European countries [5]. In recent years, European social security schemes began to target individual capabilities rather than health deficits, first and foremost in the Nordic countries [7, 8]. In this context, new questionnaires

* Correspondence: jankowiak.sylvia@baua.bund.de
Division Work and Health, Federal Institute for Safety and Health (BAuA), Noeldnerstr. 40/42, D-10317 Berlin, Germany

have been developed, such as the Norwegian Function Assessment Scale, NFAS.

To date, the standard framework for describing and organising information on functioning and disability is the International Classification of Functioning, Disability and Health (ICF). The NFAS is a 39-item self-report questionnaire whose underpinning goes back to the ICF [9]. It aims to assess the functioning based on the individual's self-perception, and was developed in 2000 by an expert group in social insurance [10]. Therefore, all categories from the activities/participation component of the ICF were considered. The expert group removed all categories that were not trusted to be relevant for the assessment of work-related functional abilities, resulting in a final list of 39 categories, which were then reformulated into questions [10].

To our knowledge, the NFAS has so far been applied in five studies, all of them conducted in Norway. Attention was drawn to sick-listed participants ($n = 386$) who showed a considerably reduced functioning [10] and to a sample of the general population aged 24 to 86 years ($n = 1620$) for obtaining normative data [11]. Furthermore, an association of NFAS values with a positive expectancy for eventually returning to work was demonstrated for disability pensioners with back pain ($n = 89$) [12]. The NFAS was also found to be a strong predictor of receiving allowances 3 years after an occupational rehabilitation due to long-term sick leave ($n = 338$) [13].

In all of these studies, a four-point scale was used for coding the responses. A trial study with a sample of the general population aged 24 to 86 years ($n = 1705$) revealed a clear superiority of a five- over a four-point scale, followed by the recommendation to use the more differentiated one in future studies [14].

The working population – a group the NFAS was also designed for – has as yet not been examined. However, an application to the working population would provide important normative data necessary for score interpretation and for defining objectives in rehabilitation. Therefore, in the Study on Mental Health at Work, S-MGA (Studie zur mentalen Gesundheit bei der Arbeit) [15] we set out to obtain normative data on the employed population in Germany as measured through the NFAS.

Germany's workforce is composed of three groups: employees, civil servants, and persons engaged in freelancing or self-employment [16]. The term 'employee' includes the entire spectrum of sectors and the full range of requirements (working tasks from very simple to highly complex). In 2011, employees accounted for 81.4% of the workforce in Germany [16]. According to German law, employees have a liability for social security contributions (such as health, nursing, pension and unemployment insurance). The German Federal Employment Agency runs the register 'Integrated Employment Biographies', which solely focuses on the employees in Germany. Civil-servants and freelancers/self-employed persons (4.9% and 13.6% in 2011, respectively) are not registered, and they are obliged to pay for their health insurance only.

The purpose of this study was to obtain normative values on the NFAS as part of the Study on Mental Health at Work. In order to examine the variability of the functional ability depending on sex, age, professional qualification, disabilities, congenital diseases, and accidents we describe and estimate the influence of these factors on the NFAS scores.

Methods

The Study on Mental Health at Work (S-MGA) is a nationwide panel study of employees in Germany with a five-year retake period [17]. The first assessment was conducted from November 2011 to June 2012 (S-MGA I) on a sample of 4511 employees. For S-MGA I employees aged 31 to 60 years were considered, because most Germans have completed their professional training/studies at this stage of their life and are not yet superannuated. The S-MGA serves two purposes: to examine the impact of employment on mental health and to analyse the association between functioning and work ability. The latter purpose constitutes the line of the present study.

S-MGA I recruitment and study procedure

The population considered for the S-MGA I comprised the birth cohorts 1951 to 1980 who were subject to social insurance contributions in Germany on December 31st 2010. At this time, Germany had 31.9 million employees [18], and 21.5 million of them were aged 31 to 60 years [16, 17]. For creating a representative sample, a two-stage cluster sampling method was used [15]. Initially, all of the 12,227 German municipalities were stratified proportionally, by region and population size. Out of these, 206 municipalities throughout Germany were randomly selected. Next, the random gross sample was built. Therefore, 13,590 individuals were drawn within the randomly selected municipalities. One week prior to the first contact attempt, a letter including information on the study was sent to the registered addresses of the selected individuals. The survey was carried out by 243 trained interviewers on the condition that the respondent was fluent in German. The employees were interviewed face-to-face at their homes via computer-assisted personal interview (CAPI). The interviews took around 60 to 70 min to complete and covered socio-demographic information, employment and working conditions, work ability and functioning, motivational, volitional and personal co-factors, and mental health [17]. The obtained data was linked to the register

'Integrated Employment Biographies' if the participants gave their written permission. The full protocol of the study has been published elsewhere [17]. The four thousand, five hundred and eleven participants of the S-MGA I constitute a representative sample as it properly displays a variety of characteristics of employees in Germany, such as sex, education, employment, occupational status, working hours, nationality, and wages. For the present study, we included employees with a current weekly working time of at least 14 h per week, resulting in a final number of 3937 employees.

The Norwegian function assessment scale (NFAS)

The NFAS consists of 39 items relevant for assessing the physical and mental functioning in the working life and in daily living. Based on a principal component analysis, the items are arranged across seven domains [10]. The physical domains are Walking/standing, Holding/picking up things, Lifting/carrying and Sitting; the mental domains cover Managing, Cooperation/communication and Senses. Each item is preceded by the following question: 'Have you had difficulty doing the following activities during the last week ...?' The NFAS was developed with a four-point scale [10] and is now recommended to be used with a five-point scale. Additionally, the original NFAS contains a 'missing data' category.

The German version of the NFAS was included in the S-MGA I [17], covering the same 39 items and its possible difficulty within the last week. The German NFAS version was generated in a five-step process. Firstly, the NFAS was translated by a bilingual Norwegian-German. Secondly, this translation was compared to the English NFAS version (as rated by four persons). Thirdly, a preliminary German NFAS was chosen. Next, it was back-translated by another bilingual person. This Norwegian back-translation was sent to the NFAS authors and users S. Brage and N. Østerås who found it remarkably similar (e-mail communication). As a last step, the very small changes suggested by the authors were adapted, and the final German NFAS was formed. As recommended by Østerås et al. [14] the German NFAS was applied by using a five-point scale: 1 = no difficulty; 2 = little difficulty; 3 = moderate difficulty; 4 = much difficulty; and 5 = could not do it. The German version aimed at differentiating the reasons for having missing items, and therefore three 'missing data' categories were applied: 'inapplicable to me', 'refused' and 'don't know'. The German version of the NFAS is provided as supplementary material [see Additional file 1].

Variable selection

The basic confounder sex was dealt with stratification. Of the factors that potentially affect a person's working life we chose the following variables as described in [3]: age, professional qualification, and the three health limitations disabilities, congenital diseases, and accidents.

Age was taken in decades, i.e. 31 to 40, 41 to 50, and 51–60 years. Professional qualification was assessed by using the three groups 'university', 'occupational training', and 'unskilled/semi-skilled'. The group 'university' includes qualification from a university or a university of applied sciences; the group 'occupational training' considered having completed i) a training; ii) a vocational or commercial school; and iii) a master or technical college.

To form the binary variable 'disabilities', the existence of an official confirmation of the individuals 'severely handicapped' status was verified. Additionally, the degree of disability was recorded (range 20% to 100%). The binary variables 'congenital diseases' and 'accidents' had to be determined by a physician. The kind of congenital disease was not enquired. Accidental injuries (e.g. to the back, limbs, or burns) refer to the life time. For reasons of readability these three conditions were labeled 'health limitations'.

Data analysis

The seven domain scores were calculated by adding up the item scores and dividing by the number of items completed. At least 50 % of the items had to be answered to calculate any particular NFAS domain. The NFAS total scores were calculated by adding all 39 item scores and dividing by the number of items completed given that none of the domain scores was missing. Missing data were calculated as percentages and displayed for the category 'inapplicable to me'. The selection of the scale's bottom value (i.e. value '1' no difficulty) was calculated as percentage per item as well.

For descriptive statistics we included the means of the item values, of the domain scores and of the total score. A low score indicates good functional ability. As we hypothesised differences in the NFAS scores for women and men, we ran stratified analyses. All tables are split by sex. Additionally, total values are given in the descriptive part.

The Norwegian studies [10, 11, 14] provided evidence that the distribution of item and domain scores is skewed to the right. Instead of providing standard deviations (SDs) for skewed data we computed 95% confidence intervals (CIs) through bootstrap estimation [19]. For this purpose a bias-corrected and accelerated method was used [19].

It was hypothesised that both the NFAS domain scores and the NFAS total score are influenced by age, professional qualification as well as disabilities, congenital disorders and accidents. Descriptive analyses show NFAS domain values with 95% CIs for each of the five factors.

For the comparison of means we used the fact that there is a very close relationship between confidence intervals and significance tests [20]. This approach uses the two separate CIs of both means to compare (as opposed to the CI of the difference of means). A conservative variant of a usual significant difference is indicated lest the CIs do not overlap. Here, the real α in probability is smaller than the nominal α of 0.05, even though the exact α is not provided.

To simultaneously estimate the partial effect of these five factors on the NFAS total score, generalised linear regression analyses were run (score value minus 1). The Tweedie function [21] served as distribution function because it covers the data's specific distribution in an appropriate manner (link function identity, initial value $p = 1.5$). Tweedie's compound Poisson distribution is a mixture of a degenerate distribution at zero and a continuous distribution on the positive real line [21]. All analyses were performed using the SPSS Statistics 23 software except for the bootstrap estimations which were calculated with SYSTAT 13.

Results

The results were based on $n = 3937$ employees in Germany with a working time of at least 14 h per week. The employees' mean (SD) age was 45.1 (4.5) years. The group age distribution was as follows: 31–40 years 21.3%, 41–50 years 39.0%, and 51–60 years 39.7%. The sample consisted of 47.5% women. Table 1 summarises the characteristics of the population.

Distribution and data quality

Table 2 depicts the percentage of inapplicability per NFAS item (column 2), the bottom value '1' per item (column 3), and the mean NFAS domain and item scores (columns 4 to 9).

Table 1 Characteristics of the study population

	Number	Percent
Full Sample	3937	100
Sex		
Women	1872	47.5
Men	2065	52.5
Age (years)		
51–60	1530	38.9
41–50	1589	40.4
31–40	818	20.8
Professional Qualification		
University	864	21.9
Occupational training	2870	72.9
Unskilled/semi-skilled	202	5.1
Health Limitations		
Disabilities	336	8.5
Congenital diseases	73	1.9
Accidents	1186	30.1

For each of the 39 items, the most frequent response was 'no difficulty' (69.5% to 98.4% of the answers per item). This resulted in an overall right-skewed distribution. Thirty-five per cent of the employees (33.0% of the women and 37.0% of the men) reported not a single difficulty on the whole questionnaire (only '1's on a five-point scale). In contrast, six abilities were affected for at least every fifth employee, i.e. 'going up and down stairs' (item no. 05; domain Walking/standing), 'remembering things' (item no. 32; domain Cooperation/communication), and four items of the domain Managing: 'staying alert and being able to concentrate', 'managing everyday stress and strains', 'managing to take criticism', and 'managing to control your anger and aggression' (items no. 25, 29, 30, 31; Table 2).

Among employees in Germany the NFAS total score was $\bar{x}_T$=1.17, CI = 1.15–1.17. Most severely affected was the ability to take criticism $\bar{x}_T$=1.42, CI = 1.38–1.44, least affected the ability to listen to the radio $\bar{x}_T$=1.02, CI = 1.01–1.02; Table 2. On the domains Managing and Walking/standing employees scored equally problematic with $\bar{x}_T$=1.26, CI = 1.23–1.27. Least difficulty was reported for the NFAS domain Senses with $\bar{x}_T$=1.03, CI = 1.02–1.04.

In general, men reported a significantly better functional ability than women (total score men $\bar{x}_M$=1.15, CI = 1.13–1.16 vs. women $\bar{x}_W$=1.19, CI = 1.17–1.20, Table 2). The in-depth results presented in Table 2 revealed 31 items where men scored better than women, apart from the eight items of the domains Cooperation/communication and Senses.

Almost all missing data (99.9%) were missing due to the fact that the activities in question were not applicable to the employees. On average, 2% of the NFAS values were not applicable. Predominant sectors included using public transport (item no. 24) and doing the laundry by oneself (item no. 21) with 16.5% and 11.2% of unconcerned employees, respectively (Table 2).

Separate effects of age, professional education and health limitations on the NFAS

Table 3 shows the mean values of the domain scores and the total score in association to age, professional education and health limitations, stratified by sex.

Age was associated with the NFAS total and domain scores of both sexes. As shown in Table 3, a significantly lower functional level became apparent for employees aged 51–60 (women $\bar{x}_W$=1.23, CI = 1.19–1.25 and men $\bar{x}_M$=1.17, CI = 1.14–1.19) as compared to those aged 31–40 years (women $\bar{x}_W$=1.15, CI = 1.11–1.17 and men $\bar{x}_M$=1.12, CI = 1.09–1.13).

Table 2 Missing data, percentage of employees without difficulty and mean NFAS domain and item scores with 95% CI for the full sample and stratified by sex ($n = 3937$). A value of 1 characterises the best possible functional ability

	Full Sample (n = 3937)				Women ($n = 1872$)		Men ($n = 2065$)	
Domains/items[a]	ia[b] (%)	nd[c] (%)	$\bar{x}_T$	95% CI	$\bar{x}_W$	95% CI	$\bar{x}_M$	95% CI
Walking/Standing	**0.7**	**65.7**	**1.26**	**1.23–1.27**	**1.28**	**1.24–1.30**	**1.24**	**1.20–1.25**
01 Standing	0.1	82.2	1.31	1.27–1.33	1.35	1.29–1.37	1.28	1.23–1.31
02 Walking less than a kilometre on flat ground	0.3	89.6	1.19	1.16–1.20	1.21	1.17–1.23	1.17	1.13–1.19
03 Walking more than a kilometre on flat ground	1.5	84.7	1.27	1.23–1.29	1.32	1.26–1.35	1.23	1.19–1.26
04 Walking on different surfaces	0.8	85.3	1.26	1.23–1.28	1.30	1.25–1.33	1.23	1.19–1.25
05 Going up and down stairs	0.2	75.2	1.41	1.37–1.43	1.44	1.39–1.47	1.39	1.34–1.41
06 Going shopping for your groceries	2.2	87.4	1.18	1.15–1.19	1.22	1.17–1.24	1.14	1.11–1.16
07 Putting on your shoes and socks	0.0	89.4	1.18	1.15–1.19	1.16	1.12–1.18	1.19	1.15–1.21
Holding/Picking up things	**1.7**	**80.8**	**1.09**	**1.08–1.10**	**1.11**	**1.09–1.12**	**1.08**	**1.06–1.09**
08 Picking up a coin from a table with your fingers	0.6	95.7	1.06	1.04–1.07	1.08	1.05–1.09	1.04	1.03–1.05
09 Holding and turning a steering wheel	3.0	94.9	1.04	1.03–1.05	1.05	1.03–1.07	1.03	1.02–1.04
10 Driving a car	4.9	92.1	1.06	1.04–1.07	1.07	1.05–1.09	1.05	1.03–1.06
11 Preparing food	3.0	94.2	1.05	1.04–1.05	1.06	1.04–1.08	1.03	1.02–1.04
12 Writing	0.2	96.2	1.05	1.04–1.06	1.07	1.05–1.08	1.04	1.02–1.05
13 Performing everyday tasks on your own	0.1	92.8	1.10	1.08–1.11	1.13	1.11–1.15	1.08	1.05–1.09
14 Engaging in your leisure activities	1.4	84.6	1.26	1.22–1.28	1.28	1.23–1.31	1.24	1.20–1.27
15 Putting on and taking off your clothes	0.0	93.6	1.10	1.08–1.11	1.10	1.07–1.11	1.10	1.07–1.11
Lifting/Carrying	**4.0**	**75.6**	**1.16**	**1.14–1.17**	**1.20**	**1.17–1.21**	**1.12**	**1.09–1.13**
16 Lifting an empty soda bottle crate from the floor	0.8	87.9	1.20	1.17–1.22	1.28	1.23–1.30	1.14	1.10–1.16
17 Carrying shopping bags in your hands	1.4	86.8	1.21	1.18–1.22	1.29	1.25–1.32	1.13	1.10–1.15
18 Carrying a little sack/backpack on your shoulders or back	2.8	87.3	1.17	1.14–1.18	1.23	1.17–1.25	1.11	1.08–1.13
19 Pushing and pulling with your arms	0.5	88.7	1.19	1.16–1.20	1.22	1.18–1.25	1.15	1.11–1.17
20 Cleaning your house	7.1	83.0	1.18	1.15–1.19	1.24	1.20–1.27	1.11	1.08–1.12
21 Washing your clothes	11.2	83.6	1.09	1.07–1.10	1.11	1.08–1.12	1.06	1.04–1.08
Sitting	**6.5**	**88.6**	**1.11**	**1.09–1.12**	**1.13**	**1.10–1.14**	**1.10**	**1.08–1.11**
22 Sitting on a kitchen chair	0.3	93.3	1.10	1.08–1.11	1.12	1.11–1.14	1.08	1.06–1.09
23 Riding as a passenger in a car	2.8	89.9	1.13	1.10–1.14	1.14	1.11–1.16	1.11	1.08–1.13
24 Riding as a passenger on public transport	16.5	79.5	1.09	1.06–1.10	1.10	1.11–1.12	1.07	1.05–1.09
Managing	**2.2**	**51.4**	**1.26**	**1.23–1.27**	**1.29**	**1.26–1.30**	**1.23**	**1.21–1.24**
25 Staying alert and being able to concentrate	0.0	79.9	1.27	1.24–1.28	1.30	1.26–1.32	1.24	1.21–1.25
26 Working in groups	4.5	87.9	1.11	1.09–1.12	1.13	1.10–1.14	1.10	1.08–1.12
27 Guiding others in their activities	7.3	84.1	1.12	1.10–1.14	1.14	1.11–1.16	1.11	1.09–1.13
28 Managing everyday responsibility	0.1	87.7	1.17	1.15–1.18	1.20	1.17–1.22	1.14	1.11–1.16
29 Managing everyday stress and strains	0.1	79.1	1.28	1.25–1.30	1.32	1.27–1.34	1.24	1.21–1.26
30 Managing to take criticism	1.1	68.7	1.42	1.38–1.44	1.47	1.43–1.50	1.37	1.33–1.40
31 Managing to control your anger and aggression	2.1	69.5	1.38	1.35–1.40	1.39	1.35–1.42	1.37	1.32–1.39
Cooperation/Communication	**0.1**	**69.2**	**1.13**	**1.11–1.13**	**1.12**	**1.11–1.13**	**1.13**	**1.11–1.14**
32 Remembering things	0.0	74.6	1.33	1.30–1.34	1.34	1.29–1.36	1.32	1.28–1.34
33 Understanding spoken messages	0.0	89.2	1.13	1.11–1.14	1.12	1.10–1.14	1.13	1.11–1.14
34 Understanding written messages	0.1	90.9	1.11	1.09–1.12	1.11	1.09–1.12	1.11	1.09–1.12
35 Speaking	0.0	95.8	1.05	1.04–1.05	1.05	1.03–1.05	1.05	1.04–1.06

Table 2 Missing data, percentage of employees without difficulty and mean NFAS domain and item scores with 95% CI for the full sample and stratified by sex ($n = 3937$). A value of 1 characterises the best possible functional ability *(Continued)*

	Full Sample (n = 3937)				Women ($n = 1872$)		Men ($n = 2065$)	
Domains/items[a]	ia[b] (%)	nd[c] (%)	$\bar{x}_T$	95% CI	$\bar{x}_W$	95% CI	$\bar{x}_M$	95% CI
36 Participating in a conversation with many people	0.3	91.1	1.12	1.10–1.12	1.11	1.09–1.13	1.12	1.09–1.13
37 Using the telephone	0.0	97.3	1.04	1.02–1.04	1.03	1.02–1.04	1.04	1.03–1.05
Senses	**0.8**	**97.2**	**1.03**	**1.02–1.04**	**1.03**	**1.02–1.04**	**1.02**	**1.01–1.03**
38 Watching television	0.9	96.8	1.03	1.02–1.03	1.04	1.02–1.05	1.03	1.02–1.03
39 Listening to the radio	0.7	97.7	1.02	1.01–1.03	1.03	1.01–1.03	1.02	1.01–1.03
Total	**2.0**	**35.1**	**1.17**	**1.15–1.17**	**1.19**	**1.17–1.20**	**1.15**	**1.13–1.16**

[a]Domains are depicted in bold. Items are based on a five-point scale with 1 = 'no difficulty', 2 = 'little difficulty', 3 = 'moderate difficulty', 4 = 'much difficulty' and 5 = 'could not do it'
[b]ia = inapplicable to me, [c]nd = no difficulty

Unskilled/semi-skilled employees showed a significantly higher NFAS total score (women $\bar{x}_W$ =1.29, CI = 1.19–1.36 and men $\bar{x}_M$ =1.21, CI = 1.13–1.27) than employees holding a university degree (women $\bar{x}_W$ =1.15, CI = 1.11–1.17 and men $\bar{x}_M$ =1.09, CI = 1.07–1.10) (Table 3).

Among the 336 disabled individuals, 39% were determined to have a degree of disability of 50% or higher. Individuals with confirmed disabilities were found to have significantly higher NFAS total scores than their counterparts without such condition, which was true for both sexes (women: cases $\bar{x}_W$ =1.47, CI = 1.37–1.53 vs. non-cases $\bar{x}_W$ =1.16, CI = 1.14–1.17; men: cases $\bar{x}_M$ =1.32, CI = 1.24–1.37 vs. non-cases $\bar{x}_M$ =1.13, CI = 1.11–1.14). For both women and men the variable disability revealed the highest NFAS total scores among the five considered variables. Likewise, being disabled resulted in the highest scores of any of the NFAS domains with a maximum of $\bar{x}_W$ =1.80, CI = 1.62–1.91 for women in the domain Walking/standing (Table 3).

Also, there were significant differences in the NFAS total scores between individuals who had an accident (women $\bar{x}_W$ =1.25, CI = 1.21–1.28 and men $\bar{x}_M$ =1.18, CI = 1.15–1.19) and those who hadn't (women $\bar{x}_W$ =1.17, CI = 1.15–1.18 and men $\bar{x}_M$ =1.13, CI = 1.11–1.14). Concerning congenital diseases there were significant differences in the NFAS total score for women (cases $\bar{x}_W$ =1.33, CI = 1.20–1.39 vs. non-cases $\bar{x}_W$ =1.18, CI = 1.16–1.19) and numerical differences for men (cases $\bar{x}_M$ =1.22, CI = 1.14–1.27 vs. non-cases $\bar{x}_W$ =1.14, CI = 1.12–1.15).

Combined effects of age, professional education and health limitations on the NFAS

Separate analyses result in raw differences of the mean, which can overestimate the effect of each variable. Therefore, for all single variables described above the effects were estimated simultaneously in a regression model (Table 4).

For both sexes the regression reconfirmed a significantly lower functional level of the oldest age group, for disabled employees and employees who had an accident. These factors resulted in an increase of the NFAS total score by up to 0.274 points for women and up to 0.165 points for men (disabilities vs. no disability, Table 4). The regression model reconfirmed that female employees with a congenital disease had a significantly higher NFAS total score, expressing a lower functional ability, which was not found for men. For women and men a university degree was significantly associated with a higher functional level referring to the NFAS total scores.

With one exception (unskilled/semi-skilled women vs. women with an occupational training) all simultaneously estimated effects on the NFAS total score (Table 4) were smaller than the single effects given by the mean differences in Table 3. This means that the considered variables have a correlated influence on the NFAS total score. For example, the difference in NFAS total scores between women with and without disabilities was 0.274 points as estimated via regression analysis, whereas the single consideration of 'disabilities' vs. 'no disabilities' resulted in a mean difference of 0.31 points (Table 3). The reason is that of the 557 women who had at least one health limitation 34 (6.1%) had a combination of disability plus accident, around 3% had a congenital disease plus accident or a congenital disease plus disability, respectively, and less than 1.5% had all three health limitations.

Discussion

The NFAS was developed as a measure of individual functioning and was applied here to the target population of employees for the first time. Relevant co-factors such as sex, age, professional qualifications, employees that suffer from disabilities, congenital diseases and accidents were considered for the analyses.

Table 3 Mean NFAS domain and total scores with 95% CI (in parenthesis) by age decades, professional qualification, and for employees with disabilities, congenital diseases and accidents; stratified by sex (n = 1872 women and n = 2065 men). A value of 1 characterises the best possible functional ability

	Walking/standing	Holding/picking up things	Lifting/carrying	Sitting	Managing	Cooperation/ communication	Senses	Total scores
Women								
Age (years)								
51–60 (*n* = 778)	1.39 (1.32–1.42)	1.13 (1.10–1.15)	1.26 (1.20–1.29)	1.17 (1.12–1.20)	1.30 (1.23–1.32)	1.15 (1.12–1.17)	1.03 (1.02–1.04)	1.23 (1.19–1.25)
41–50 (*n* = 744)	1.21 (1.16–1.25)	1.09 (1.06–1.11)	1.16 (1.12–1.18)	1.10 (1.06–1.12)	1.28 (1.24–1.31)	1.11 (1.09–1.13)	1.04 (1.02–1.05)	1.16 (1.13–1.18)
31–40 (*n* = 350)	1.21 (1.13–1.25)	1.09 (1.05–1.10)	1.14 (1.09–1.16)	1.11 (1.06–1.13)	1.27 (1.19–1.30)	1.10 (1.06–1.11)	1.02 (1.00–1.03)	1.15 (1.11–1.17)
Professional qualification								
Unskilled/semi-skilled (*n* = 97)	1.53 (1.32–1.66)	1.18 (1.07–1.25)	1.32 (1.17–1.42)	1.15 (1.04–1.24)	1.33 (1.19–1.41)	1.15 (1.08–1.20)	1.03 (1.01–1.05)	1.29 (1.19–1.36)
Occupational training (*n* = 1378)	1.30 (1.25–1.32)	1.11 (1.08–1.12)	1.21 (1.16–1.22)	1.14 (1.11–1.16)	1.29 (1.25–1.30)	1.13 (1.11–1.14)	1.04 (1.02–1.04)	1.20 (1.17–1.20)
University (*n* = 396)	1.18 (1.12–1.22)	1.09 (1.05–1.11)	1.14 (1.09–1.18)	1.07 (1.04–1.10)	1.27 (1.22–1.31)	1.12 (1.09–1.14)	1.01 (1.00–1.03)	1.15 (1.11–1.17)
Disabilities								
Cases (*n* = 148)	1.80 (1.62–1.91)	1.29 (1.19–1.34)	1.58 (1.41–1.68)	1.39 (1.24–1.48)	1.55 (1.41–1.63)	1.22 (1.14–1.26)	1.08 (1.02–1.12)	1.47 (1.37–1.53)
Non-cases (*n* = 1708)	1.23 (1.19–1.25)	1.08 (1.07–1.10)	1.16 (1.13–1.17)	1.10 (1.08–1.11)	1.26 (1.23–1.27)	1.12 (1.10–1.13)	1.03 (1.02–1.03)	1.16 (1.14–1.17)
Congenital Diseases								
Cases (*n* = 79)	1.52 (1.32–1.63)	1.20 (1.10–1.26)	1.39 (1.18–1.51)	1.24 (1.08–1.36)	1.44 (1.27–1.55)	1.13 (1.06–1.18)	1.07 (1.00–1.15)	1.33 (1.20–1.39)
Non-cases (*n* = 1791)	1.27 (1.22–1.29)	1.10 (1.08–1.11)	1.19 (1.16–1.20)	1.12 (1.10–1.14)	1.28 (1.25–1.29)	1.12 (1.11–1.13)	1.03 (1.02–1.04)	1.18 (1.16–1.19)
Accidents								
Cases (*n* = 414)	1.38 (1.30–1.44)	1.17 (1.12–1.20)	1.27 (1.20–1.31)	1.17 (1.10–1.20)	1.34 (1.29–1.38)	1.16 (1.12–1.18)	1.06 (1.02–1.08)	1.25 (1.21–1.28)
Non-cases (*n* = 1457)	1.26 (1.21–1.28)	1.09 (1.07–1.10)	1.18 (1.14–1.20)	1.12 (1.09–1.13)	1.27 (1.24–1.29)	1.12 (1.10–1.13)	1.02 (1.01–1.03)	1.17 (1.15–1.18)
Men								
Age (years)								
51–60 (*n* = 752)	1.30 (1.24–1.34)	1.09 (1.06–1.10)	1.13 (1.10–1.16)	1.10 (1.07–1.13)	1.23 (1.19–1.26)	1.15 (1.11–1.16)	1.03 (1.02–1.04)	1.17 (1.14–1.19)
41–50 (*n* = 845)	1.22 (1.17–1.25)	1.08 (1.05–1.09)	1.12 (1.09–1.14)	1.11 (1.07–1.13)	1.23 (1.19–1.25)	1.12 (1.10–1.14)	1.02 (1.01–1.04)	1.14 (1.12–1.16)
31–40 (*n* = 468)	1.14 (1.08–1.17)	1.07 (1.03–1.09)	1.08 (1.05–1.10)	1.08 (1.04–1.10)	1.23 (1.18–1.26)	1.11 (1.08–1.12)	1.01 (1.00–1.02)	1.12 (1.09–1.13)
Professional qualification								
Unskilled/semi-skilled (*n* = 105)	1.36 (1.18–1.45)	1.11 (1.04–1.15)	1.17 (1.09–1.24)	1.13 (1.05–1.20)	1.29 (1.18–1.36)	1.22 (1.12–1.27)	1.00 (1.00–1.00)	1.21 (1.13–1.27)
Occupational training (*n* = 1492)	1.26 (1.23–1.29)	1.09 (1.07–1.10)	1.14 (1.11–1.16)	1.12 (1.09–1.13)	1.24 (1.21–1.25)	1.13 (1.11–1.16)	1.03 (1.02–1.04)	1.16 (1.14–1.17)
University (*n* = 467)	1.11 (1.07–1.14)	1.04 (1.03–1.05)	1.04 (1.02–1.05)	1.03 (1.01–1.04)	1.19 (1.15–1.21)	1.10 (1.07–1.12)	1.01 (1.00–1.02)	1.09 (1.07–1.10)
Disabilities								
Cases (*n* = 188)	1.62 (1.45–1.72)	1.19 (1.12–1.24)	1.31 (1.21–1.38)	1.22 (1.12–1.29)	1.40 (1.31–1.46)	1.18 (1.13–1.23)	1.04 (1.01–1.07)	1.32 (1.24–1.37)
Non-cases (*n* = 1848)	1.19 (1.16–1.20)	1.06 (1.05–1.07)	1.09 (1.07–1.10)	1.08 (1.06–1.09)	1.21 (1.19–1.23)	1.12 (1.11–1.13)	1.02 (1.01–1.03)	1.13 (1.11–1.14)

Table 3 Mean NFAS domain and total scores with 95% CI (in parenthesis) by age decades, professional qualification, and for employees with disabilities, congenital diseases and accidents; stratified by sex (n = 1872 women and n = 2065 men). A value of 1 characterises the best possible functional ability *(Continued)*

	Walking/standing	Holding/picking up things	Lifting/carrying	Sitting	Managing	Cooperation/ communication	Senses	Total scores
Congenital Diseases								
Cases (*n* = 96)	1.42 (1.24–1.54)	1.12 (1.05–1.16)	1.18 (1.08–1.24)	1.12 (1.03–1.19)	1.31 (1.20–1.38)	1.16 (1.08–1.20)	1.05 (1.00–1.12)	1.22 (1.14–1.27)
Non-cases (*n* = 1965)	1.23 (1.19–1.24)	1.08 (1.06–1.08)	1.11 (1.09–1.12)	1.10 (1.08–1.11)	1.23 (1.20–1.24)	1.13 (1.11–1.14)	1.02 (1.01–1.03)	1.14 (1.12–1.15)
Accidents								
Cases (*n* = 772)	1.29 (1.23–1.32)	1.10 (1.08–1.12)	1.15 (1.11–1.17)	1.13 (1.09–1.15)	1.27 (1.23–1.29)	1.15 (1.12–1.16)	1.02 (1.00–1.03)	1.18 (1.15–1.19)
Non-cases (*n* = 1289)	1.20 (1.16–1.22)	1.06 (1.05–1.07)	1.10 (1.08–1.11)	1.08 (1.06–1.10)	1.21 (1.18–1.22)	1.12 (1.10–1.13)	1.02 (1.01–1.03)	1.13 (1.11–1.14)

Table 4 Generalised linear regression model of the NFAS total score by sex

	Women ($n = 1866$)		Men ($n = 2060$)	
Variable	Beta coefficients	95% CI	Beta coefficients	95% CI
Intercept	0.558***	0.450–0.665	0.357***	0.286–0.428
Age (years)				
51–60	0.054***	0.027–0.081	0.023*	0.002–0.044
41–50	0.006	−0.018 – 0.031	0.008	−0.011 – 0.028
31–40 (ref.)	0		0	
Professional qualification				
Unskilled/semi-skilled	0.110**	0.043–0.178	0.032	−0.017 – 0.081
Occupational training (ref.)	0		0	
University	−0.027*	−0.049 – −0.005	−0.053***	−0.070 – −0.036
Disabilities vs. no disabilities	0.274***	0.193–0.355	0.165***	0.111–0.220
Congenital diseases vs. no congenital diseases	0.084*	0.008–0.159	0.044	−0.008 – 0.095
Accidents vs. no accidents	0.080***	0.050–0.110	0.031**	0.013–0.050

*$p < 0.05$, **$p < 0.01$, *** $p < 0.001$

Overall, the level of functioning as indicated by a NFAS total score of 1.17 was very high. This positive tendency was further underscored by the fact that 35% of the employees reported the best possible functional ability regarding the 39 queried activities.

Considering single factors, we found that men generally rated a significantly better functioning than women, except for the items of the domains Cooperation/communication and Senses. A better self-reported functional ability of men compared to women was expected on the basis of previous NFAS studies [11–14], as was the well-known age-dependency on functional ability that was found in our study, too. We found positive effects of higher professional education on the NFAS total score, and negative effects in case of being an unskilled or semi-skilled employee. Effects of education as shown previously in [22] and in line with the NFAS literature [11–14] were reconfirmed by the NFAS-results at hand. Employees with disabilities and serious accidents showed significantly more functional problems than their unaffected counterparts – a result that also fits well with previous findings [10, 12]. Additionally, suffering from a confirmed disability revealed the most problems on each of the NFAS domains, and is plausible, well-described and proof of the NFAS scale in itself [23].

Two methods were used to estimate the effects of the factors on the NFAS scores. The first method – calculation of the NFAS scores with confidence intervals for each factor, stratified by sex – revealed slightly higher differences of the NFAS total score for not taking into account co-factors that can be correlated. The second method – running a generalised linear regression with all five co-factors for women and for men – in general resulted in slightly smaller regression coefficients (these coefficients accord to the differences of the NFAS total score). The use of both methods resulted in two effect estimates which provide the range of evidence for normative values of functional ability among employees. Referring to our data, the largest difference of these two effect estimates was 0.04 NFAS points. The important essential is that both methods revealed the same general result: there were more functional difficulties for older employees, females, employees with low professional qualification, and for employees suffering from accidents and confirmed disabilities.

The NFAS score values of the present study can be compared to the Norwegian general population aged 24 to 86 ($n = 1705$) and their NFAS total score of 1.31 [14]. In detail, the Norwegian subgroup of individuals with no sickness absence in the previous year resulted in a NFAS total score of 1.13, as compared to 1.17 for all employees of the German sample and to 1.10 for the German subgroup of always healthy employees (36% of the S-MGA I sample). Among the German sample, 38% had one to 9 days of sick-leave in the year preceding the survey, resulting in a NFAS score of 1.13, just as the very healthy Norwegian subsample. For the remaining third German subsample with 10 or more days of sick-leave a NFAS total score of 1.30 was obtained, exactly replicating the score of the Norwegian individuals that were sick-listed for at least 1 week in the previous year. Very close to these subpopulations ranges the Norwegian general population with their NFAS total score of 1.31. Thus, the combination of age, sickness and the demands of work [2] seem to be key factors for functional ability as measured by the NFAS. Interestingly, the observed pattern of the NFAS domain scores among employees in

Germany was very similar to the Norwegian NFAS pattern for almost all NFAS domains: the most severe difficulties appeared for the domains Managing and Walking/standing, the least for the domain Senses with NFAS with values of 1.43, 1.37 and 1.09 for the Norwegian general population and values of 1.26, 1.26 and 1.03 for the employee sample in Germany [14].

Concerning missing data, the study addressed a limitation noted in a previous study [11] by providing the options 'inapplicable to me', 'refused' and 'don't know'. The last two categories were literally irrelevant as they accounted for only 0.01% of the unanswered items. This signifies a high acceptance of the NFAS, potentially further strengthened by having conducted personal interviews instead of questionnaires as in all other applications of the NFAS. The mean level of missing values was similarly low for the Norwegian and the German sample (2.6% and 2.0%, respectively). For further applications of the NFAS, one missing category 'inapplicable to me' seems to be sufficient.

To our knowledge, there are no cut-off values which are relevant for a process at the interface of workforce participation and rehabilitation. Having seen that more than one-third of the employees showed the ideal point of 39 times a value of 1, it still remains an open question to determine a maximum level of non-functioning for participating at work. From our perspective, this issue has to be addressed through longitudinal studies, having return-to-work as an outcome.

As a main strength of the study we consider its large sample size based on random sampling within a nationwide sampling frame. Furthermore, this data base provides normative values of the NFAS for a reference population of employees, taking into account sex, age, professional qualification, and health limitations. It takes only 10 min to respond to the items, and the frequency of item non-response appears to have a negligible effect. Hence, it is assumed that the NFAS is highly accepted by employees. With the longitudinal data of the S-MGA survey that will repeatedly include the NFAS, it will be possible to recommend NFAS domains and to find out levels for a premature exit of older employees from the labour market. The present study is limited by the participant group. On the one hand it solely includes persons with a dependent employment, and on the other hand their age is restricted to 31 to 60 years.

Conclusions

This study presents stratified NFAS scores of a representative sample of employees by age, profession qualification, and for individuals with confirmed disabilities, congenital disorders and accidents. The main findings were that women, elder employees and individuals who are unskilled or semi-skilled reported more functional problems than men, younger employees and persons with a university degree. Employees with disabilities, congenital diseases and accidents had significantly more functional problems than their counterparts without such conditions. Disabled employees showed most functional problems, scoring highest on each of the NFAS domains. While considering all five variables simultaneously, the single effects were reconfirmed. One third of employees reported no difficulty for all the items. Most problems with functional abilities were reported within the domains Walking/standing and managing. The data constitute a basis of normative values of functional ability for the workforce.

Abbreviations

CAPI: Computer-assisted personal interview; CI: Confidence interval; ICF: International Classification of Functioning, Disability and Health; NFAS: Norwegian Function Assessment Scale; SD: Standard deviation; S-MGA: Studie zur mentalen Gesundheit bei der Arbeit; Study on Mental Health at Work; SPSS: Statistical Package for the Social Sciences

Acknowledgements

We would like to acknowledge Dr. F. Thalau† for his conceptual contribution to the use of the NFAS in the S-MGA I and Dr. F. Liebers for a methodical suggestion. For the process of translation we wish to thank I. Osterberg, Dr. S. Neumer, L. M. Evertsen, Dr. S. Brage and N. Østerås.

Funding

The project F2387 was funded by the German Federal Institute for Occupational Safety and Health (BAuA).

Authors' contributions

SJ and NK developed the project and selected the variables. SJ coordinated the project, interpreted the data and drafted the manuscript. NK was in charge of the data repository, checked the data, and selected and run the analyses. UR was involved in the composition of the NFAS questionnaire and the organisation of the data collection. All authors contributed to the discussion. All authors gave final approval of the version to be published and agreed to be accountable for all aspects of the work in ensuring that questions related to the accuracy or integrity of any part of the work are appropriately investigated and resolved.

Consent for publication

Not applicable.

Competing interests

The authors declare that they have no competing interests.

References

1. Kirch W. Encyclopedia of public health: volume 1: A-H volume 2: I-Z. New York: Springer Science+Business Media; 2008.
2. Nordenfelt L. The concept of work ability. Brussels: PIE Peter Lang; 2008.
3. Badura B, Ducki A, Schröder H, Klose J, Meyer M. Fehlzeiten-Report 2015. Berlin Heidelberg: Springer; 2015.
4. De Boer WEL, Brenninkmeijer W, Zuidam W. Long-term disability arrangement. A comparative study of assessments and quality control. Hoofddrop, the Netherlands: The Netherlands Organisation for Applied Scientific Research; 2004.
5. Statistics Norway. Statistical yearbook of Norway 2013. Oslo: Statistics Norway; 2014.
6. Robert Koch-Institut (Hrsg). Gesundheit in Deutschland. Gesundheitsberichterstattung des Bundes. Berlin: RKI; 2015.
7. Brage S, Donceel P, Falez F. Development of ICF core set for disability evaluation in social security. Disabil Rehabil. 2008;30:1392–6.
8. Cerniauskaite M, Quintas R, Boldt C, Raggi A, Cieza A, Bickenbach JE, et al. Systematic literature review on ICF from 2001 to 2009: its use, implementation and operationalisation. Disabil Rehabil. 2011;33:281–309.
9. Organization WH. International classification of functioning, disability and health: ICF. Geneva: World Health Organization; 2001.
10. Brage S, Fleten N, Knudsrød O, Reiso H, Ryen A. Norwegian functional scale - a new instrument in sickness certification and disability assessments. Tidsskrift for den Norske laegeforening: tidsskrift for praktisk medicin, ny raekke. 2004;124:2472–4.
11. Osteras N, Brage S, Garratt A, Benth JS, Natvig B, Gulbrandsen P. Functional ability in a population: normative survey data and reliability for the ICF based Norwegian function assessment scale. BMC Public Health. 2007;7:278.
12. Magnussen LH, Strand LI, Eriksen HR. Physical and mental functioning in disability pensioners with back pain. J Musculoskelet Pain. 2009;17:37–47.
13. Oyeflaten I, Midtgarden IJ, Maeland S, Eriksen HR, Magnussen LH. Functioning, coping and work status three years after participating in an interdisciplinary, occupational rehabilitation program. Scand J Public Health. 2014;42:425–33.
14. Osteras N, Gulbrandsen P, Garratt A, Benth JS, Dahl FA, Natvig B, et al. A randomised comparison of a four- and a five-point scale version of the Norwegian function assessment scale. Health Qual Life Outcomes. 2008;6:14.
15. Schröder H, Schiel S, Schulz S, Kleudgen M. Mentale Gesundheit bei der Arbeit (S-MGA): Methodenbericht zur Repräsentativerhebung an Erwerbstätigen in Deutschland. 2. überarbeitete Auflage ed. Bundesanstalt für Arbeitsschutz und Arbeitsmedizin: Dortmund/Berlin/Dresden; 2015.
16. Bundesamt S. Bevölkerung und Erwerbstätigkeit. Haushalte und Familien. Ergebnisse des Mikrozensus. Wiesbaden: Statistisches Bundesamt; 2011.
17. Rose U, Schiel S, Schröder H, Kleudgen M, Tophoven S, Rauch A, et al. The study on mental health at work: design and sampling. Scand J Public Health. 2017;45:584–94.
18. Bundesamt S. Statistisches Jahrbuch Deutschland und Internationales 2016. Wiesbaden: Statistisches Bundesamt; 2016.
19. SYSTAT Inc. SYSTAT 13. Statistics I. Chicago: SYSTAT Software, Inc.; 2009.
20. Rüschendorf L. Mathematische Statistik. Berlin: Springer; 2014.
21. Tweedie MCK. An index which distinguishes between some important exponential families. Statistics: Applications and New Directions - Proceedings of the Indian Statistical Institute Golden Jubilee International Conference. Calcutta: Indian Statistical Institute. 1984;579–604.
22. Grammenos S. Illness, disability and social inclusion. Dublin: European Foundation for the Improvement of Living and Working Conditions; 2003.
23. Falvo D. Medical and psychosocial aspects of chronic illness and disability. Burlington, MA: Jones & Bartlett; 2014.

18

Olfactory dysfunction revisited: a reappraisal of work-related olfactory dysfunction caused by chemicals

Sabine Werner* and Eberhard Nies

Abstract

Occupational exposure to numerous individual chemicals has been associated with olfactory dysfunction, mainly in individual case descriptions. Comprehensive epidemiological investigations into the olfactotoxic effect of working substances show that the human sense of smell may be impaired by exposure to metal compounds involving cadmium, chromium and nickel, and to formaldehyde. This conclusion is supported by the results of animal experiments. The level of evidence for a relationship between olfactory dysfunction and workplace exposure to other substances is relatively weak.

Keywords: Chemically induced anosmia, Formaldehyde, Metals, Occupational exposure, Olfaction disorders

Background

Many occupational groups are reliant upon intact olfactory function in order to perform their work and for their safety. Examples are chefs, gas fitters, firefighters, perfumers, sommeliers, coffee and tea tasters, grocers, workers in the chemical industry, and domestic helpers. The importance of the olfactory function for early detection of hazardous substances with an odour is illustrated by the specific case of an anosmic who lit a cigarette whilst in close proximity to a leaking petrol pipe, thereby causing an explosion [1]. Muttray et al. [2] report the case of a patient who did not become aware of his olfactory dysfunction until his colleagues fled their workplace, to him for no apparent reason, owing to an intense solvent smell. In Germany, an assessment of olfactory function is a requirement for persons applying for certification of their fitness to perform fumigation [3], and loss of olfactory function constitutes grounds for example for the discharge of members of the US military, including reservists, and of coastguard employees [4].

* Correspondence: Sabine.Werner@dguv.de
Institute for Occupational Safety and Health of the German Social Accident Insurance, Unit Toxicology of Industrial Chemicals, Alte Heerstrasse 111, 53757 Sankt Augustin, Germany

Diagnosis and assessment of olfactory dysfunction

Assessment of olfactory function and diagnosis of olfactory dysfunction requires, firstly, a detailed medical history and examination by an otolaryngologist [5, 6]. The medical history should include information on the triggering events, development, complementary symptoms, surgical operations, medication and toxicants. The ENT diagnosis comprises medical status, endoscopy of nose and nasopharyngeal space and evaluation of the olfactory cleft. If a neurological disorder is suspected, an examination by a neurologist including tests of cognition and memory could be necessary. Secondly, a validated test method is needed that enables subjective sensory perceptions to be quantified objectively. This is essential for a standardised distinction between normosmia (normal olfactory function), hyposmia and anosmia (impaired olfactory function and its complete loss, respectively), and hyperosmia (olfactory oversensitivity). A screening of global taste function (retronasal smelling) is also advantageous owing to the close connection between smell and taste (patients complaining of a dysfunctional sense of taste are in fact often suffering from olfactory impairment).

Only in the last three decades have standardised and practicable psychophysical tests for humans been developed. Of these, UPSIT (University of Pennsylvania Smell

Identification Test [7]) and the "Sniffin' Sticks" test widely used in Europe [8, 9], are important examples.

"Sniffin' Sticks" are felt sticks that release aromatic substances when the cap of the stick is removed. In conventional form, they permit threshold, discrimination and identification tests; the last two of these are above-threshold tests. The threshold test indicates the concentration above which an odour is sensed (the sensory threshold). As standard, n-butanol or phenyl ethyl alcohol (rose scent) are used for testing. The non-verbal discrimination test examines the ability to distinguish between odours. In the identification test, 16 odours are tested for recognition [10]. This is a structured, reliable and validated test system that is widely used in Europe and is readily available. Extensive validation studies and defined standard values exist for this test [11, 12]. Regularly updated standardised values are published for example on the website of the Interdisciplinary Center Smell & Taste (University Clinic Dresden) [13].

A similar identification test used in America is the UPSIT method, in which up to 40 odorants, microencapsulated on a sheet of paper, are released by scratching with the point of a pencil. In this test, the various odorants must be identified with reference to a list of four terms per substance. The test kit has a long shelf life, is very well validated and is widely used. The UPSIT test does not require clinician supervision and is therefore very convenient. International versions are also available; they have however rarely been validated specifically for individual countries. A drawback of the test is that it studies only the identification of odours.

Where patients might not be able to comply with psychophysical testing, or in medico-legal assessments, the olfactory dysfunction can be assessed objectively by recording electrical activity of the brain (olfactory event-related potentials, OERPs) following presentation of odours. This method requires virtually no active participation on the part of the test subject, and has been used since the 1970s. It involves the application of olfactory stimuli to the nose of the test subject with the aid of an olfactometer. The stimuli trigger corresponding OERPs, which can then be registered on electrodes applied to the test subject's head. The use of an electro-olfactograph (the recording of generator potential via an electrode in contact with the olfactory epithelium) is limited to research. Olfactory functional imaging methods such as PET (positron emission tomography) and fMRI (functional magnetic resonance imaging) are also largely limited to research applications [5, 6].

Important information on the toxic properties of inhaled substances that may affect olfaction has been obtained from experiments on animals. Besides histological analyses of the olfactory epithelium, the results of behavioural tests are also relevant. Since the laboratory animal is not able to communicate actively to the researcher whether or not it senses an odour, an operant conditioning test is usually performed. In such a test, mice for example are first taught to expect a reward (such as water following restricted access to water) after sensing a certain olfactory stimulus. The animals are then presented with other odours that are not followed by a reward, in addition to the odour that they have learnt to associate with the reward. Where the animal has recognised the correct odour and looks for its reward, this can be registered, for example by means of a light barrier (for a detailed description, see Kuner and Schaefer 2011 [14]; an up-to-date overview with detailed test protocols can be found in Zou et al. 2016 [15]).

Work-related olfactory dysfunction

The prevalence of olfactory dysfunction in the wider population is estimated at around 5% (for functional anosmia) [16]. It is considerably more common among older people, and around a quarter of the population aged over 50 exhibit an impaired sense of smell. The results of recent studies suggest that specific anosmias, the failure to sense a specific odour, are far more prevalent than was previously assumed and are the norm rather than the exception [16, 17]. The proportion of olfactory dysfunction caused by occupational exposure remains unclear. Figures for olfactory dysfunction caused by exposure to the effects of chemicals and pharmaceuticals fluctuate between 0.5 and 5% of all cases [18]. According to a large-scale survey of all ear, nose and throat clinics in the German-speaking world, covering 79,000 patients, 2% of the cases had toxic causes [19]. A recent Belgian publication covering a substantially smaller collective of 496 patients with exclusively non-sinusoidal complaints from a specialist clinical centre assumed that 3.4% were toxic in origin [20]. "Idiopathic" cases of olfactory dysfunction, which are put at between 10 and 25%, may however include cases of chemically induced damage caused by workplace exposure not classified as such [21, 22]. In his paper on functional testing and dysfunction of olfaction, Herberhold [23] assumed several decades ago that pathologically elevated olfactory thresholds were present in around 30% of workers in the metals and chemical industry, possibly rising to around 50% with increasing age and increasing duration of exposure to the hazardous substances. Today's working conditions and exposures are clearly not comparable with those of the 1970s; in her review however, Dalton 2010 [24] also cites a questionnaire and survey conducted in 1995 among 712,000 individuals in Canada and the USA which revealed that factory workers of all ages reported a weaker sense of smell and performed significantly worse in an olfactory test than members of other occupational groups.

According to Herberhold [23], thermal, mechanical and chemical noxae may lead to olfactory dysfunction, the effects triggered by chemicals being more pronounced the more active the chemical substance, the smaller the particles, and the longer the duration of exposure of the sensory apparatus to them. Occupational exposure to numerous industrial chemicals, notably those that are irritative and corrosive to the mucous membranes or harmful to the nerves, is associated with the incidence of olfactory dysfunction (see for example Klimek et al. 1999 [25] and Muttray et al. 2006 [26]). In his overview, Amoore [27] lists over 100 substances presumed capable of causing olfactory dysfunction. This information is based almost entirely upon case reports rather than on large-scale studies. The discussion below therefore gives consideration to the substances associated with occupational olfactory dysfunction that have been studied under standardised conditions in epidemiological studies and studies of test subjects. The results of relevant animal experiments concerning the substances identified in this way that to some extent permit conclusions regarding the possible mechanism of action are also presented.

Industrial chemicals with a potential impact upon olfaction

In order to identify industrial chemicals exposure to which may potentially lead to olfactory dysfunction, a literature survey was conducted in the Pubmed database in order to identify substances characterised as olfactotoxic primarily on the basis of epidemiological studies and studies of test subjects conducted under standardised conditions. The terms "anosmia", "hyposmia", "dysosmia", "smell disorders", "olfactory function", "olfactory dysfunction" and "olfaction disorders" were each combined in the search with "occupational", "professional" and "workplace". In the second step, the substances identified in this way were used as search terms in combination with the relevant clinical pictures (see above) in order to identify animal experiments. Relevant studies in the bibliographies of the identified literature were considered. Pharmacological and environmental studies associated with the identified industrial chemicals were also included. Case reports, for example concerning accident-type events involving very high exposures, were disregarded.

A comprehensive overview of long-term effects of occupational exposures to metals and olfactory toxicity can be found in the reviews by Gobba 2006 and Sunderman 2001 [21, 28]. One aspect addressed by the recent review in Doty 2015 is likewise the influence of exposure to neurotoxic substances in the environment or at the workplace upon the sense of smell [4]. Accordingly, the studies referred to in these publications will not be considered in further detail in the present paper. The focus here lies on the epidemiological and animal studies not stated there. The latter will be described in detail. Human studies on olfactotoxic effects caused by chemicals are summarised in Table 1.

Cadmium and nickel

A considerable number of epidemiological studies demonstrate an association between exposure to metals in the form of dusts and vapours, and occupational olfactory dysfunction. Anosmia and hyposmia were diagnosed for example among workers exposed to dust containing nickel or cadmium in plants for the production of alkaline batteries, nickel refineries, and the cadmium industry.

Human studies

Cadmium exposure Nine epidemiological studies published in the period from 1950 to 2003 [29–37] address the association between workplace cadmium/nickel exposure and olfactory impairment. The older studies lack clear information on the test methods and comparisons with non-exposed subjects [29–32]. Anosmia/hyposmia was detected in a significantly high proportion of the exposed workers in all human studies. Differentiated sensory and identification tests were conducted in three studies [34–37]; Rydzewski et al. and Sulkowski et al. [35, 36] describe the same data, which can therefore also be counted as one. Whereas Rose et al. and Mascagni et al. [34, 37] demonstrated that the values obtained in the sensory threshold test were considerably higher among the workers than in the control group, the identification test revealed no significant differences. The sensory threshold test for n-butanol or phenyl ethyl alcohol is regarded as an instrument for diagnosing the function of the peripheral olfactory receptor neurons. According to this interpretation, the ability to identify odours is based primarily upon the processing of olfactory information in the cerebral cortex. This absolute distinction is problematic however, since the sensory threshold test also encompasses complex functions of the central nervous system, and the identification of odours is dependent upon the activity of the olfactory receptor neurons.

Many of the epidemiological studies that describe the incidence of olfactory dysfunction following exposure to cadmium are older. In the 1950s and 1960s, occupational exposure to cadmium was appreciably higher than it is today, for example 0.6–236 mg/m^3 in a battery factory [31]. The threshold limit values (TLVs) proposed by the American Conference of Governmental Industrial Hygienists (ACGIH) stated a limit concentration of 50 $\mu g/m^3$ in 1975 and 10 $\mu g/m^3$ as of 1995. Conversely, more recently published measured exposure values of 0.004–0.187 mg/m^3 [32], 0.3 mg/m^3 [34] and 1.53 mg/m^3 (1975) and 0.0171 mg/m^3 (1995) [37] demonstrate that damage to olfactory function may arise even at low concentrations.

Table 1 Work-related olfactory dysfunction: Human studies (in chronological order)

Human studies Reference	Occupation	Exposure (mg/m³)	Exposed workers, residents, patients	Controls	Test method	Results
Cadmium/nickel						
[a]Friberg 1950 [29]	Battery factory	3–15 Cd 10–150 Ni	43 (group 1: longer employment 9–34 years) 15 (group 2: shorter employment 1–4 years)	–	Test with odour samples (coffee, perfume, peppermint and petrol)	Group 1: 37% impaired sense of smell (32.6%: anosmia). Group 2: 6.7% (one case) partially impaired sense of smell.
[a]Baader 1951 [30])	Battery factory	N. i.	8	–	Test with odour samples (no further details)	4 hyposmic or anosmic.
[a]Potts 1965 [31]	Battery factory	Cd dust and fumes: 0.6–236 (1949) < 0.5 (1950) < 0.1 (1956)	70	–	N. i.	64% anosmic.
[a]Liu et al. 1985 [32]	Cadmium smelters	Cd oxide: 0.004–0.187	65	–	N. i.	21.5% anosmic.
[a]Adams and Crabtree 1961 [33]	Battery factory	Cd: 0.028–2.76 Ni: 0.0016–0.056	106	84	Threshold test with phenol	27.3% anosmic (Co: 4.8% anosmic)
[a]Rose et al. 1992 [34]	Factory producing refrigerating coils	Cd fumes up to 0.3	55	16	Threshold test with n-butanol. Identification test with 10 different olfactory stimuli	13% severe hyposmia (Co: 0%), 44% weakly hyposmic (Co: 31%). Identification test: no significant difference.
[a]Rydzewski et al. 1998 [35] [a]Sulkowski et al. 2000 [36]	Battery factory	Atmospheric cadmium concentrations: 0.05–2.1	73	43 forestry workers	Threshold identification test with modified Elsberg-Levys method	Significantly impaired ability to detect and identify odours. Overall result: 26% hyposmia, 17.8% parosmia, 1.4% anosmia (Co: 30.2% parosmia, 69.8 normosmia).
[a]Mascagni et al. 2003 [37]	Workers in a cadmium foundry and sintering plant	Cadmium concentrations (max.): 1.530 (1975) -0.0171 (1995); by 1978, the measurement results had already dropped substantially below 1 (at 0.207)	33	39 drivers and storekeepers, 23 welders	Threshold test with phenyl ethyl alcohol Identification test with Wright's confusion matrices	Olfactory threshold significantly higher in Cd workers than in controls. Identification test: no significant difference (a non-significant impairment in cadmium workers). Overall results: 3.1% anosmic, 3.1% severely hyposmic, 24.1% mildly/moderately hyposmic (welders: 0% anosmic, 4.3% severely hyposmic, 8.7% mildly/moderately hyposmic; Co: 0% anosmic, 0% severely hyposmic, 7.7% mildly/moderately hyposmic).

Table 1 Work-related olfactory dysfunction: Human studies (in chronological order) *(Continued)*

Human studies Reference	Occupation	Exposure (mg/m^3)	Exposed workers, residents, patients	Controls	Test method	Results
[a]2 studies from USSR cited in Sunderman [28]: (Tatarskaya 1960) (Kucharin 1970)	Electrolytic Ni refinery Electrolytic Ni refinery	N. i. N. i.	N. i. 458	N. i. N. i.	N. i. N. i.	Frequent olfactory impairment, atrophic nasal mucosa, nasal septal ulceration and sinusitis. Anosmia in 114/251 workers (46%) with chronic sinusitis; less severe loss of smell in other Ni-exposed workers.
Chromium						
Seeber et al. 1976 [53]	Chrome paint plant (manufacture of basic zinc chromate (zinc yellow))	Values exceeded 0.1 CrO_3 air, and rose at certain points to up to 20 CrO_3. More precise values are not stated.	5 chronically exposed workers, 14 intermittently exposed workers (not longer than 2 h per day), 5 mask-wearing workers (wearing fine-dust filter masks for the full duration)	9 office workers at the same company, 23 employees at hospital	Test with odour strips (6 different stimuli in 8 concentrations)	Olfactory sensitivity of control group and non-exposed individuals substantially higher than that of exposed individuals. "Significant" relationship between chromium exposure and loss of olfaction. Chronically exposed individuals: damage to the nasal mucous membrane. Intermittently exposed group and workers with a mask: damage to the nasal mucous membrane only in a part.
Seeber and Fikentscher 1980 [54]	See above	Occupational exposure "substantially reduced" by suitable measures (not specified)	3 chronically exposed workers, 9 intermittently exposed workers (not longer than 2 h per day) 4 mask-wearing workers (wearing fine-dust filter masks for the full duration)	7 office workers at the same company, 23 employees at hospital	See above	Confirmation of the relationship between the pathological nasal mucous membrane findings and olfactory dysfunction in 16 workers exposed to different levels. No improvement in the mucous membrane or olfaction.
[a]Watanabe and Fukuchi (1981) [55]	Chromate production plant	Air Cr concentration of 20.17 according to [56]	33	–	T&T olfactometer (odour detection threshold and odour recognition)	"Middle and high grade decrease of odor recognition faculty" in 18 workers (54.5%) including 2 anosmiac, one of whom also complained of a taste disorder. 51% exhibited nasal septum perforations. Relation between degree of olfaction loss and duration of employment in the chromate producing factory.
[a]Kitamura et al. 2003 [56]	Cr plating factory	Average atmospheric concentration was 0.0228	27	34	T&T olfactometer (odour detection threshold and odour recognition) Olfactory perception threshold test	No significant differences for sensory and perception threshold. Significantly higher values for the odour recognition test than those for controls, positive correlation with duration of exposure. None of Cr workers showed nasal septum perforation or ulceration.

Table 1 Work-related olfactory dysfunction: Human studies (in chronological order) *(Continued)*

Human studies Reference	Occupation	Exposure (mg/m^3)	Exposed workers, residents, patients	Controls	Test method	Results
Aiyer et al. 2003	Chromium plating industry	N. i.	28	–	N. i.	11 workers anosmic (nasal septal perforation of different magnitudes on all exposed workers, majority with initial symptom of nasal irritation).
Manganese						
[a]Lucchini et al. 1997 [58]	Ferroalloy production plant	Manganese dust exposure: 0.026–0.750 (geometric mean: 0.193)	35	37	Olfactory perception threshold to PM-carbinol (3-methyl-1-phenylpentan-3-ol dilution series)	No significant differences (although it was negatively associated with Mn levels in urine in the exposed group)
[a]Mergler et al. 1994 [59]	Ferromanganese and silicomanganese alloy plant	Manganese dust exposure: 0.014–11.48 Total Mn levels in dust: 0.89 (geometric mean) Manganese content of respirable dust fraction: 0.001 and 1.273 (geometric mean: 0.04)	74 (matched pairs)	74	Olfactory perception threshold to PM-carbinol	Significantly increased olfactory perception among workers compared to controls.
[a]Antunes et al. 2007 [60] [a]Bowler et al. 2007 [61]	San Francisco/ Oakland Bay Bridge welders	Atmospheric manganese levels lay between 0.11 and 0.46 (55% > 0.20)	43 welders	43 (matched by age, sex, education and smoking status from the database of the University of Pennsylvania Smell and Taste Center)	UPSIT identification test	Significantly weaker olfactory function of welders than in controls. Score of 88% of the workers below their individually matched controls. 3% of the welders were anosmic. Better olfactory function in workers with the highest Mn blood levels than those with the lowest Mn blood levels.
Bowler et al. 2011 [62]	Follow-up study three and a half years later	–	26 welders from the San Francisco/Oakland Bay Bridge welder study (13 study participants were no longer working as welders)	–	UPSIT identification test	No significant differences from earlier findings. The blood-manganese levels of the former workers were significantly lower than those of their colleagues.
Sen et al. 2011 [63]	Welders	Cumulative Mn exposure (mg/m^{3}x years): Welders 0.881 (± 0.567) Controls 0.002 (± 0.0003)	7 welders	7	MRI	Increased manganese deposition in the olfactory bulb and in other regions of the brain. No statistically significant differences in the olfactory test between the two groups (data not shown).
Guarneros et al. (2013)	Persons living in proximity to a manganese plant	Elevated manganese hair concentration (mean 0.00973 vs. 0.00101)	30 persons living within a one-kilometre radius of a Mexican manganese mine	30 controls living more than 50 km away	Sniffin' Sticks olfactory test series (threshold, discrimination and identification tests)	Significantly diminished olfactory function in those living close to the manganese mine (in threshold, discrimination and identification tests).

Table 1 Work-related olfactory dysfunction: Human studies (in chronological order) *(Continued)*

Human studies Reference	Occupation	Exposure (mg/m^3)	Exposed workers, residents, patients	Controls	Test method	Results
Lucchini et al. 2012 [65]	Residents of Valcamonica: Italian region, marked by ferrous alloy plants until 2001	Average Mn atmospheric and soil values at the time of the study: 0.0495, 958	154 young people aged between 11 and 14	157 young people from Lake Garda region	Sniffin' Sticks (identification test)	Significantly poorer olfactory function associated with Mn content in the soil.
Iannilli et al. 2016	Valcamonica (see above) and Bognolo Mella: regions with a history of high Mn contamination	–	9 young people from Valcamonica and Bagnolo Mella exposed to manganese	4 young people from the Lake Garda region	Sniffin' Sticks (identification test), fMRT (response activity to olfactory tasks)	No significantly different results of the identification test between the two groups. Reduction in activity in relevant olfactory brain regions. In comparison with a larger control group from a database, significant differences were observed with regard to the size of the olfactory bulb and in the olfactory test involving Sniffin' Sticks.
Casjen et al. 2017 [67]	Blue collar workers	Median: 58.3 $\mu g/m^3$ x years (interquartile range 19–185 $\mu g/m^3$ x years)	354	1031	Sniffin' Sticks (identification test)	No relevant association of former Mn exposure at relatively low levels with impaired olfaction.
Zinc						
Pyatayev et al. 1971 [73]	Zinc production plant	Zinc oxide, zinc sulfate and metal dusts. Co-exposure to further strongly corrosive and irritant substances	301	63	Olfactometer employing mint and dilute acetic acid	Significant elevations of sensory thresholds. Elevations were highest among workers responsible for roasting the zinc ore.
Anonymous 1938, [a]Tisdall et al. 1938 [74, 75]	(Treatment in special clinics with zinc in nasal spray for prevention of poliomyelitis infection)	Nasal spray solution containing 1% zinc sulfate and 0.5% tetracaine	5233 children (4713 (received two sprayings) + 520 (received one spraying))	6300	N. i.	No more than a quarter exhibited temporary anosmia.
[a]Tisdall et al. 1938 [75]	(Patients treated by the same otolaryngologists, but in their private practices)	See above	5000 children and adults	–	N.i.	6 months following treatment: 44 of the patients were permanently anosmic (52 with disturbances of smell and taste).
Davidson et al. 2010 [76]	(Nasal Dysfunction Clinic of the University of California in San Diego)	Intranasal zinc gluconate gel	10 patients	–	n-Butanol threshold UPSIT (identification test)	3 subjects with anosmia and 7 with hyposmia.
Alexander et al. 2006 [77]	(See above)	Intranasal zinc gluconate gel	17 patients	–	n-Butanol threshold,	Impaired olfaction in all patients: 7 patients anosmic, 10 hyposmic.

Table 1 Work-related olfactory dysfunction: Human studies (in chronological order) *(Continued)*

Human studies Reference	Occupation	Exposure (mg/m^3)	Exposed workers, residents, patients	Controls	Test method	Results
					identification test employing seven known odorants and one substance for testing the trigeminal function, UPSIT (9 patients)	Trauma and infection were ruled out as causes of hyposmia and anosmia diagnosed in 15 of these patients in the relevant tests.
Jafek et al. 2004 [78]	(Special "Taste and Smell Center" at the University of Colorado School of Medicine)	Use of zinc gluconate gel	10 patients	–	N. i.	Suffering of severe hyposmia in conjunction with parosmia or anosmia following use of zinc gluconate gel.
"Pesticides"						
[a]Calvert et al. 1998 [102]	Structural fumigation workers	Lifetime duration of methyl bromide and sulfuryl fluoride exposure: 1.2 and 2.85 years Sulfuryl fluoride values of earlier NIOSH measurements: below 20	123	120	UPSIT (identification test)	Significantly weaker olfactory function in workers with high sulfuryl fluoride exposure over the year preceding examination.
Quandt et al. 2016 [104]	Latino farmworkers	Lifetime exposure. Total years in jobs involving pesticide exposure: farmworkers 13.11 (mean), non-farmworkers 3.84 (mean)	304	247	Sniffin' Sticks Kit (identification test and threshold test with n-butanol)	No difference in odour identification performance but significantly higher odour thresholds.
Formaldehyde						
[a]Holmström and Wilhelmsson 1988 [111]	Workers at a chemical plant where formaldehyde and products based on formaldehyde were produced	0.05–0.5 formaldehyde (for the group of workers impregnating paper up to 1)	70	36 (office workers with 0.9 mean exposure to formaldehyde)	Sensory threshold test employing pyridine	Significantly reduced olfactory function.
[a]Holmström and Wilhelmsson 1988 [111]	Work with glued wood in the production of furniture	0.2–0.3 (formaldehyde) 1–2 (wood dust)	100	36	See above	Significantly reduced olfactory function (but no difference between the formaldehyde and the formaldehyde-wood dust groups).
[a]Hisamitsu et al. 2011 [112]	Medical students during cadaver dissection	0.64–1.2 (middle of the laboratory), 0.28–0.88 (in the corners)	41	–	Nagashima jet nebulising olfaction test with bromine (detection threshold)	Significantly diminished olfactory function (32%, temporary).

Table 1 Work-related olfactory dysfunction: Human studies (in chronological order) *(Continued)*

Human studies Reference	Occupation	Exposure (mg/m³)	Exposed workers, residents, patients	Controls	Test method	Results
Kilburn et al. 1985 [113]	Histology technicians	0.25–2.38 (exposure to other solvents such as xylene, toluene and also chloroform)	76	56	Questionnaire	Significantly more self-reported frequent reduced sense of smell in histology technicians (32% of the women who were exposed to formaldehyde for 1 to 3 h and likewise 32% of the women who were exposed for over 4 h stated that their olfactory function was diminished, 5% Co).
Edling et al. 1988 [114]	Workers at different plants (laminate plants, particle board plants)	0.1–1.1 with exposure peaks of up to 5 (formaldehyde), 0.6–1.1 (wood dust)	75	25	Histological examination	Pathological changes of the nasal mucous membrane in 72 individuals.
Acrylates						
[a]Schwartz et al. 1989 [119]	Workers at a chemical facility manufacturing acrylates and methacrylates	0.0416–232.96 ethyl acrylate and acrylic acid (mostly around 30 for acrylic acid and 20.8 for ethyl acrylate)	55 (high) 164 (low)	512	UPSIT (identification test)	No association in the first instance between exposure and results of olfactory tests.
[a]Schwartz et al. 1989 [119] embedded case-control study	See above	See above	77	77		Dose-effect relationship between olfactory dysfunction and cumulative exposure; the effect appeared to be reversible. Workers who had never smoked had the highest relative risk of olfactory dysfunction.
Muttray et al. 1997 [120]	Chemical workers in acrylic sheet production	Methyl methacrylate (MMA): 104–416 (1988), 41.6–208 (1989–1994), 9.6 ±7.1 years (mean duration of MMA exposure)	175	88	Rhino Identification Test (6 tested aromas, very similar in design to the UPSIT test)	No significant difference between exposed workers and control group.
Muttray et al. 2007 [121]	Healthy volunteers	208 MMA and room air in an exposure chamber at an interval of one week, in each case for 4 h	20	–	Olfactory threshold for n-butanol (Sniffin' Sticks)	Olfactory threshold: no changes.
Styrene						
[a]Cheng et al. 2004 [123]	Injection-moulding workers exposed to acrylonitrile-butadiene-styrene (mainly manufacture of computer shells)	–	52	72	Olfactory threshold test employing 1-butanol, CCCRC olfactory test (identification)	Slight but significant reduction in olfactory function (threshold) at the end of the shift (whereas the initial situation at the beginning of the shift had been the same). The identification test revealed no differences before and after the shift.

Table 1 Work-related olfactory dysfunction: Human studies (in chronological order) *(Continued)*

Human studies Reference	Occupation	Exposure (mg/m^3)	Exposed workers, residents, patients	Controls	Test method	Results
[a]Dalton et al. 2003 [124]	Workers in the reinforced-plastics industry	Mean airborne styrene concentrations: 89.2 (day 1), 106.1 (day 2) Means and ranges of historic exposures to airborne styrene for individual workers (*n* = 52): 57.37 (15.16–134.23) Cumulative mean exposure: 675.48 (59.75–1420.24) Peak year exposure: 112.58 (22.52–331.25)	52	52	Olfactory threshold for phenyl ethyl alcohol and styrene, retronasal odour identification test with five stimuli, identification test with 20 odorants	No significant differences between styrene-exposed workers and matched controls in the results of the phenylethyl alcohol threshold test, retronasal test, or odour identification test. Significantly different odour detection thresholds for styrene among exposed and unexposed groups.
[a]Dalton et al. 2007 [125]	Workers in a reinforced plastics boat-manufacturing facility	Calculated effective mean concentration of styrene in air: 43.3–108.25 (measured airborne styrene concentration for this group: 303.1–346.4)	15	15	Olfactory threshold for phenyl ethyl alcohol (PEA) and styrene, identification test with 18 odorants	No significant difference in olfactory threshold for PEA. Significant difference in the threshold test involving styrene among exposed and unexposed groups. Significant difference in the identification test between workers with high vs. low exposure (possible explanations: more individuals with poor values in both groups than in normal population, cultural and educational differences between the two groups).
Organic solvents and mineral oil products						
[a]Schwartz et al. 1990 [130]	Workers in paint manufacturing facilities	Solvents: toluene, xylene and methyl ethyl ketone Lifetime hydrocarbon dose in ppm years (averages at the two production plants): 180 (±128), 97 (±70)	187	–	UPSIT identification test	Significant dose-dependent deterioration in olfactory function with rising lifetime exposure among workers who had never smoked.
[a]Sandmark et al. 1989 [131]	Painters	No quantitative exposure measurement (described as "low to moderate")	54	42	UPSIT identification test	No statistically significant impairment of olfactory function after adjustment for age and smoking habits.
Studies cited in Muttray et al. 1998 [133]: (Dragomitretzky et al. 1970) (Kmita 1953) (Latkowski et al. 1981 [134])	Workers at a shoe factory, petroleum chemistry workers	A petroleum mixture ("Galoscha"), ethyl acetate and butyl acetate (solvent concentration: 220–300), rubber adhesive containing petroleum (up to 3000) N. i.	216 205 547	N. i. N. i. 100 (cotton industry workers)	N. i. N. i. Smell and taste tests	31% suffered the loss of olfactory function, and among the remainder, olfactory function was impaired in comparison to a control group. Olfactory dysfunction as a result of rhinitis arose after a few years. Hyposmia in 238 (43.5%) and anosmia in 50 (9.2%) subjects. Dysgeusia in 319 (58.3%).

Table 1 Work-related olfactory dysfunction: Human studies (in chronological order) *(Continued)*

Human studies Reference	Occupation	Exposure (mg/m^3)	Exposed workers, residents, patients	Controls	Test method	Results
						(Co: dysgeusia in 69%, anosmia in 24% of subjects).
[a]Ahlstrom et al. 1986 [132]	Tank cleaners	Mineral oil products (heavy and light oils, hydrocarbon content: 240–1615)	20	40	Threshold test, perceived odour intensity test (pyridine, dimethyl disulfide, n-butanol and heated oil vapour)	Elevated olfactory threshold values for heated oil vapour and n-butanol in comparison to controls (for n-butanol within the normal range, oil vapour had not been studied in this respect before). Higher threshold values for all tested substances exhibited by tank cleaners exposed one day prior to the test in comparison to individuals exposed earlier. Lower odour intensity values at the lowest stimulus concentrations for all 4 substances in comparison to those of control subjects ("odour intensity recruitment").

N.i. not indicated, *Co* control group, [a]studies which have already been discussed in the reviews by Sunderman, Gobba and Doty [4, 21, 28]

Nickel exposure With the exception of the studies stated by Sunderman, we are not aware of any studies into the association between workplace nickel exposure and olfactory dysfunction. Sunderman [28] cites two studies from the former Soviet Union from 1960 and 1970, according to which workers exposed to nickel in electrolytic nickel refineries exhibited olfactory dysfunction/anosmia in addition to atrophy of the nasal mucous membrane, chronic sinusitis and ulceration of the nasal septum.

In the studies cited concerning cadmium, the workers were often exposed not only to cadmium, but also to nickel (see above). Whereas in the 1940s, occupational nickel exposure of 10–150 mg/m^3 for example was possible [29], considerably lower values of up to 0.056 mg/m^3 were measured in the publication by Adams and Crabtree in 1961 [33]. ACGIH currently sets a TLV of 1.5 mg/m^3 for the inhalable fraction of nickel.

Animal experimental studies

Cadmium exposure Following inhalation tests on rats (250 and 500 $\mu g/m^3$ CdO, 5 h per day, 5 days per week for 20 weeks), an elevated cadmium level was determined in the olfactory bulb. This was accompanied neither by significant histopathological changes in the mucous membrane, nor by a reduction in the olfactory function [38].

In another animal experiment, administration of 400 μg of $CdCl_2$ to mice by intranasal instillation resulted in partial damage to the olfactory epithelium, reversible loss of olfactory discrimination, and specific cadmium deposition in the olfactory bulb but not in other parts of the central nervous system [39]. Czarnecki et al. [40] also observed anosmia in a behavioural test following intranasal instillation of a cadmium chloride solution in mice. They further demonstrated a dose-dependent reduction in the odour-induced release of neurotransmitters from the olfactory nerve into the olfactory bulb. Moreover, a 20% drop in the dendrite density of the olfactory epithelium was described at the highest dose (20 μg $CdCl_2$). In further experiments, Czarnecki et al. demonstrated a clear cadmium accumulation on mice specifically in the olfactory bulb by bilateral instillation of a buffer solution of 20 μg of $CdCl_2$ per nostril. The accumulation was still measurable 4 weeks after exposure. A reduction in the axonal terminals of the olfactory receptor neurons was also demonstrated histologically. A decrease in neurotransmitter release in response to olfactory stimulation was detected in vivo on the mice exposed to cadmium (intranasal instillation with 0.2, 2 and 20 μg $CdCl_2$) 2, 7 and 28 days after exposure. After the laboratory animals treated with cadmium had exhibited significant olfactory deficits in a behavioural test, these deficits disappeared after two weeks of olfactory training; however, the mice with restored olfaction continued to exhibit damaged projections of the olfactory receptor neurons in the results of optical imaging. Czarnecki et al. conclude from this that restoration of olfactory function is attributable to neuroplasticity: the brain, they assume, has learnt to reinterpret the reduced stimuli appropriately. Such processes of neuronal plasticity could mask severe damage by neurotoxic substances [41].

Cadmium-induced olfactory impairment was also confirmed in fish [42]: after 8-h exposure to 347 ppb of Cd in fresh seawater, coho salmon exhibited not only histological changes to the olfactory epithelium and diminished olfaction in the behavioural test (for example loss of the tonic immobility response to olfactory alarm signals), but also significantly reduced expression of olfactory receptors and increased expression of enzymes involved in the antioxidant reaction in relation to metals. During 48-h exposure to 3.7 ppb, tonic immobility responses were diminished and histological changes to the olfactory epithelium likewise occurred that were not as pronounced as in the highly exposed fish group.

Nickel exposure Inhalation of $NiSO_4$ (0.635 mg, 6 h per day, 16 days) caused atrophy of the olfactory epithelium in rats, α-Ni_3S_2 additional chronic inflammation of the nasal tissue. Significant impairment of olfaction was not recorded [43–47]. Studies on rats and apes confirm the transport of nickel into the olfactory bulb following inhalation of soluble $NiSO_4$ [47]. Following intranasal instillation of $^{63}Ni^{2+}$ in rats, the uptake pathway was tracked from the olfactory epithelium, via the axons of the primary olfactory neurons, into the glomeruli in the olfactory bulb and into further parts of the brain [48]. A maximum $^{63}Ni^{2+}$ transport rate of 0.13 mm/h was measured in the olfactory neurons of pike [49]. In a recent examination by Jia et al. [50], intranasal instillation of nickel sulfate (0.5 and 2.5 mg/kg) in mice led to dose-dependent and time-dependent atrophy of the olfactory epithelium of the turbinate bone, but not of the septum. The sustentacular cells were affected first by apoptotic cell loss on the first day post exposure, the olfactory receptor neurons on the third day; a significant increase in cell proliferation in the olfactory epithelium was detected after 5 to 7 days.

Neuronal signal transduction by calcium and apoptosis is a factor in olfactory impairment by nickel: according to Zhao et al. [51], $NiSO_4$ is capable of inducing apoptosis by activation of the death receptor 3 and caspase-8 and subsequent activation of caspase-3; Jia et al. suspect $NiSO_4$-induced apoptosis of the olfactory receptor neurons to be attributable to this mechanism. Moreover, according to Gautam et al. [52], Ni^{2+} can reduce the odour-induced calcium influx by inhibition of the T-type

Ca^{2+} channels in the olfactory receptor neurons, thereby impairing signal transduction.

Chromium

Human studies

Exposure to chromium is frequently encountered in combination with nickel and other metals. According to Seeber et al. [53], ulcers on the skin and mucous membrane and perforation of the nasal septum caused by chromium were known as long ago as 1826. Few epidemiological studies exist of a possible association between chromium exposure and olfactory dysfunction.

In all 5 human studies known to us, deficits in the olfactory function of the exposed workers were detected that were associated significantly with the chromium exposure and the duration of employment [53–57]. The study by Seeber et al. and the follow-up research by Seeber and Fikentscher of 1976 and 1980 were not mentioned in the reviews by Gobba, Sunderman and Doty, and are described accordingly in more detail here: Seeber et al. (1976) and Seeber and Fikentscher (1980) reported on damage to the nasal mucous membrane and olfactory dysfunction among workers at a chrome paint plant in the German Democratic Republic (GDR) in which basic zinc chromate (zinc yellow) was manufactured [53, 54]. In their comparison between chronically exposed workers (5), intermittently exposed workers (14, not longer than 2 h per day), mask-wearing workers (5, wearing fine-dust filter masks for the full duration), non-exposed individuals (9 office workers at the same company) and a control group (23 employees at a hospital), they determined by means of rhinoscopic examinations that damage to the nasal mucous membrane was evident on all five of the chronically exposed individuals, but occurred only in a part of the intermittently exposed group and among the workers wearing masks, and not at all in the other groups. Olfactory tests involving odour strips for ascertaining the sensitivity to certain substances showed the olfactory sensitivity of the control group and the non-exposed individuals to be substantially higher than that of the exposed individuals. The authors considered this relationship between chromium exposure and loss of olfaction to be "significant". According to the authors, the dust values measured at the points at which zinc chromate dust was produced clearly exceeded the occupational exposure limit for chromium (VI) applicable in the GDR at this time of 0.1 mg CrO_3/m^3 air, and rose at certain points to up to 200 times the occupational exposure limit. More precise values are not stated. Four years later, after violation of the occupational exposure limit in this plant had been "substantially reduced" by suitable measures (not specified), the workforce was examined once again. It was found that in 16 workers exposed to different levels, the relationship between the pathological nasal mucous membrane findings and olfactory dysfunction was confirmed, and that on average, no improvement in the mucous membrane or olfaction was detected [54].

Besides the results obtained by Watanabe and Fukuchi (1981) and Kitamura et al. (2003), in which an impaired olfactory function in workers in the chromate and galvanising industry was detected by means of the T&T olfactometer and which have already been described in detail in Gobba 2006, workers in galvanising are also shown to be affected by olfactory dysfunction in an Indian publication from 2003: the authors reported on 28 workers in the chromium industry aged between 22 and 37 and exposed to chromium for between 5 and 14 years. Of these, all 28 employees exhibited nasal septum perforations, and 11 were anosmic. Information on the level of exposure and on the test method was not provided [57].

Kitamura et al. reported chromium-induced olfactory dysfunction at low workplace concentrations [56]. The exposure values for chromium measured in this study were 0.0047 to 0.059 mg/m^3. ACGIH set a TLV of 0.05 mg/m^3 for water-soluble Cr (VI) compounds and 0.01 mg/m^3 for insoluble Cr (VI) compounds.

Animal experimental studies

In his review of the relationship between exposure to metals and nasal toxicity, Sunderman cites an animal experiment on rats. Following 40 days' inhalation of sodium dichromate (0.2 mg/m^3, 6 h per day, 40 days), the rats exhibited no morphological nasal changes. Olfaction was not tested [28].

Manganese

Human studies

According to the results of our searches, 10 human studies are available to date that examine the association between manganese exposure and impairment of the sense of smell [58–67]. The study populations encompass not only exposed workers, but also persons living close to a manganese mine and young people living in a region in which manganese emissions of industrial origin were very high prior to 2001. In the two studies conducted on workers in the metals industry [58, 59], in which only the sensory test method was employed, the results were either not significant [58] or, surprisingly, revealed a significantly increased olfaction perception among the workers in measurements of the sensory olfactory threshold [59]. By comparison, use of the olfactory identification test employing Sniffin' Sticks on welders or the inhabitants of an area with elevated background manganese values revealed significantly poorer values [60–62, 64–66]. In further magnetic or functional resonance imaging studies, elevated manganese deposition in the olfactory bulb was measured on welders [63] and a reduction in activity in relevant olfactory brain regions was measured in young people living in a region exhibiting elevated manganese values [66].

The following recent studies have not yet been discussed in the reviews by Sunderman, Gobba and Doty and will therefore be presented in more detail here:

In a follow-up survey, 26 welders who had participated in the San Francisco/Oakland Bay Bridge welder study [60, 61] were examined three and a half years later by the same methods. Although 13 participants were no longer working as welders, the results obtained in the UPSIT did not differ significantly from the earlier findings. The blood-manganese levels of the workers who were no longer welding were significantly lower than those of their colleagues [62].

For seven welders, increased manganese deposition in the olfactory bulb and in other regions of the brain was demonstrated by means of functional magnetic resonance tomography [63].

Guarneros et al. (2013) conducted a Sniffin' Sticks olfactory test series encompassing threshold, discrimination and identification tests on persons living in proximity to a manganese plant and exhibiting an elevated manganese concentration (mean 9.73 µg/g vs. 1.01 µg/g) in their hair [64]. Significant differences between the subjects were observed. In this study, 30 persons (non-smokers) living within a one-kilometre radius of a Mexican manganese mine were compared with 30 controls living more than 50 km away. The groups were matched by age, sex and school education; none had previously worked in a job involving manganese exposure. The results of the Sniffin' Sticks test revealed substantially diminished olfactory function in those living close to the manganese mine.

By means of the identification test employing Sniffin' Sticks, Lucchini et al. also documented significantly poorer olfactory function associated with the Mn content in the soil on 154 young people aged between 11 and 14 in Valcamonica (Italy). Up until 2001, this region was marked by ferrous alloy plants and the emissions from them (average Mn atmospheric and soil values at the time of the examination: 49.5 ng/m^3 and 958 ppm respectively). Young people from the region around Lake Garda were tested as the control group [65]. In a further study employing functional magnetic resonance tomography, the activity of the brain in 9 young people from Valcamonica and Bagnolo Mella exposed to manganese was compared with that of 4 young people from the Lake Garda region. In the exposed young people, a reduction in activity in relevant olfactory brain regions was detected, for example in the orbitofrontal cortex and piriform cortex and in further brain regions typically associated with olfactory function, such as the middle frontal gyrus and cerebellum. In comparison with a larger control group from a database, significant differences were also monitored with regard to the size of the olfactory bulb and in the olfactory test involving Sniffin' Sticks. Reduced activity in comparison with that of the controls was also noted in the regions of the limbic system [66].

In a recent prospective cohort study, Casjens et al. examined the influence of work-related manganese exposure upon the olfactory function. The study population comprised 1385 men, of whom 354 had potentially been exposed to manganese in their earlier occupations. No relevant association was determined between manganese exposure and a deterioration in olfactory function [67].

Animal experimental studies

Experiments on pikes and rats showed that following intranasal application of a dilute $^{54}MnCl_2$ solution, manganese is absorbed by the olfactory epithelium and transported on into the brain. In the process, manganese accumulates in the olfactory bulb and can be detected after 12 weeks throughout the brain and spinal cord [68–71]. Transport of the manganese from the nasal cavities into the brain requires the axonal projections of the olfactory epithelium's receptor neurons to be intact [72]. Foster et al. also evaluated the transport of manganese from the olfactory epithelium to the olfactory bulb: a bilateral instillation of 40 µl 200 mM $MnCl_2$ in rats leads to an increase in manganese levels in both the olfactory epithelium and the olfactory bulb, and the rats exposed to manganese exhibit decreased performance in the olfactory discrimination task. Manganese accumulation in the olfactory bulb and in other regions of the brain was also demonstrated by MRT studies on non-human primates exposed to aerosolised $MnSO_4$ ($\geq$ 0.06 mg Mn/m^3) [71].

Zinc

Exposure to zinc in the form of fumes and dust frequently occurs during the manufacture and processing of metals. With the exception of one study published in 1971 in Russian [73], we are not aware of any studies of a possible relationship between the incidence of olfactory dysfunction and occupational zinc exposure. Studies do exist of the frequent incidence of anosmia following medical intranasal application of sprays or gels containing zinc, as do studies on animals demonstrating an association between intranasal exposure to zinc salts and adverse influence upon olfactory function [74–94].

Human studies

In 1971, 301 workers at a zinc production plant were examined with regard to their olfactory and trigeminal function and compared with a control group comprising 63 workers at a machine factory [73]. The olfactory tests were performed by means of an olfactometer employing mint and dilute acetic acid (trigeminal stimulation). In comparison with the sensory threshold values of the control group the sensory thresholds of the exposed workers were statistically significantly elevated. The elevations were highest among the workers responsible for roasting the zinc ore. High concentrations – according to the author several times higher (without closer specification) than the limits in force at the time – of further strongly corrosive and irritant substances such as sulfur dioxide, sulfur anhydride, sulfuric acid, chlorine, hydrogen fluoride and others were however released in all three working areas (roasting, leaching, electrolysis) covered by the study, besides zinc oxide, zinc sulfate and metal dusts. Assessing the impact upon health to a particular substance is therefore difficult.

The link postulated by Seeber and Fikentscher between the effects of olfactory impairment observed among workers in a zinc chromate plant and exposure to chromium may perhaps equally be associated with zinc. This possibility was not examined in these studies [53, 54].

The suspicion that zinc in the form of a pharmaceutical component was capable of triggering olfactory dysfunction dates back to the 1930s. The suitability of a solution containing 1% zinc sulfate and 0.5% tetracaine (a topical anaesthetic) for use as a nasal spray for prevention of poliomyelitis infection was studied in Toronto in 1938 [28]. It was found not only that the desired protection was not achieved, but that some children and adults also developed anosmia. According to reports by the British Medical Journal and the Journal of Pediatrics, of 5233 children (for the most part aged between 3 and 10) treated in special clinics by otolaryngologists, approximately a quarter exhibited temporary anosmia [74, 75]. Unfortunately, the documentation contains no description of the diagnostic method, quantitative details of temporary and permanent olfactory dysfunction, or any indication whatsoever of systematic olfaction testing in the control group [74, 75]. Information on the control group and the test method were relevant insofar as recent studies indicate that olfaction is poorer in children than in adults: in the study by Sorokowska et al. of 1422 test subjects (aged between 4 and 80), children aged under 10 and adults aged over 70 performed worst in an identification test involving Sniffin' Sticks with 16 different odours [95]. Tisdall et al. (1938) were in possession of data from a collective of an estimated 5000 further patients (children and adults) treated with zinc sulfate of which 44 were permanently anosmic as a consequence of the treatment. However, in this collective the 44 patients identified as having permanent olfactory dysfunction accounted for fewer than 1%, which is below the estimated figure for olfactory dysfunction in the wider population [16, 96].

Olfactory dysfunction occurring in patients following intranasal use of Zicam gel, claimed by the manufacturer to be "homeopathic" (according to Mossad, Zicam nasal gel contains 33 mmol/l zinc gluconate [97]) for prophylactic or therapeutic purposes against the symptoms of colds, was documented by Davidson and Smith, Alexander and Davidson, and Jafek et al. [76–78].

In 2009, the US Food and Drug Administration (FDA) issued warnings to consumers against three intranasal "Zicam" products containing zinc owing to the suspicion that they "may cause a loss of sense of smell", possibly permanent [98]. The products concerned were then taken off the market in 2009.

The possible olfactory effect of a nasal insulin spray containing zinc as an additive was also the subject of recent discussion [99, 100]. Indeed, it is unclear how much of the zinc spray actually reaches the olfactory cleft. Notable in this context are the results of experiments by Herranz Gonzalez-Botas and Padin Seara, who examined the efficacy of the nasal gel form of application and ascertained that pigmented nasal gel is not detectable in the olfactory cleft following self-application by 16 test subjects [101].

Animal experimental and in vitro studies

The cytotoxic effect of Zicam was also demonstrated in vivo on mice and in vitro on human nasal tissue. Following instillation of Zicam by injection in the nasal cavities (15 µl per cavity), the olfactory epithelium was especially affected. The results of the behavioural test showed that treatment of the mice with Zicam led to olfactory dysfunction that still persisted two months after treatment. In the human nasal tissue samples, necrosis of the epithelial and subepithelial structures was observed following the application of Zicam [80].

Numerous further histological studies have been performed that illustrate the degenerative effect of zinc salts upon the olfactory epithelium in mice and fish [81–86]. Several studies in which $ZnSO_4$ is used for experimental induction of anosmia in laboratory animals demonstrate that direct treatment of the olfactory mucous membrane with zinc sulfate solution impairs olfaction in mice, rats, hamsters and pigeons [81, 84, 87–91]. McBride et al. (2003) provide an overview of 22 behavioural studies on mice in which olfactory dysfunction was induced by means of intranasal irrigation with $ZnSO_4$ [81].

Following intranasal zinc gluconate instillation on mice (33 mM, 50–100 µl per nostril), Duncan-Lewis et al. (2011) were able to demonstrate, by means of a behavioural test, a significant reduction in olfaction compared to control mice treated only with phosphate-buffered saline (PBS) [92]. Significantly weaker olfaction was also exhibited by mice following treatment with copper gluconate. Irrigation with magnesium gluconate yielded no differences. The olfactory dysfunction was reversible, since no differences in olfactory behaviour were observed in a further behavioural test performed one month after treatment.

Electroolfactograms and patch-clamp tests on isolated rat olfactory epithelia showed that exposure to zinc metal nanoparticles in the picomolar range had a significantly reinforcing effect upon the reaction of the olfactory neurons following olfactory induction, whereas Zn^{2+} ions in the same concentration led to a reduced response to olfactory stimulation [93].

The toxic properties of zinc oxide nanoparticles in the olfactory system of rats are presented by Gao et al.: once-off instillation of a suspension of zinc oxide nanoparticles led to significant damage of the olfactory epithelium and to inflammation reactions [94]. In addition, the exposed rats exhibited a change in sniffing behaviour and appeared no longer able to distinguish between vanillin diluted with distilled water and distilled water alone. In an in-vitro assay on primary human olfactory cells, Osmond-McLeod et al. demonstrated that zinc oxide nanoparticles are able to induce cellular stress reactions, inflammation reactions and apoptosis, but do not activate DNA repair mechanisms [79]. They established that the cellular reactions to zinc oxide nanoparticles with a coated surface were weaker.

"Pesticides"

Human studies

As already reported by Doty the neurological functions of workers employed in structural fumigation involving the pesticides of methyl bromide and sulfuryl fluoride were compared in 2015 in a cross-sectional study with those of control persons [102]. Significantly weaker olfactory function tested with UPSIT was observed among the workers subject to high sulfuryl fluoride exposure. A corresponding observation was not made for the workers with high exposure to methyl bromide. It should be noted here that with the exception of 11 individuals, the majority of workers were subject to coexposure with methyl bromide. Clear distinction between the effects of methyl bromide and those of sulfuryl fluoride is therefore difficult, not least since division of the workers by the criteria of "high exposure to sulfuryl fluoride" and "high exposure to methyl bromide" is based upon statements made by the workers themselves in a questionnaire. Methyl bromide is highly toxic and harmful to the central nervous system. In animal experiments it also causes damage to the olfactory epithelium. According to the authors, further pesticides (including chlorpyrifos, organophosphates, carbamates, pyrethrins, organochlorine pesticides) with which the test subjects had come into contact during work or leisure revealed no significant association with the results of the olfactory test and the memory test involving patterns. During work, the fumigators were also exposed to "small amounts" of chloropicrin, which was used as an irritant warning substance during fumigation with sulfuryl fluoride and methyl bromide (no concentration stated). Chloropicrin is a highly irritant gas [103].

In one recently published study an impaired olfactory function was demonstrated in Latino farmworkers exposed to pesticides [104]. 304 farmworkers exposed to pesticides were compared with 247 non-farmworkers. At significantly greater self-reported lifetime pesticide exposure, the farmworkers required significantly higher concentrations for odour detection; the odour identification did not differ between the groups (Sniffin' Sticks). Unfortunately, it is not specified which types of pesticides the farmers worked with. In this context it is interesting that an impaired olfactory function could be an early symptom of Parkinson's disease (PD), and that pesticides are also suspected of inducing symptoms of Parkinson's. A strong association between farmers with a PD diagnosis and a reduced sense of smell is shown by Shrestha et al. 2017 [105].

Animal experimental studies

Whereas methyl bromide can strongly damage the olfactory epithelium in animal tests [106], the available literature provides no clear indication of the effect of sulfuryl fluoride upon olfaction. Inflammation of the nasal tissue was reported after high exposure to sulfuryl fluoride (inhalation of 300–600 ppm) in rats and rabbits [107, 108].

Formaldehyde

Olfactory dysfunction in humans caused by formaldehyde was described relatively early. Spealman [109] provides an indirect indication in that he cites the medical department of an airline that had rejected the use of deodorants containing formaldehyde in airliners on the grounds that formaldehyde was known to impair olfaction. Lehnhardt and Rollin mention the strange case of a company emergency response officer who developed anosmia allegedly owing to compulsive sniffing of a therapeutic agent that released formaldehyde [110].

Human studies

Four human studies involving formaldehyde and its association with olfactory dysfunction were identified [111–114].

In an epidemiological cross-sectional study by Holmström et al. of workers at a factory producing formaldehyde and formaldehyde-based products and workers exposed to both formaldehyde and wood dust, significantly reduced olfactory function was measured (sensory threshold test employing pyridine) [111]. Hisamitsu et al. demonstrated a significantly diminished olfactory function in medical students who were exposed to formaldehyde vapours during an anatomy course in Japan. It must be emphasised that all affected individuals already had a preexisting history of allergic rhinitis. Olfactory function was fully restored after a year [112]. The publications of Holmström et al. and Hisanitsu et al. [111, 112] are mentioned by Doty 2015 [4] and will not be presented in greater detail here.

Kilburn et al. describe the result of a survey involving 76 female histology technicians (average age 40.8) who were exposed to formaldehyde (0.2–1.9 ppm) and to other substances such as xylene and toluene during their work with histological preparations [113]. 22 of these women were exposed to formaldehyde for 1 to 3 h, 47 for over 4 h. In a survey, 32% of the women in each subgroup stated that their olfactory function was diminished. Among a control group of 56 non-exposed women (average age 39.5), this was stated by only 5%.

A study of 75 male workers (average age: 38) with occupational exposure either to formaldehyde alone (0.1–1.1 mg/m^3 with exposure peaks of up to 5 mg/m^3) or to formaldehyde and wood dust (0.6–1.1 mg/m^3) detected pathological changes of the nasal mucous membrane in 72 individuals [114]. No differences in the histological findings were observed between the workers exposed solely to formaldehyde and those who had also been exposed to wood dust.

Based upon the results of long-term toxicological inhalation studies on laboratory animals, an NOAEL for nasal damage of 1 ppm formaldehyde was determined in the literature [115]. In their cross-sectional study, Holmström and Wilhelmsson observed a significant worsening of the sensory threshold even at formaldehyde concentrations below 0.37 mg/m^3 (= 0.3 ppm, and corresponding to the German OEL) [111]. Irreversible damage to the sensory tissue need not however be anticipated below the irritation threshold, upon which the OEL is based.

Animal experimental studies

Inhaled formaldehyde (3.2 ppm) and acrylic aldehyde (0.67 ppm) led to degeneration of the respiratory epithelium in rats, inhaled acetaldehyde (750 ppm) to degeneration of the olfactory epithelium. It was demonstrated on the same species of laboratory animal that the effects of a combined exposure to these aldehydes can increase exponentially [116].

10 rats were exposed for 4 h per day for 7 days to 12.5 mg/m^3 formaldehyde by Li et al. [117]. Examination of the olfactory bulbs and hippocampi of the exposed rats revealed severe morphological damage compared to an untreated control group. Reduced production of glutamate, gamma-aminobutyric acid and nitrogen oxide synthase was also detected in this damaged tissue. Since the publication was in Chinese, only the English abstract could be evaluated here.

Diminished olfactory function was determined in rats that had been subject for 30 min twice a day for 14 days to inhalative exposure to a formaldehyde concentration of 13.5 ± 1.5 ppm [118].

Acrylates

Human studies

Gobba and Doty have already described the study by Schwartz et al. in their reviews: hundreds of workers were studied in a cross-sectional analysis at a factory producing acrylates and methacrylates [119]. The workers were divided into four classes according to their exposure. No association was established in the first instance between exposure and the results of olfactory tests (UPSIT, $p = 0.09$). By means of an embedded case-control study, a dose-effect relationship was observed between olfactory dysfunction and cumulative exposure; the effect appeared to be reversible. The risk of developing olfactory dysfunction was greatest in the group of non-smokers.

Two studies were, however, not mentioned by Gobba or Doty:

In a cross-sectional study of 175 workers exposed to methyl methacrylate and a control group of 88 non-exposed workers employed in the same production unit for acrylic glass sheet casting, performance of the Rhino Identification Test (6 tested aromas, very similar in design to the UPSIT test) revealed only a single hyposmic case in the exposed group [120]. At 58.3%, the proportion of smokers was higher in the exposed group than in the control group (34.1%). Over an 8-h shift, exposure lay between 25 and 100 ml/m^3 in 1988 and between 10 and 50 ml/m^3 in the period from 1989 to 1994. The average exposure duration was 9.6 ±7.1 years. With the exception of 2 workers who were additionally exposed briefly to formaldehyde up to 1990 and 4 workers who additionally had contact with acrylonitrile, and a further 2 workers who were additionally exposed to both formaldehyde and acrylonitrile, all workers were exposed solely to methyl methacrylate. These results permit the conclusion that at exposures of up to 50 ml/m^3 methyl methacrylate, olfactory function is not harmed.

In a more recent exposure study, 20 healthy male volunteers (non-smokers, aged 20–62) were exposed in an exposure chamber once to 49.2 (±1.4) ppm methyl methacrylate for 4 h. Following exposure, no changes occurred in the olfactory threshold for n-butanol, which was measured by means of Sniffin' Sticks, nor had the measured mucociliary transit time (time from introduction of a saccharin particle in the lower nasal vestibule to perception of a sweet taste in the throat) changed. Also unchanged were the measured concentrations of protein and mRNA markers of inflammation in the nasal secretion and respiratory epithelium. Furthermore, only minor differences were observed in the mental state, which was evaluated by questionnaire. The authors concluded from this that acute exposure to 50 ppm methyl methacrylate causes no inflammatory changes to the respiratory nasal mucous membrane, and that in view of the absence of a rise in the olfactory threshold following exposure to 50 ppm methyl methacrylate, this dose is not sufficient to cause toxic damage to the olfactory epithelium. These results of acute exposure cannot be readily transferred to chronic conditions [121].

Animal experimental studies

Chronic exposure to 100 ppm methyl methacrylate can cause degeneration and atrophy of the olfactory epithelium in rats. It must be considered that the activity of the carboxylesterase in the olfactory epithelium of the nasal mucous membrane is considerably higher in rats than in humans. The unspecific carboxylesterase hydrolyses methyl methacrylate to methyl acrylic acid, which is responsible for the local toxicity [122].

Styrene

Human studies

Three studies have already been listed by Doty [4]:

Cheng et al. [123] compared injection moulding workers exposed to styrene with non-exposed workers. At the end of a working day, a slight but significant reduction in olfactory function was detected in the olfactory threshold test employing 1-butanol, whereas the initial situation at the beginning of the shift had been the same. An identification test employing 7 odours (Connecticut Chemosensory Clinical Research Center (CCCRC) olfactory test) revealed no differences before and after the shift. According to Doty [4] these results support the "concept that the olfactory thresholds reflect adaptation rather than sustained neurological damage". Unfortunately, no exposure measurements were performed in this study.

Other epidemiological studies of workers in the glass fibre reinforced plastic industry revealed no relationship between styrene exposure and a general deterioration in olfactory function [124, 125]. In both studies the olfactory threshold for styrene was significantly higher among the exposed workers. According to Dalton et al., this is also explained by an adaptation effect, which leads to a reversible reduction in sensitivity. This has already been frequently observed for volatile substances in industry or the laboratory and is correspondingly well documented [126]. Whereas the identification test revealed no differences between exposed and non-exposed individuals in the study published in 2003, the identification test published in 2007 resulted in a significant difference between the workers with high vs. low exposure [125]. Dalton et al. state that the proportion of individuals showing poor values in the identification test is substantially higher in both groups (40 and 20%) than in the normal population (10%) [125]. Even with the aid of multiple regression analysis, no association was demonstrated between the results of the identification test and the exposure values measured at present or in the past in the group of workers subject to high exposure. The authors therefore suspect that the high proportion of immigrants in the exposed group had influenced the results of the test, and they do not consider the results to be valid evidence of impairment of human olfactory function by workplace exposure to styrene.

Animal experimental studies

In two studies on rodents conducted in 1997 and 1998, already cited by Doty 2015, styrene exposure of between 20 and 50 ppm led to lesions of the olfactory epithelium [127, 128]. Green et al. assumed that the nasal lesions induced in mice by exposure to styrene were caused by styrene oxide, which cannot be detected in the human nasal epithelium [129].

Organic solvents and mineral oil products

Human studies

The publications by Schwartz et al. [130], Sandmark et al. [131] and Ahlstrom [132] are epidemiological studies evaluating a possible association between solvent exposure and impairment of olfaction. They are also cited by Gobba and Doty:

With consideration for smoker status, the UPSIT identification test performed by Schwartz et al. [130] yielded a significant dose-dependent deterioration in olfactory function of workers exposed to solvent in paint manufacture with rising lifetime exposure among workers who had never smoked. This effect was not observed among workers who had always smoked. The results remained the same when the confounders of age and cultural background (vocabulary testing) were taken into account. Schwartz et al. suspect that the induction of cytochrome P450 enzymes by cigarette smoke leads to an increase in the metabolism and thereby to detoxification of organic olfactotoxins before they reach the olfactory epithelium. The exposed workers who had always smoked performed worse in the UPSIT olfactory test compared to reference values, albeit not with dose dependency. The best olfactory function was exhibited by the workers with the lowest exposure who had never smoked.

In an UPSIT identification test on painters, no impairment of olfactory function was observed following multiple regression analysis including consideration for age and smoker status [131]. Quantitative exposure measurement was not performed; the exposure was described as low to moderate. Tank cleaners studied by Ahlstrom et al. exposed to mineral oil products exhibited elevated olfactory threshold values for heated oil vapour and n-butanol; these were still within the normal range for n-butanol. Oil vapour had not been studied in this respect before. To determine whether a relationship existed between the elevated threshold values and the interval between the most recent exposure and the olfactory test, the exposed workers were assigned to three groups with intervals of different duration (1 day to over 30 days) between exposure and the olfactory test. It was found that the tank cleaners who had been exposed just one day prior to the test exhibited higher threshold values for all tested substances than those who had not. A further test of the subjectively perceived odour intensity of all 4 substances tested (pyridine, dimethyl disulfide, n-butanol and heated oil vapour) revealed that at the lowest stimulus concentrations, the exposed persons exhibited lower odour intensity values than the control subjects [132].

Muttray et al. refer to one Russian and two Polish studies of the olfactotoxic effect of adhesives containing petroleum: of workers at a Russian shoe factory who had been exposed to an adhesive containing a petroleum mixture ("Galoscha"), ethyl acetate and butyl acetate (solvent concentration: 220–300 mg/m^3), over 25% suffered atrophy of the nasal mucous membrane owing to inflammatory processes, 31% suffered the loss of olfactory function, and among the remainder, olfactory function was impaired in comparison to a control group [133]. Among 205 workers who used a rubber adhesive containing petroleum and were exposed to it up to a level of approximately 3000 mg/m^3, olfactory dysfunction as a result of rhinitis arose after only a few years. Muttray also cited a study of 547 petroleum chemical workers. According to the abstract of this publication (article in Polish, [134]) the senses of smell and taste were examined. Hyposmia was found in 238 (43.5%) and anosmia in 50 (9.2%) subjects. Dysgeusia (distortion of the sense of taste) was identified in 319 (58.3%) subjects, with no reaction at all in 102 (18.6%) persons. In the control group (100 cotton industry workers) dysgeusia was determined in 69%, anosmia in 24% of subjects. According to Muttray the exposure was described insufficiently.

Animal experimental studies

In an experiment conducted by the US National Toxicology Program (NTP), no conspicuous lesions of the olfactory epithelium were observed in rodents following inhalation of tetrahydrofurane [135]. In a further NTP study, degeneration of the olfactory epithelium was observed in all exposed mice following exposure to cyclohexanone in drinking water [136].

The capacity of 2-ethylhexanol to impair both the olfactory epithelium and the olfactory bulb in mice is demonstrated by Miyake et al. [137]: subchronic inhalation of 2-ethylhexanol induced degeneration of the olfactory epithelium at a lowest observed adverse effect level of 20 ppm. Following exposure for three months, changes in the olfactory bulb (such as a reduction in the glomeruli diameter, increase in the microglia) were also observed.

Mechanism of olfactory dysfunction

Odorants enter the nose orthonasally or retronasally and bind to receptors on the cilia of the olfactory sensory neurons in the olfactory epithelium. The stimulus is converted here into signals and forwarded to the brain. Whereas the respiratory epithelium lines the greater part of the respiratory tract, possesses no sensory neurons, and as the epithelium of the respiratory tract has the functions of keeping the tract clean and of moistening and warming the breathing air, the human olfactory epithelium is limited to a small area of approximately 2 × 5 square centimetres in the superior turbinate bone [138, 139]. Besides the approximately 10–30 million olfactory (bipolar) neurons, the olfactory epithelium consists of basal cells and supporting cells. The functions of the supporting cells (sustentacular cells) include biotransformation of xenobiotics [140].

Olfactory dysfunction can be caused by impairment of transport of the odorant molecules to the olfactory epithelium (conductive cause) and/or by sensorineural dysfunction.

Exclusively conductive or sensorineural dysfunction are rare; a combination of both is common. A possible conductive cause is for the transport of odours to the olfactory epithelium to be obstructed: in sufficient doses and with sufficiently long exposure, allergens and substances irritative and corrosive to the mucous membrane may cause rhinitis accompanied by inflammatory swelling of the mucous membrane. By obstructing nasal breathing, this can lead to anosmia, which is reversible once inflammation has subsided [141]. Conductive olfactory dysfunction may also be caused by chronic irritation by dusts such as calcium carbonate or cement [110].

Sensorineural causes can be broken down further according to the affected olfactory structure into damage to the olfactory epithelium, damage to the olfactory fibres, and central nervous effects.

The neurons of the olfactory epithelium are directly exposed to environmental influences. Their apical end is in direct contact with the external environment and not separated from it by synapses, and at their basal end they have direct access to the brain via their nerve fibre (axon): inhaled hazardous substances may therefore lead to impairment of the olfactory epithelium and, owing to the intracranial connection, consequently to damage to the bulbus olfactorius and higher brain regions [142].

Compared to all other neurons, those of the olfactory epithelium in the nose of vertebrates are unique in a further respect: they are able to self-renew after a certain lifespan (approximately 30–60 days in the case of rodents; data for human beings are not available [140]) by the differentiation of basal cells. The capacity for regeneration probably decreases with increasing age.

Of the industrial chemicals discussed in the present article, exposure to cadmium, nickel, zinc, cyclohexanone, styrene, acrylates and formaldehyde resulted in damage to the olfactory epithelium in animal experiments. Acute high exposure to reactive and soluble gas such as formaldehyde, chlorine and ammonia may directly damage the respiratory and sensory epithelium in the nose and induce lesions up to and including necroses, resulting in olfactory dysfunction [143]. In animal experiments, it was observed histologically that the olfactory epithelium appears "naked" following toxic exposure. It is described in these terms in one textbook of olfactory dysfunction and dysgeusia [142]. The textbook documents the histological finding of an olfactory biopsy of an anosmic patient following exposure to chlorine gas, by way of a photograph on which the loss of the olfactory receptor neurons is clearly visible.

The spectrum of histological changes that can occur following chronic exposure to irritants encompasses inflammation reactions, degeneration, atrophy, necrosis, keratinisation, hyperplasia, metaplasia and neoplasia [22]. Specific observations include both regeneration of the damaged epithelium by basal cells and metaplastic processes, besides a reduction in the number of olfactory cilia, degeneration of sensory and sustentacular cells and of the Bowman's glands and nerve fascicles, and necrosis of individual cells. The olfactory epithelium can therefore be replaced by respiratory/squamous epithelium.

Unspecific necrosis of cells of the olfactory epithelium can be caused by reactive irritative substances such as chlorine and sulfur dioxide, whereas cell-specific toxicity, affecting for example the sustentacular cells or sensory cells, can be induced by dibasic esters and methyl bromide. Methyl methacrylate is known to be metabolised by a non-specific esterase in the olfactory mucus to methanol and to methacrylic acid, which destroys the receptor cells [120]. The effect may be reversible when the basal cells, from which new receptor cells can form, remain intact.

In the olfactory epithelium itself, enzymes, particularly of the cytochrome P450 family (CYP), are expressed which metabolise toxic substances and can therefore both detoxify and toxify. The sustentacular cells express CYP proteins, which are responsible for the oxidation of xenobiotics. If these cells are damaged or destroyed, the metabolic activity of the CYP enzymes is also inhibited. Further factors, such as genetic polymorphisms, tobacco smoke and other exogenous substances (diallyl sulfide, m-xylene, 8-methoxypsoralen) may also have an inhibiting effect upon the respiratory CYP isoenzymes [22].

The activity of these enzymes decisively influences the toxic effects of many inhaled substances upon the respiratory and olfactory mucous membrane. Whereas, following inhalation, many toxic substances can be converted by metabolisation with the aid of these enzymes to intermediate products of lower toxicity, xenobiotic substances also exist that do not become toxic reactive intermediates until after metabolisation, as in the example of metabolic activation of carcinogenic nitrosamines from tobacco smoke catalysed by CYP2A13. CYP2A13 is strongly expressed in the nasal mucous membrane and is able to catalyse a range of atmospheric hazardous substances such as naphthalene, styrene and toluene [22].

The induction by cigarette smoke of CYP proteins (including CYP1A1) in the olfactory mucous membrane has been demonstrated in rats [144, 145]. Metabolisation to more toxic vs. less toxic products or intermediates may also potentially explain the apparently partly contradictory results regarding the impairment of olfactory function by inhaled substances in smokers. In an exposure study involving acrylates and methacrylates for example, the risk of developing olfactory dysfunction was greater in the non-smoker group [119]. Since tobacco smoke damages the sustentacular cells and thus inhibits enzymatic biotransformation, the creation of toxic intermediary products can also be prevented as a result, and the nasal function thus protected. Conversely, it is also conceivable that inhibition of the enzymes reduces detoxification of the substances, resulting in greater damage to the olfactory mucous membrane.

Altogether, little is known of central nervous effects leading to toxic olfactory dysfunction by substances. Following binding of the odorant molecules to the olfactory receptors, the stimulus information is further transmitted along the bundled axons of the olfactory receptor neurons (nervus olfactorius) through holes in the cribriform plate (lamina cribrosa) into the brain to specific glomeruli in the bulbus olfactorius. The glomeruli consist of the projections of the receptor neurons, which form synapses with the dendrites of pyramid-like mitral cells and of interneurons. Over 1000 axons of olfactory receptor neurons with the same receptor type project onto the dendrites of a single mitral cell [138]. Cadmium and manganese can be detected in the bulbus olfactorius of animals (see above, [38, 39, 63, 68, 72]) and in humans: Baader (1952) was able to determine atrophy of the nasal mucous membrane and an intensive yellow colouring of the olfactory bulb following the autopsy of an affected worker exposed to cadmium, which led him to suspect that cadmium reached the brain via the olfactory pathway [146]. After MRT research on non-human primates exposed to aerosolised manganese sulfate (particle diameter: 1.04–2.12 μm) had already demonstrated transport of manganese via the olfactory pathway and accumulation of manganese in the olfactory bulb [147], increased deposition of manganese in the olfactory bulb was also detected on 7 welders by means of functional magnetic resonance tomography [63].

Over a decade ago, Oberdörster et al. voiced their suspicion that inhaled nanoparticles were able to penetrate the brain through the olfactory nerve [148]. It was shown recently that following inhalative exposure on mice, "quantum dots" (cadmium selenide and zinc sulfate nanocrystals) enter the brain and olfactory bulb by direct axonal transport from the nose; activation of microglia in the olfactory bulb was observed at the same time [149]. In humans, the progress of direct transfer of a substance – in this instance following application of thallium-201 (^{201}TI) – from the nose, via the olfactory epithelium and the olfactory nerve, into the brain was first demonstrated in 2010 by a Japanese team with the aid of SPECT computer tomography and magnetic resonance tomography [150]. Interestingly, this method was also used recently to document that significantly lower migration of ^{201}TI into the olfactory bulb occurred in patients with an olfactory dysfunction [151]. Neurodegeneration was also observed following exposure to manganese: intranasal exposure of mice to manganese chloride in saline solution led to increased necrosis of the granule cells in the bulbus olfactorius. Generally acting as inhibitory interneurons, the granule cells contribute to lateral inhibition and thus to contrast intensification of the activity patterns, sharper discrimination between different odours [138, 152].

At molecular level, a toxin-mediated reduction in the release of neurotransmitters could contribute to olfactory dysfunction: following intranasal application of a dilute cadmium chloride solution in mice, Czarnecki et al. demonstrated anosmia by means of a behavioural test, and a dose-dependent reduction in the odour-induced release by the olfactory nerve of neurotransmitters into the olfactory bulb [40]. Regarding the possible mechanism of action, Czarnecki et al. speculate that as a divalent cation, Cd^{2+} disrupts calcium-mediated neuronal signal transduction by blockage of the transmembrane calcium channels. Earlier studies had shown that release of neurotransmitters from the presynaptic terminals of the olfactory receptor neurons requires an influx of calcium ions via N-type calcium channels. This permits the presumption that owing to the mechanism of amplifying signal transduction, even a minor cadmium-mediated reduction in the presynaptic calcium influx may have a major influence upon the entire release of transmitters by the olfactory nerve.

Diminished release of neurotransmitters following exposure to manganese was also demonstrated by Moberly et al. and Guilarte et al. in the olfactory bulb and in the basal ganglia [153, 154]. Whereas no histopathological changes were evident, the study by Moberly et al. showed that intranasal instillation of as little as 2 μg $MnCl_2$ in mice was sufficient to cause significant changes in odour-induced neurotransmitter release from the olfactory nerve [153]. At 200 μg, the reduction was 90%. This effect may be presumed attributable to a central nervous effect of the manganese, since the release of neurotransmitters was reduced not only after odour stimulation, but also after electrical stimulation.

Evaluation

As yet, few reasonably reliable epidemiological studies have been produced of the olfactotoxic effect of industrial chemicals. Interpretation of these publications revealed that cadmium, nickel, chromium and formaldehyde encountered under workplace conditions can be assumed with reasonable certainty to impair the human olfactory function. This finding is supported for the most part by the results of animal experiments.

The level of evidence for an empirically demonstrated relationship between the development of olfactory dysfunction and exposure to potentially olfactotoxic substances at workplaces can be considered comparatively weak in the majority of cases for the following reasons:

The majority of epidemiological studies of this specific occupational problem are cross-sectional involving heterogeneous collectives in which the individual levels and durations of exposure often differ widely. Despite high variance in olfactory function within the wider population, the studies discussed in this article consider comparatively small groups of people. Aside from the large-scale poliomyelitis prevention campaign employing zinc sulfate nasal spray, only Pyatayev [73] and Casjens et al. [67] have studied several hundred individuals. According to Mücke and Lemmen [126], olfactory sensitivity in a population approximately follows a normal distribution: "(...) although the breadth of perceived concentrations may differ by a factor of up to a hundred within the group (...)". To our knowledge, no valid specific prospective cohort studies of work-related olfactory dysfunction other than Casjens et al. are available. However cross sectional analysis of data collected in large nationwide surveys such as the US National Health and Nutrition Examination Survey (NHANES) provides estimates representative at national level of the prevalence of taste and smell impairment in the US population and also identifies exposure variables correlating with olfactory dysfunction [155–158]. In the German National Cohort (GNC), a random sample of the general population will be taken by 18 German regional study centres, including a total of 100,000 women and 100,000 men aged 20–69 years, with the aim of increasing understanding of the role of particular risk factors in the development of major forms of chronic disease. Special emphasis will be placed on selected lifestyle factors, but also on occupational and environmental influences. One functional measurement that will be performed is of olfactory function [159].

Details of the reversibility or persistence of olfactory dysfunction induced by working substances are often unavailable. More follow-up studies of workers who have changed jobs could be useful. Olfactory dysfunction is not easily quantified. Standardised olfactory tests were not developed until recent decades. Comparison between the study results is rendered more difficult by differences between the test methods employed. Olfactory self-assessment tends to be unreliable and it has been shown that people do not perform well when compared with psychophysical testing [6].

Monitoring of all relevant confounders is difficult in workplace assessments. Olfactory function is known to decrease with increasing age. Indications exist of differences between the sexes, and differences in ethnic background may also be associated with differences in olfactory function. Olfactory function may be affected by alcoholism and smoking behaviour, medication, hormonal impacts, hunger and environmental influences [160–162].

The problem of mixed exposure exists at many workplaces, as described for example in Chapter 2 with regard to the metals industry. Firefighters, paramedics and police officers may be exposed to a range of different dusts and fumes in disaster situations. An impressive example is provided by Altman et al. and Dalton [24, 163]: following the terror attack on the World Trade Center in New York in 2001, many responders and local residents exhibited impairment of olfactory function, in addition to the symptoms of other conditions. Workers are also exposed in day-to-day operations in sewage works and landfills to a range of irritants and agents corrosive to the mucous membrane which may lead to impairment of the sense of smell [164].

Comparison of the concentrations in the studies cited with the current situation at workplaces in central Europe is hampered by the gaps in the information provided by the studies on the sampling and analysis methods. Convincing evidence that the olfactory dysfunction triggered by olfactotoxic industrial chemicals is the critical, namely most sensitive toxicological effect of these substances, has not yet been provided.

In general, relevant physiological differences, and also anatomical differences, must be considered when the results of animal experiments are transferred to humans. Whereas humans are oronasal breathers, rodents are obligate nasal breathers. In humans, the olfactory epithelium covers approximately 3% of the nasal cavity; in rats for example, it covers as much as 50%. The situation is similar for mice, rabbits and dogs. Owing to the olfactory epithelium's sheltered location in human beings, less than 15% of the air inhaled through the nose reaches it – substantially less than for example in rodents [22].

Certain differences are observed in the activity of metabolic enzymes in laboratory animals and humans. High concentrations of the two cytochrome P450 isoforms which are required for the conversion of styrene to styrene oxide were for example detected in respiratory fractions of rats and mice, but not in those of humans [165]. At styrene exposure concentrations resembling those of occupational exposure, mice and rats exhibit extensive damage, whilst humans exhibit no indication of a dose-dependent long-term change in olfactory function [124, 125, 127, 128].

Conclusion and future prospects

An impaired olfactory function not only diminishes the quality of life of those affected, but can also present a workplace hazard for the workers and the company if it results in hazardous substances no longer being detected sufficiently quickly.

Isolated indications that chronic occupational exposure to comparatively low levels of the substances stated above has a harmful impact upon olfactory function should be examined more closely, as should the issue of the effects' reversibility. In this context, the significance of neuroplasticity must be considered, which seeks to compensate for failures in the sensory apparatus.

Since many affected individuals are shown not to be aware of their olfactory dysfunction, greater consideration should be given to regular check-ups of the olfactory function of workers at certain workplaces. At present, olfactory check-ups are performed only in very few working areas. In Germany, tasks associated with room fumigation and room disinfection are an example [3, 166]. SUVA, the Swiss accident insurance institution, recommends olfactory tests as part of occupational health monitoring for persons working with smellable toxic and explosive hazardous substances [167]. The substances occurring at the workplace concerned should be included in the olfactory test, in order for selective anosmia for certain industrial chemicals also to be detected [126]. Normal accustomisation effects such as adaptation and habituation that may impair the sensing of possible hazardous substances at the workplace should be considered at the same time.

An olfactory test not only ensures that the employees with potential contact with smellable hazardous substances are able to sense them and their warning function, but could also serve as a means of early detection of pathological changes. Rose et al. and Mascagni et al. for example discuss the possible use of olfactory dysfunction as an early indicator of toxic effects induced by cadmium [34, 37]. It is also possible that other neurotoxic substances not only cause direct damage to the olfactory epithelium, but also damage the central nervous system following transport through the nose into the brain. Accordingly, olfactory dysfunction could have an early-warning function for potential damage to the brain induced by the same neurotoxins. Olfactory dysfunction also serves as a marker for certain neurodegenerative diseases. In conjunction with the idiopathy of Parkinson's syndrome, olfactory dysfunction may arise as early as four to six years before the first motor dysfunction typical of Parkinson's, such as shaking and muscular rigidity [16, 168].

Not only must employees with severe olfactory dysfunction be advised that they are able to detect smellable hazardous substances only poorly, if at all, suitable measures must also be taken at work and in private life to prevent a hazard arising.

Acknowledgements

We wish to thank Professor Thomas Hummel, head of the Interdisciplinary Center Smell & Taste (University Hospital Carl Gustav Carus, Dresden), for his critical review of the first version of the manuscript.

Authors' contributions

S.W. produced the first draft which was revised by E.N. Evaluation and conclusion were jointly written by both authors. Both authors read and approved the final manuscript.

Competing interests

The authors declare that they have no competing interests.

References

1. Doty RL. A review of olfactory dysfunctions in man. Am J Otolaryngol. 1979; 1(1):57–79.
2. Muttray A, Konietzko J. Störungen des Riechvermögens durch und für Arbeitsstoffe. Arbeitsmed Sozialmed Umweltmed. 1994;29:409–13.
3. BMAS (Federal Ministry of Labour and Social Affairs). Neufassung der Empfehlung des BMA zur Durchführung der Eignungsuntersuchung von Befähigungsscheinbewerbern für Begasungen gemäß Anhang V Nr. 5.2 Abs. 2 Ziffer 2 GefStoffV. BArbBl. 1995;12:41–4. berichtigt in BArbBl. 1996. 4:46.
4. Doty RL. Neurotoxic exposure and impairment of the chemical senses of taste and smell. Handb Clin Neurol. 2015;131:299–324.
5. AWMF – The Association of the Scientific Medical Societies (Arbeitsgemeinschaft der Wissenschaftlichen Medizinischen Fachgesellschaften e.V.): S2k-Leitlinie 017/050: Riech- und Schmeckstörungen; 2016. https://www.awmf.org/uploads/tx_szleitlinien/017-050l_S2k_Riech-und-Schmeckst%c3%b6rungen_2017-03.pdf. Accessed 25 Jan 2018.
6. Hummel T, Whitcroft KL, Andrews P, Altundag A, Cinghi C, Costanzo RM, et al. Position paper on olfactory dysfunction. Rhinol Suppl. 2017;54(26):1–30.
7. Doty RL, Shaman P, Dann M. Development of the University of Pennsylvania Smell Identification Test: a standardized microencapsulated test of olfactory function. Physiol Behav. 1984;32(3):489–502.
8. Kobal G, Hummel T, Sekinger B, Barz S, Roscher S, Wolf S. "Sniffin' sticks": screening of olfactory performance. Rhinology. 1996;34(4):222–6.
9. Hummel T, Sekinger B, Wolf SR, Pauli E, Kobal G. Sniffin' sticks': olfactory performance assessed by the combined testing of odor identification, odor discrimination and olfactory threshold. Chem Senses. 1997;22(1):39–52.
10. Hummel T, Welge-Lüssen A. Erfassung des Riech-und Schmeckvermögens. In: Hummel T, Welge-Lüssen A, editors. Riech-und Schmeckstörungen. Stuttgart: Thieme; 2009; p. 43–59.
11. Stuck B, Beule A, Damm M, Gudziol H, Hüttenbrink KB, Landis B, et al. Positionspapier "Die chemosensorische Testung bei der gutachterlichen Abklärung von Riechstörungen". Laryngo-Rhino-Otologie. 2014;93(05):327–9.
12. Hummel T, Kobal G, Gudziol H, Mackay-Sim A. Normative data for the "Sniffin' sticks" including tests of odor identification, odor discrimination, and olfactory thresholds: an upgrade based on a group of more than 3,000 subjects. Eur Arch Otorhinolaryngol. 2007;264(3):237–43.
13. University Hospital Carl Gustav Carus: Normative data for Sniffin Sticks 2012.; https://www.uniklinikum-dresden.de/de/das-klinikum/kliniken-polikliniken-institute/hno/forschung/interdisziplinaeres-zentrum-fuer-riechen-und-schmecken/downloads/downloads/SDI_Normwerte_2012.pdf (2016). Accessed 25 Jan 2018.
14. Kuner T, Schaefer AT. Moleküle, Zellen und Netzwerke für die Verarbeitung von Geruchsreizen im Riechkolben der Maus. e-Neuroforum. 2011;17(3):102–9.
15. Zou J, Wang W, Pan YW, Lu S, Xia Z. Methods to measure olfactory behavior in mice. Curr Protoc Toxicol. 2015;63:11 8 1–21.
16. Hüttenbrink KB, Hummel T, Berg D, Gasser T, Hähner A. Riechstörungen: Häufig im Alter und wichtiges Frühsymptom neurodegenerativer Erkrankungen. Dtsch Arztebl Int. 2013;110:1–7.
17. Croy I, Olgun S, Mueller L, Schmidt A, Muench M, Hummel C, et al. Peripheral adaptive filtering in human olfaction? Three studies on prevalence and effects of olfactory training in specific anosmia in more than 1600 participants. Cortex. 2015;73:180–7.
18. Mott AE, Leopold DA. Disorders in taste and smell. Med Clin North Am. 1991;75(6):1321–53.
19. Damm M, Temmel A, Welge-Lüssen A, Eckel H, Kreft MP, Klussmann J, et al. Riechstörungen HNO. 2004;52(2):112–20.
20. Fonteyn S, Huart C, Deggouj N, Collet S, Eloy P, Rombaux P. Non-sinonasal-related olfactory dysfunction: a cohort of 496 patients. Eur Ann Otorhinolaryngol Head Neck Dis. 2014;131(2):87–91.
21. Gobba F. Olfactory toxicity: long-term effects of occupational exposures. Int Arch Occup Environ Health. 2006;79(4):322–31.
22. Dalton P. Olfactory toxicity in humans and experimental animals. In: Morris JBSD, editor. Toxicology of the nose and upper airways. New York: Informa Healthcare; 2010. p. 215–41.
23. Herberhold C. Funktionsprüfungen und Störungen des Geruchssinnes. Arch Otorhinolaryngol. 1975;210(1):67–164.
24. Dalton PH, Opiekun RE, Gould M, McDermott R, Wilson T, Maute C, et al. Chemosensory loss: functional consequences of the world trade center disaster. Environ Health Perspect. 2010;118(9):1251–6.
25. Klimek L, Muttray A, Moll B, Konietzko J, Mann W. Riechstörungen durch inhalative Schadstoffexposition. Laryngo-Rhino-Otologie. 1999;78(11):620–6.
26. Muttray A, Haxel B, Mann W, Letzel S. Anosmie und Rhinitis durch eine berufliche Lösungsmittelexposition. HNO. 2006;54(11):883–7.
27. Amoore J. Effects of chemical exposure on olfaction in humans. In: Barrow CS, editor. Toxicology of the nasal passages. New York: Hemisphere Publishing Corp; 1986. p. 155–90.
28. Sunderman FW Jr. Nasal toxicity, carcinogenicity, and olfactory uptake of metals. Ann Clin Lab Sci. 2001;31(1):3–24.
29. Friberg L. Health hazards in the manufacture of alkaline accumulators with special reference to chronic cadmium poisoning; a clinical and experimental study. Acta Med Scand Suppl. 1950;240:1–124.

30. Baader EW. Die chronische Kadmiumvergiftung. Dtsch Med Wochenschr. 1951;76(14):484–7.
31. Potts CL. Cadmium proteinuria - the health of battery workers exposed to cadmium oxide dust. Ann Occup Hyg. 1965;8:55–61.
32. Liu YZ, Huang JX, Luo CM, Xu BH, Zhang CJ. Effects of cadmium on cadmium smelter workers. Scand J Work Environ Health. 1985;11(Suppl 4):29–32.
33. Adams RG, Crabtree N. Anosmia in alkaline battery workers. Br J Ind Med. 1961;18:216–21.
34. Rose CS, Heywood PG, Costanzo RM. Olfactory impairment after chronic occupational cadmium exposure. J Occup Med. 1992;34(6):600–5.
35. Rydzewski B, Sulkowski W, Miarzynska M. Olfactory disorders induced by cadmium exposure: a clinical study. Int J Occup Med Environ Health. 1998; 11(3):235–45.
36. Sulkowski WJ, Rydzewski B, Miarzynska M. Smell impairment in workers occupationally exposed to cadmium. Acta Otolaryngol. 2000;120(2):316–8.
37. Mascagni P, Consonni D, Bregante G, Chiappino G, Toffoletto F. Olfactory function in workers exposed to moderate airborne cadmium levels. Neurotoxicology. 2003;24(4–5):717–24.
38. Sun TJ, Miller ML, Hastings L. Effects of inhalation of cadmium on the rat olfactory system: behavior and morphology. Neurotoxicol Teratol. 1996; 18(1):89–98.
39. Bondier JR, Michel G, Propper A, Badot PM. Harmful effects of cadmium on olfactory system in mice. Inhal Toxicol. 2008;20(13):1169–77.
40. Czarnecki LA, Moberly AH, Rubinstein T, Turkel DJ, Pottackal J, McGann JP. In vivo visualization of olfactory pathophysiology induced by intranasal cadmium instillation in mice. Neurotoxicology. 2011;32(4):441–9.
41. Czarnecki LA, Moberly AH, Turkel DJ, Rubinstein T, Pottackal J, Rosenthal MC, et al. Functional rehabilitation of cadmium-induced neurotoxicity despite persistent peripheral pathophysiology in the olfactory system. Toxicol Sci. 2012;126(2):534–44.
42. Williams CR, Gallagher EP. Effects of cadmium on olfactory mediated behaviors and molecular biomarkers in coho salmon (Oncorhynchus kisutch). Aquat Toxicol. 2013;140-141:295–302.
43. National Toxicology Program. NTP toxicology and carcinogenesis studies of nickel subsulfide (CAS No. 12035–72-2) in F344 rats and B6C3F1 mice (Inhalation Studies). Natl Toxicol Program Tech Rep Ser. 1996;453:1–365.
44. National Toxicology Program. NTP toxicology and carcinogenesis studies of nickel sulfate hexahydrate (CAS No. 10101–97-0) in F344 rats and B6C3F1 mice (Inhalation Studies). Natl Toxicol Program Tech Rep Ser. 1996;454:1–380.
45. Evans JE, Miller ML, Andringa A, Hastings L. Behavioral, histological, and neurochemical effects of nickel (II) on the rat olfactory system. Toxicol Appl Pharmacol. 1995;130(2):209–20.
46. Miller ML, Andringa A, Evans JE, Hastings L. Microvillar cells of the olfactory epithelium: morphology and regeneration following exposure to toxic compounds. Brain Res. 1995;669(1):1–9.
47. Lewis J, Hahn F, Dahl A. Transport of inhaled toxicants to the central nervous system. Characteristics of a nose-brain barrier. The vulnerable brain and environmental risks. 1994;3:77–103.
48. Henriksson J, Tallkvist J, Tjälve H. Uptake of nickel into the brain via olfactory neurons in rats. Toxicol Lett. 1997;91(2):153–62.
49. Tallkvist J, Henriksson J, d'Argy R, Tjalve H. Transport and subcellular distribution of nickel in the olfactory system of pikes and rats. Toxicol Sci. 1998;43(2):196–203.
50. Jia C, Roman C, Hegg CC. Nickel sulfate induces location-dependent atrophy of mouse olfactory epithelium: protective and proliferative role of purinergic receptor activation. Toxicol Sci. 2010;115(2):547–56.
51. Zhao J, Bowman L, Zhang X, Shi X, Jiang B, Castranova V, et al. Metallic nickel nano- and fine particles induce JB6 cell apoptosis through a caspase-8/AIF mediated cytochrome c-independent pathway. J Nanobiotechnology. 2009;7:2.
52. Gautam SH, Otsuguro KI, Ito S, Saito T, Habara Y. T-type Ca2+ channels mediate propagation of odor-induced Ca2+ transients in rat olfactory receptor neurons. Neuroscience. 2007;144(2):702–13.
53. Seeber H, Fikentscher R, Roseburg B. Geruchs- und Geschmacksstörungen bei Chromfarbenarbeitern. Z Gesamte Hyg. 1976;22(11):820–2.
54. Seeber H, Fikentscher R. Schäden der Nasenschleimhaut und Riechstörungen durch berufliche Chromstaubexposition. Z Gesamte Hyg. 1980;26(7):506–8.
55. Watanabe S, Fukuchi Y. Occupational impairment of the olfactory sense of chromate producing workers (in Japanese). Sangyo Igaku. 1981;23(6):606–11.
56. Kitamura F, Yokoyama K, Araki S, Nishikitani M, Choi JW, Yum YT, et al. Increase of olfactory threshold in plating factory workers exposed to chromium in Korea. Ind Health. 2003;41(3):279–85.
57. Aiyer RG, Kumar G. Nasal manifestations in chromium industry workers. Indian J Otolaryngol Head Neck Surg. 2003;55(2):71–3.
58. Lucchini R, Bergamaschi E, Smargiassi A, Festa D, Apostoli P. Motor function, olfactory threshold, and hematological indices in manganese-exposed ferroalloy workers. Environ Res. 1997;73(1–2):175–80.
59. Mergler D, Huel G, Bowler R, Iregren A, Belanger S, Baldwin M, et al. Nervous system dysfunction among workers with long-term exposure to manganese. Environ Res. 1994;64(2):151–80.
60. Antunes MB, Bowler R, Doty RL. San Francisco/Oakland Bay bridge welder study: olfactory function. Neurology. 2007;69(12):1278–84.
61. Bowler RM, Roels HA, Nakagawa S, Drezgic M, Diamond E, Park R, et al. Dose-effect relationships between manganese exposure and neurological, neuropsychological and pulmonary function in confined space bridge welders. Occup Environ Med. 2007;64(3):167–77.
62. Bowler RM, Gocheva V, Harris M, Ngo L, Abdelouahab N, Wilkinson J, et al. Prospective study on neurotoxic effects in manganese-exposed bridge construction welders. Neurotoxicology. 2011;32(5):596–605.
63. Sen S, Flynn MR, Du G, Troster AI, An H, Huang X. Manganese accumulation in the olfactory bulbs and other brain regions of "asymptomatic" welders. Toxicol Sci. 2011;121(1):160–7.
64. Guarneros M, Ortiz-Romo N, Alcaraz-Zubeldia M, Drucker-Colín R, Hudson R. Nonoccupational environmental exposure to manganese is linked to deficits in peripheral and central olfactory function. Chemical senses. 2013;38(9):783–91.
65. Lucchini RG, Guazzetti S, Zoni S, Donna F, Peter S, Zacco A, et al. Tremor, olfactory and motor changes in Italian adolescents exposed to historical ferro-manganese emission. Neurotoxicology. 2012;33(4):687–96.
66. Iannilli E, Gasparotti R, Hummel T, Zoni S, Benedetti C, Fedrighi C, et al. Effects of manganese exposure on olfactory functions in teenagers: a pilot study. PLoS One. 2016;11(1):e0144783.
67. Casjens S, Pesch B, Robens S, Kendzia B, Behrens T, Weiss T, et al. Associations between former exposure to manganese and olfaction in an elderly population: results from the Heinz Nixdorf recall study. Neurotoxicology. 2017;58:58–65.
68. Tjalve H, Henriksson J. Uptake of metals in the brain via olfactory pathways. Neurotoxicology. 1999;20(2–3):181–95.
69. Tjalve H, Henriksson J, Tallkvist J, Larsson BS, Lindquist NG. Uptake of manganese and cadmium from the nasal mucosa into the central nervous system via olfactory pathways in rats. Pharmacol Toxicol. 1996;79(6):347–56.
70. Tjalve H, Mejare C, Borg-Neczak K. Uptake and transport of manganese in primary and secondary olfactory neurones in pike. Pharmacol Toxicol. 1995; 77(1):23–31.
71. Foster ML, Rao DB, Francher T, Traver S, Dorman DC. Olfactory toxicity in rats following manganese chloride nasal instillation: a pilot study. Neurotoxicology. 2018;64:284–90.
72. Thompson KJ, Molina RM, Donaghey T, Savaliya S, Schwob JE, Brain JD. Manganese uptake and distribution in the brain after methyl bromide-induced lesions in the olfactory epithelia. Toxicol Sci. 2011;120(1):163–72.
73. Pyatayev GE. The state of olfactory function in zinc production workers, in Russian. Zh Ushn Nos Gorl Bolezn. 1971;31:17–21.
74. Anonymous. Zinc Sulphate spray for prevention of poliomyelitis. Br Med J. 1938;1(4034):953–4.
75. Tisdall F, Brown A, Defries R. Persistent anosmia following zinc sulfate nasal spraying. J Pediatr. 1938;13(1):60–2.
76. Davidson TM, Smith WM. The Bradford Hill criteria and zinc-induced anosmia: a causality analysis. Arch Otolaryngol Head Neck Surg. 2010;136(7):673–6.
77. Alexander TH, Davidson TM. Intranasal zinc and anosmia: the zinc-induced anosmia syndrome. Laryngoscope. 2006;116(2):217–20.
78. Jafek BW, Linschoten MR, Murrow BW. Anosmia after intranasal zinc gluconate use. Am J Rhinol. 2004;18(3):137–41.
79. Osmond-McLeod MJ, Osmond RI, Oytam Y, McCall MJ, Feltis B, Mackay-Sim A, et al. Surface coatings of ZnO nanoparticles mitigate differentially a host of transcriptional, protein and signalling responses in primary human olfactory cells. Part Fibre Toxicol. 2013;10(1):54.
80. Lim JH, Davis GE, Wang Z, Li V, Wu Y, Rue TC, et al. Zicam-induced damage to mouse and human nasal tissue. PLoS One. 2009;4(10):e7647.
81. McBride K, Slotnick B, Margolis FL. Does intranasal application of zinc sulfate produce anosmia in the mouse? An olfactometric and anatomical study. Chem Senses. 2003;28(8):659–70.

82. Burd GD. Morphological study of the effects of intranasal zinc sulfate irrigation on the mouse olfactory epithelium and olfactory bulb. Microsc Res Tech. 1993;24(3):195–213.
83. Cancalon P. Degeneration and regeneration of olfactory cells induced by $ZnSO_4$ and other chemicals. Tissue Cell. 1982;14(4):717–33.
84. Harding JW, Getchell TV, Margolis FL. Denervation of the primary olfactory pathway in mice. V. Long-term effect of intranasal $ZnSO_4$ irrigation on behavior, biochemistry and morphology. Brain Res. 1978;140(2):271–85.
85. Matulionis DH. Light and electron microscopic study of the degeneration and early regeneration of olfactory epithelium in the mouse. Am J Anat. 1976;145(1):79–99.
86. Smith CG. Changes in the olfactory mucosa and the olfactory nerves following intranasal treatment with one per cent zinc sulphate. Can Med Assoc J. 1938;39(2):138–40.
87. Benvenuti S, Gagliardo A. Homing behaviour of pigeons subjected to unilateral zinc sulphate treatment of their olfactory mucosa. J Exp Biol. 1996; 199(11):2531–5.
88. Hansen LF, Hammer M, Petersen SH, Nielsen GD. Effects of intranasal $ZnSO_4$ irrigation on olfactory and trigeminal cues. Physiol Behav. 1994;55(4):699–704.
89. Mayer AD, Rosenblatt JS. Peripheral olfactory deafferentation of the primary olfactory system in rats using $ZnSO_4$ nasal spray with special reference to maternal behavior. Physiology Behav. 1993;53(3):587–92.
90. Winans SS, Powers JB. Olfactory and vomeronasal deafferentation of male hamsters: histological and behavioral analyses. Brain Res. 1977;126(2):325–44.
91. Alberts JR, Galef BG Jr. Acute anosmia in the rat: a behavioral test of a peripherally-induced olfactory deficit. Physiol Behav. 1971;6(5):619–21.
92. Duncan-Lewis CA, Lukman RL, Banks RK. Effects of zinc gluconate and 2 other divalent cationic compounds on olfactory function in mice. Comp Med. 2011;61(4):361–5.
93. Viswaprakash N, Dennis JC, Globa L, Pustovyy O, Josephson EM, Kanju P, et al. Enhancement of odorant-induced responses in olfactory receptor neurons by zinc nanoparticles. Chem Senses. 2009;34(7):547–57.
94. Gao L, Yang ST, Li S, Meng Y, Wang H, Lei H. Acute toxicity of zinc oxide nanoparticles to the rat olfactory system after intranasal instillation. J Appl Toxicol. 2013;33(10):1079–88.
95. Sorokowska A, Schriever VA, Gudziol V, Hummel C, Hähner A, Iannilli E, et al. Changes of olfactory abilities in relation to age: odor identification in more than 1400 people aged 4 to 80 years. Europ Arch Otorhinolaryngol. 2015; 272(8):1937–44.
96. Muttray A, Moll B, Letzel S. Die sozialmedizinische Bedeutung von Riechstörungen am Beispiel einer Kasuistik. Arbeitsmed Sozialmed Umweltmed. 2003;38:428–34.
97. Mossad SB. Effect of zincum gluconicum nasal gel on the duration and symptom severity of the common cold in otherwise healthy adults. QJM. 2003;96(1):35–43.
98. FDA: Warnings on Three Zicam Intranasal Zinc Products. https://wayback.archive-it.org/7993/20170113083935/http://www.fda.gov/ForConsumers/ConsumerUpdates/ucm166931.htm. Accessed 25 Jan 2018.
99. Hamidovic A. Position on zinc delivery to olfactory nerves in intranasal insulin phase I-III clinical trials. Contemp Clin Trials. 2015;45(Pt B):277–80.
100. Brunner YF, Benedict C, Freiherr J. Intranasal insulin reduces olfactory sensitivity in normosmic humans. J Clin Endocrinol Metab. 2013;98(10):E1626–30.
101. Herranz Gonzalez-Botas J, Padin SA. Nasal gel and olfactory cleft. Acta Otorrinolaringol Esp. 2012;63(5):370–5.
102. Calvert GM, Mueller CA, Fajen JM, Chrislip DW, Russo J, Briggle T, et al. Health effects associated with sulfuryl fluoride and methyl bromide exposure among structural fumigation workers. Am J Public Health. 1998;88(12):1774–80.
103. DFG (Deutsche Forschungsgemeinschaft). Chlorpikrin [MAK Value Documentation in German language, 1974]. In: DFG, editor. The MAK-Collection for Occupational Health and Safety. Weinheim: Wiley-VCH Verlag GmbH & Co. KGaA; 1974.
104. Quandt SA, Walker FO, Talton JW, Summers P, Chen H, McLeod DK, et al. Olfactory function in Latino farmworkers: subclinical neurological effects of pesticide exposure in a vulnerable population. J Occup Environ Med. 2016; 58(3):248–53.
105. Shrestha S, Kamel F, Umbach DM, Beane Freeman LE, Koutros S, Alavanja M, et al. Nonmotor symptoms and Parkinson disease in United States farmers and spouses. PLoS One. 2017;12(9):e0185510.
106. Schwob JE, Youngentob SL, Mezza RC. Reconstitution of the rat olfactory epithelium after methyl bromide-induced lesion. J Comp Neurol. 1995; 359(1):15–37.
107. Eisenbrandt DL, Nitschke KD. Inhalation toxicity of sulfuryl fluoride in rats and rabbits. Fundam Appl Toxicol. 1989;12(3):540–57.
108. Mattsson JL, Albee RR, Eisenbrandt DL, Chang LW. Subchronic neurotoxicity in rats of the structural fumigant, sulfuryl fluoride. Neurotoxicol Teratol. 1988;10(2):127–33.
109. Spealman CR. Odors, odorants, and deodorants in aviation. Ann N Y Acad Sci. 1954;58(2):40–3.
110. Lenhardt E, Rollin H. Berufsbedingte Riechstörungen. HNO. 1969;17:104–6.
111. Holmström M, Wilhelmsson B. Respiratory symptoms and pathophysiological effects of occupational exposure to formaldehyde and wood dust. Scand J Work Environ Health. 1988;14(5):306–11.
112. Hisamitsu M, Okamoto Y, Chazono H, Yonekura S, Sakurai D, Horiguchi S, et al. The influence of environmental exposure to formaldehyde in nasal mucosa of medical students during cadaver dissection. Allergol Int. 2011; 60(3):373–9.
113. Kilburn KH, Seidman BC, Warshaw R. Neurobehavioral and respiratory symptoms of formaldehyde and xylene exposure in histology technicians. Arch Environ Health. 1985;40(4):229–33.
114. Edling C, Hellquist H, Odkvist L. Occupational exposure to formaldehyde and histopathological changes in the nasal mucosa. Br J Ind Med. 1988; 45(11):761–5.
115. Arts JH, Rennen MA, de Heer C. Inhaled formaldehyde: evaluation of sensory irritation in relation to carcinogenicity. Regul Toxicol Pharmacol. 2006;44(2):144–60.
116. Cassee FR, Groten JP, Feron VJ. Changes in the nasal epithelium of rats exposed by inhalation to mixtures of formaldehyde, acetaldehyde, and acrolein. Fundam Appl Toxicol. 1996;29(2):208–18.
117. Li Y, Chen H, Yin Y, Han F, Ye X, Ling S. Formaldehyde inhalation may damage olfactory bulb and hippocampus in rats. Zhejiang da xue xue bao Yi xue ban Journal of Zhejiang University Medical Sciences. 2010;39(3):272–7.
118. Zhang Q, Yan W, Bai Y, Zhu Y, Ma J. Repeated formaldehyde inhalation impaired olfactory function and changed SNAP25 proteins in olfactory bulb. Int J Occup Environ Health. 2014;20(4):308–12.
119. Schwartz BS, Doty RL, Monroe C, Frye R, Barker S. Olfactory function in chemical workers exposed to acrylate and methacrylate vapors. Am J Public Health. 1989;79(5):613–8.
120. Muttray A, Schmitt B, Klimek L. Effects of methyl methacrylate on the sense of smell. Cent Eur J Occup Environ Med. 1997;3:58–66.
121. Muttray A, Gosepath J, Brieger J, Faldum A, Zagar C, Mayer-Popken O, et al. V17 Zur Wirkung von 50 ppm Methylmethacrylat auf die oberen Atemwege gesunder Probanden. Arbeitsmed Sozialmed Umweltmed. 2007;42(3):105.
122. DFG (Deutsche Forschungsgemeinschaft). Methyl methacrylate [MAK Value Documentations, Vol. 26, 2010]. In: DFG, editor. The MAK-Collection for Occupational Health and Safety. Weinheim: Wiley-VCH Verlag GmbH & Co. KGaA; 2010.
123. Cheng SF, Chen ML, Hung PC, Chen CJ, Mao IF. Olfactory loss in poly(acrylonitrile-butadiene-styrene) plastic injection-moulding workers. Occup Med (Lond). 2004;54(7):469–74.
124. Dalton P, Cowart B, Dilks D, Gould M, Lees PS, Stefaniak A, et al. Olfactory function in workers exposed to styrene in the reinforced-plastics industry. Am J Ind Med. 2003;44(1):1–11.
125. Dalton P, Lees PS, Gould M, Dilks D, Stefaniak A, Bader M, et al. Evaluation of long-term occupational exposure to styrene vapor on olfactory function. Chem Senses. 2007;32(8):739–47.
126. Mücke W, Lemmen C. Duft und Geruch: Wirkungen und gesundheitliche Bedeutung von Geruchsstoffen. Heidelberg, München, Landsberg, Frechen, Hamburg: ecomed-Storck GmbH; 2010.
127. Cruzan G, Cushman JR, Andrews LS, Granville GC, Miller RR, Hardy CJ, et al. Subchronic inhalation studies of styrene in CD rats and CD-1 mice. Fundam Appl Toxicol. 1997;35(2):152–65.
128. Cruzan G, Cushman JR, Andrews LS, Granville GC, Johnson KA, Hardy CJ, et al. Chronic toxicity/oncogenicity study of styrene in CD rats by inhalation exposure for 104 weeks. Toxicol Sci. 1998;46(2):266–81.
129. Green T, Lee R, Toghill A, Meadowcroft S, Lund V, Foster J. The toxicity of styrene to the nasal epithelium of mice and rats: studies on the mode of action and relevance to humans. Chem Biol Interact. 2001;137(2):185–202.
130. Schwartz BS, Ford DP, Bolla KI, Agnew J, Rothman N, Bleecker ML. Solvent-associated decrements in olfactory function in paint manufacturing workers. Am J Ind Med. 1990;18(6):697–706.
131. Sandmark B, Broms I, Lofgren L, Ohlson CG. Olfactory function in painters exposed to organic solvents. Scand J Work Environ Health. 1989;15(1):60–3.

132. Ahlstrom R, Berglund B, Berglund U, Lindvall T, Wennberg A. Impaired odor perception in tank cleaners. Scand J Work Environ Health. 1986;12(6):574–81.
133. Muttray A, Klimek L, Jung D, Rose D, Mann W, Konietzko J. Die toxische Hyp- und Anosmie – eine "vergessene" Berufskrankheit. Zentralbl Arbeitsmed. 1998;48:66–71.
134. Latkowski B, Zalewski P, Najwer K, Zbrzezny K, Czyzewski I. Evaluation of the senses of taste and smell in petroleum chemistry workers based on 3-year observations, in Polish. Med Pr. 1981;32(1):51–7.
135. National Toxicology Program. NTP toxicology and carcinogenesis studies of tetrahydrofuran (CAS No. 109-99-9) in F344/N rats and B6C3F1 mice (Inhalation Studies). Natl Toxicol Program Tech Rep Ser. 1998;475:1–244.
136. National Toxicology Program. NTP toxicity studies of cyclohexanone oxime administered by drinking water to B6C3F1 mice (CAS No. 100-64-1). NTP toxicity studies of cyclohexanone oxime administered by drinking water to B6C3F1 mice (CAS No 100-64-1). Toxic Rep Ser. 1996;50:1–E8.
137. Miyake M, Ito Y, Sawada M, Sakai K, Suzuki H, Sakamoto T, et al. Subchronic inhalation exposure to 2-ethyl-1-hexanol impairs the mouse olfactory bulb via injury and subsequent repair of the nasal olfactory epithelium. Arch Toxicol. 2016;90(8):1949–58.
138. Hatt H. Geschmack und Geruch. In: Schmidt R, Lang F, Heckmann M, editors. Physiologie des Menschen. Heidelberg: Springer Medizin Verlag; 2010. p. 386–400.
139. Patel RM, Pinto JM. Olfaction: anatomy, physiology, and disease. Clin Anat. 2014;27(1):54–60.
140. Witt M, Hansen A. Strukturelle und funktionelle Grundlagen des Riechens. In: WL HT, editor. Riech-und Schmeckstörungen. Stuttgart, New York: Thieme; 2009. p. 11–26.
141. Muttray A, Klimek L, Letzel S. Toxische Hyposmie und Rhinitis eines Karosseriebauers und Lackierers. Ergo Med. 2003;27:106–11.
142. Welge-Lüssen A, Hummel T. Riechstörungen postinfektiöser, posttraumatischer, medikamentöser, toxischer, postoperativer und anderer Ätiologien. In: Hummel T, Welge-Lüssen A, editors. Riech-und Schmeckstörungen. Stuttgart, New York: Thieme; 2009. p. 77–94.
143. Feron VJ, Arts JH, Kuper CF, Slootweg PJ, Woutersen RA. Health risks associated with inhaled nasal toxicants. Crit Rev Toxicol. 2001;31(3):313–47.
144. Wardlaw SA, Nikula KJ, Kracko DA, Finch GL, Thornton-Manning JR, Dahl AR. Effect of cigarette smoke on CYP1A1, CYP1A2 and CYP2B1/2 of nasal mucosae in F344 rats. Carcinogenesis. 1998;19(4):655–62.
145. Gebel S, Gerstmayer B, Bosio A, Haussmann HJ, Van Miert E, Muller T. Gene expression profiling in respiratory tissues from rats exposed to mainstream cigarette smoke. Carcinogenesis. 2004;25(2):169–78.
146. Baader EW. Chronic cadmium poisoning. Ind Med Surg. 1952;21(9):427–30.
147. Dorman DC, Struve MF, Wong BA, Dye JA, Robertson ID. Correlation of brain magnetic resonance imaging changes with pallidal manganese concentrations in rhesus monkeys following subchronic manganese inhalation. Toxicol Sci. 2006;92(1):219–27.
148. Oberdörster G, Sharp Z, Atudorei V, Elder A, Gelein R, Kreyling W, et al. Translocation of inhaled ultrafine particles to the brain. Inhal Toxicol. 2004; 16(6–7):437–45.
149. Hopkins LE, Patchin ES, Chiu PL, Brandenberger C, Smiley-Jewell S, Pinkerton KE. Nose-to-brain transport of aerosolised quantum dots following acute exposure. Nanotoxicology. 2014;8(8):885–93.
150. Shiga H, Taki J, Yamada M, Washiyama K, Amano R, Matsuura Y, et al. Evaluation of the olfactory nerve transport function by SPECT-MRI fusion image with nasal thallium-201 administration. Mol Imaging Biol. 2011;13(6):1262–6.
151. Shiga H, Taki J, Washiyama K, Yamamoto J, Kinase S, Okuda K, et al. Assessment of olfactory nerve by SPECT-MRI image with nasal thallium-201 administration in patients with olfactory impairments in comparison to healthy volunteers. PLoS One. 2013;8(2):e57671.
152. Colin-Barenque L, Souza-Gallardo LM, Fortoul TI. Toxic effects of inhaled manganese on the olfactory bulb: an ultrastructural approach in mice. J Electron Microsc. 2011;60(1):73–8.
153. Moberly AH, Czarnecki LA, Pottackal J, Rubinstein T, Turkel DJ, Kass MD, et al. Intranasal exposure to manganese disrupts neurotransmitter release from glutamatergic synapses in the central nervous system in vivo. Neurotoxicology. 2012;33(5):996–1004.
154. Guilarte TR, Burton NC, McGlothan JL, Verina T, Zhou Y, Alexander M, et al. Impairment of nigrostriatal dopamine neurotransmission by manganese is mediated by pre-synaptic mechanism(s): implications to manganese-induced parkinsonism. J Neurochem. 2008;107(5):1236–47.
155. Hoffman HJ, Rawal S, Li CM, Duffy VB. New chemosensory component in the U.S. National Health and nutrition examination survey (NHANES): first-year results for measured olfactory dysfunction. Rev Endocr Metab Disord. 2016;17(2):221–40.
156. Liu G, Zong G, Doty RL, Sun Q. Prevalence and risk factors of taste and smell impairment in a nationwide representative sample of the US population: a cross-sectional study. BMJ Open. 2016;6(11):e013246.
157. Bello G, Dumancas G. Association of 2,4-dichlorophenol urinary concentrations and olfactory dysfunction in a national sample of middle-aged and older U.S. adults. Int J Environ Health Res. 2017;27(6):498–508.
158. Noel J, Habib AR, Thamboo A, Patel ZM. Variables associated with olfactory disorders in adults: a U.S. population-based analysis. World J Otorhinolaryngol Head Neck Surg. 2017;3(1):9–16.
159. The German National Cohort. Aims, study design and organization. Eur J Epidemiol. 2014;29(5):371–82.
160. Sorokowska A, Sorokowski P, Frackowiak T. Determinants of human olfactory performance: a cross-cultural study. Sci Total Environ. 2015;506-507:196–200.
161. Greenberg MI, Curtis JA, Vearrier D. The perception of odor is not a surrogate marker for chemical exposure: a review of factors influencing human odor perception. Clin Toxicol. 2013;51(2):70–6.
162. Palouzier-Paulignan B, Lacroix MC, Aime P, Baly C, Caillol M, Congar P, et al. Olfaction under metabolic influences. Chem Senses. 2012;37(9):769–97.
163. Altman KW, Desai SC, Moline J, de la Hoz RE, Herbert R, Gannon PJ, et al. Odor identification ability and self-reported upper respiratory symptoms in workers at the post-9/11 world trade center site. Int Arch Occup Environ Health. 2011;84(2):131–7.
164. Dżaman K, Wojdas A, Rapiejko P, Jurkiewicz D. Taste and smell perception among sewage treatment and landfill workers. Int J Occup Med Environ Health. 2009;22(3):227–34.
165. Green T, Toghill A, Foster JR. The role of cytochromes P-450 in styrene induced pulmonary toxicity and carcinogenicity. Toxicology. 2001;169(2):107–17.
166. TRGS 522 - technical rule for hazardous substances. Raumdesinfektionen mit Formaldehyd GMBl. 2013;15(1):298–320.
167. Glück U. Macht der Gerüche - krank machend oder belästigend. Schweiz Med Wochenschr. 1996;126:958–66.
168. Haehner A, Hummel T, Reichmann H. Olfactory dysfunction as a diagnostic marker for Parkinson's disease. Expert Rev Neurother. 2009;9(12):1773–9.

Occupational exposure to ultrafine particles in police officers: no evidence for adverse respiratory effects

G. Jordakieva[1], I. Grabovac[2*], E. Valic[3], K. E. Schmidt[4], A. Graff[5], A. Schuster[5], K. Hoffmann-Sommergruber[6], C. Oberhuber[6], O. Scheiner[6], A. Goll[7] and J. Godnic-Cvar[1]

Abstract

Background: Inhalation exposure to fine and ultrafine particles (UFPs) has been associated with respiratory diseases. However, little is known on the quality, threshold levels and concentration of these particles causing adverse health effects.

Methods: The impact of occupational exposure to submicrometer and UFPs was assessed in 30 healthy police shooting instructors by clinical investigation, self-assessment questionnaire, sputum and spirometry and compared to a control group. General laboratory chemistry parameters, circulating cytokines (interleukin [IL]-2, IL-4, IL-5, IL-6, IL-8, interferon-gamma [IFN-γ]), and granulocyte macrophage colony-stimulating factor (GM-CSF) in serum were measured. UFP exposure was recorded by Scanning Mobility Particle Sizer.

Results: Concentrations of submicrometer sized airborne particles (< 700 nm) measured between $3.34 \times 10^5/cm^3$ and $7.58 \times 10^5/cm^3$ at shooting sites, with highest concentrations found in the UFP range (< 100 nm). The size of the monodispersed particles ranged from 54.74 ± 16.25 nm to 98.19 ± 22.83 nm. Short term exposure (4 h) to high levels of UFPs caused an increase of IFN-γ in exposed subjects ($p = 0.022$). 24 h after exposure a significant decrease of IgG, albumin fibrinogen and factor VII was found. Neither directly after 4 h of high levels UFPs exposure nor 24 h after exposure subjective complaints or objective measurements indicating adverse respiratory effects in exposed subjects were found.

Conclusions: No consistent indications for adverse respiratory or inflammatory effects directly following exposure and 24 h after exposure to high levels of UFPs in our study group were detected. However we showed the assessment of short-term exposure effects at a genuine occupational setting, which might is relevant when a risk assessment of high level occupational exposures to UFPs is considered.

Keywords: Adverse health effects, Airway obstruction, Inflammation, Occupational exposure, Ultrafine particles, Indoor shooting range

Background

A relationship between increased ambient air pollution and adverse health effects has been postulated. Exposure to ultrafine particles (UFPs, defined as < 100 nm [nm] in diameter) has been reported to increase respiratory symptoms, decrease lung function, cause asthma exacerbations, increased medication use and increased hospital admissions related to respiratory diseases [1–7]. UFPs predominantly emerge from industrial (welding and metal smoke, technical carbon-particulate emissions, amorphous silica acid) and traffic emissions. Their adverse health effects have been attributed to high particle number per unit mass and reactive surface [7–13] and associated with airway inflammation with a subsequent release of chemical mediators and cytokines [14–18]. Adjuvant effects have also been observed, e.g. diesel particles have been shown

* Correspondence: igor.grabovac@meduniwien.ac.at
[2]Department of Social and Preventive Medicine, Centre for Public Health, Medical University of Vienna, Kinderspitalgasse 15/1, A-1090 Vienna, Austria
Full list of author information is available at the end of the article

to enhance and/or intensify sensitization to common allergens [9, 11, 12, 19–26].

Most of the current knowledge on pathophysiological mechanisms associated with UFPs is derived from cell cultures and animal models. Only a few groups investigated their effects on human subjects [7–10, 12–14, 16–21, 23–25, 27, 28].

While acute respiratory effects of exposure to fine particles have been established experimentally and epidemiologically, the contribution of fine particles to the development of chronic disease is less clear [29].

The measurement of UFPs at workplaces in Germany has shown that especially high number concentrations (ranging from a few 1000 to several 100,000 particles/cm^3) are associated with combustion processes such as; welding, soldering and metal grinding [30]. Firearm usage generates particulate emissions, which may accumulate in ambient air, particularly in closed spaces such as indoor shooting ranges. Airborne particles originate from explosion and vapour generation during bullet discharge, further releasing metallic components, like lead, barium and antimony. Particle diameters emitted from gunshots were reported to be mostly < 10 µm in diameter [31]. Work-site measurements conducted at indoor shooting ranges revealed a clear accumulation of UFPs ranging up to 420,000/cm^3 in Swiss and German workplace assessments, depending on exhaust availability [32, 33].

It remains to be established whether exposure to submicrometer and UFPs triggers adverse respiratory effects only in susceptible or in all exposed subjects. Even more so, adverse health effects of UFPs in an occupational setting after several years of exposure have not been evaluated thoroughly.

The aim of this study was to determine whether a defined occupational exposure to UFPs causes adverse health effects in frequently inhalation exposed shooting instructors.

Methods

Subjects

Sixty male subjects ($n = 60$) employed as federal police officers in Vienna, Austria, were included in this study and divided in two groups depending on the level of UFP exposure. The exposed group consisted of 30 police officers working as instructors at a shooting range with an average work history of 4.7 years. The control group comprised 30 police officers working in administration.

Study design

Measurements in subjects were conducted at a) three time points in the exposed group: time point "0^{exp}" = before exposure, time point "1^{exp}" = at the day of exposure (after 4 h of UFP exposure) and time point "2^{exp}" = 24 h after UFP exposure; and at b) two time points in the control group (no occupational UFP exposure) on two separate days (time point "0^{con}" and time point "1^{con}"). At each of these test points an occupational self-reporting questionnaire was completed and a diagnostic workup performed (spirometry and blood sampling).

Exposure to UFPs and metals

Shooting ranges have been identified as places with high levels of submicrometer and UFPs [32, 34, 35]. The measurements were conducted at 5 modern police shooting ranges (designated as "A", "B", "C", "D" and "E"), where UFPs arise from combustion of the explosion in the percussion-cap and metal fumes originating from the metal coat of the bullets (lead, barium, copper and antimony).

The average size of airborne particles (in nm), the metal content (in mg/m^3) of the inhalable dust and the gaseous pollutants were measured at 5 locations (Table 2). At location A and B the measurements were repeated twice and three times, respectively, on separate days to control for the repeatability of the measured values. The number and size of submicrometer and UFPs under normal working conditions while the ventilation (exhaust) system was operating (air turnover between 22 and 31 air changes/h, air flow from ceiling to target plates) was measured by the stationary Scanning Mobility Particle Sizer (SMPS™, TSI Type 3936 L; Flow Controller Model 120FC TSI; impactor diameter 0,0457 cm) and expressed as particles/cm^3 (concentrations indicated as means +/− SD). Measurement range was restricted to particle sizes 15–700 nm and measured values were presented every 2 min and 30 s.

Sampling was conducted between 2 and 4 h (see Table 2) in a total of eight shooting episodes, during which constant target practice was performed by up to 3 persons. The distance between SMPS and shooting person as well as between sampling inlet and pistol outlet were less than a meter, respectively. The study subjects, being shooting instructors, were constantly present at the shooting range and in close proximity to the shooting persons.

All aerosol exposure measurements were performed under normal working conditions with an activated ventilation system. The different particle sizes were determined using a high-voltage area resulting from particle diameter-dependent mobility of the submicrometer and ultrafine aerosol particles in the surrounding gas. First of all the aerosol passes an impactor, which prevents larger particles than those of interest arriving in the system. Subsequently, ionization of the particles takes place using a Kr^{87} source. In a high-voltage area (DMA 3081 Differential Mobility Analyser) the particles are selected according to their electrical mobility, which is a measure for their size. Mono-dispersive aerosol is supplied to a CPC (Condensation Particle Counter

3022A), where the particles are brought to the same size with the help of evaporating butanol, in order to be able to count them using a laser. The entirely controlling of the SMPS as well as the data measurement recording was conducted by PC.

Inhalable dust was measured by the personal air sampler (Gilian HFS 513 A Gilian - PAS SG10, GSA building of measure devices GmbH using a standard kit; Filter type: 10 μ nylon; holder: "O-ring seal"), the high volume sampler Gravikon PM4 (Ströhlein) and the portable dust monitor (Grimm Aerosol Technik GmbH using standard equipment). Personal sampling time was approximately 3 h. Measurements were performed 6 m and 8 m away from the shooter and 0 and 2 m away from the targets; additionally personal sampling was conducted on the shooting instructors themselves. The variability of these measurements was below 6% (calculated by GRIMM Aerosol Technik GmbH Windows).

Following gaseous pollutants: CO, NO, NO_2 - were measured by the gas monitor VRAE (RAE Systems). At ranges "A" and "B" the measurements were repeated twice and three times respectively.

To estimate baseline (non-occupational) exposure to UFPs we measured particles with the same methods at a nearby school twice for 16 h (mainly at nighttime).

Spirometry

Lung function was assessed by FVC, FEV_1, MEF_{50} and MEF_{25} measurements (American Thoracic Society 1995) with a "Flow Screen Pro" spirometer (Jäger, Germany) according to the ATS criteria [36].

Blood sample analysis

Blood was drawn from periphery veins of participating subjects. After centrifugation (4000 rpm/10 min/room temperature) serum samples were stored at − 20 °C. Two kinds of analyses were performed:

a) Blood cell count (total and differential), biochemical parameters (albumin, C-reactive protein [CRP]), haemostasis parameters (fibrinogen, prothrombin test, coagulation factor VII), immunoglobulins (IgA, IgG, IgE), and lead concentrations in blood were measured in a clinical laboratory.
b) Cytokines (interleukin (IL-)2, IL-4, IL-6, IL-8, interferon (IFN-)γ, granulocyte macrophage colony-stimulating factor (GM-CSF)) were assessed by commercial ELISA (enzyme-linked immunosorbent assay) kits (R&D Systems, Inc., Minneapolis, USA) according to manufacturer's instructions following the construction of standard curves for each ELISA system. All serum samples were applied in duplicates and undiluted. The tests were performed in an immunological laboratory of the Department of Pathophysiology and Allergy Research of the Medical University of Vienna.

Statistical methods

This study was planned as a feasibility study. Descriptive statistics (percentages, means, ranges and standard deviation) were calculated. To investigate the differences in values between the two groups at baseline (before exposure) t-tests, Wilcoxon tests or Chi Square tests were performed as appropriate.

To analyse a possible temporal impact of exposure to submicrometer and UFPs, analyses of covariance was performed for the first measurement after baseline (which is available in exposed and controls) including a fixed grouping factor (exposed/controls) and the baseline value, age and package years as co-variables. A significant grouping factor here indicated a different time course between exposed subjects and controls.

Only within the group of exposed persons, mixed models accounting for time as fixed factor (with three levels) and exposed subjects as a random factor were calculated. No correction for multiple testing was applied in this pilot study. Statistical analyses were performed using SAS Version 9.1.

Results

Demographic data

A total of sixty ($n = 60$; 100% male subjects) police officers with ($n = 30$) and without ($n = 30$) occupational UFP exposure were examined. The exposed group consisted of 30 police officers working as instructors at a shooting range with an average work history of 4.7 years. The control group comprised 30 police officers working in administration. Control group subjects were older (41.9 vs. 34.1 years, respectively; $p < 0.0001$) and had a longer (13.17 vs. 6.83 years, respectively; $p = 0.020$) and more intensive (14.47 vs. 5.53 package years, respectively; $p = 0.014$) smoking history than the exposed subjects (Table 1).

UFPs exposure load

The size of monodispersed particles ranged from 54,74 ± 16,25 nm (SD) nm at location A1 to 98.19 ± 22.83 (SD) nm at location E (Table 2). The metal content of inhalable dust was on average as follows: lead 0.01 ± 0.2 (SD), barium 0.05 ± 0.04 (SD), copper 0.01 ± 0.01 (SD), and antimony 0.002 ± 0.01 (SD). Exposure to gaseous pollutants was neglectable: CO 4.86 ± 4.87 (SD) ppm, NO and NO_2 expressed as NOx was < 0.1 ppm. Baseline (non-occupational) measurements at the control site with the same methods (nearby school) were 0.007 and 0.009 mg/m^3 for inhalable dust, whereas the metal content on average was as follows: lead 0.02 μg/m^3, barium 0.02 μg/m^3 and copper 0.5 μg/m^3.

Table 1 Characteristics of 30 shooting instructors occupationally exposed to UFPs for 4.7 years on average and 30 control participants

	Exposed to UFPs	Controls	*p*-value (t-test)
Age, years (mean)	34.1 ± 8.0	41.9 ± 5.1	< 0.0001
Current smokers %	29	34	0.65[b]
Ex-smokers %	29	31	0.87[b]
Years	6.83 range (0–25)	13.17 range (0–36)	0.02[a]
Pack-years	5.53 range (0–30)	14.47 range (0–60)	0.01[a]
Body height in cm	179.3 ± 5.5	181.6 ± 7.3	0.18
Body weight in kg	80.5 ± 11.2	84.5 ± 13.2	0.08
Systolic BP in mmHg	128.0 ± 14.1	128.0 ± 14.9	0.83
Diastolic BP in mmHg	82.3 ± 10.6	82.8 ± 10.1	0.71
VC (L)	5.01 ± 0.93	5.45 ± 0.97	0.0165
FVC %	95.6 ± 15.6	90.1 ± 13.4	
FEV_1%	96.8 ± 13.2	92.8 ± 17.0	
MEF_{50} (%)	94.7 ± 25.7	90.0 ± 32.0	
MEF_{25} (%)	85.7 ± 34.8	72.3 ± 36.8	

Data expressed in mean ± standard deviation
BP blood pressure, *VC* vital capacity, *FEV_1* forced expiratory volume in one second, *MEF_{50}* maximum expiratory flow at 50% of forced VC, *MEF_{25}* maximum expiratory flow at 25% of forced VC
[a]Wilcoxon test
[b]ChiSquare test

Self-reported symptoms

No health complaints, neither local (airways) nor systemic, were reported acutely (after 4 h of UFP exposure) or belatedly (24 h after exposure). Subjects who were occupationally exposed to submicrometer and UFPs did not report more airway or general health complaints at baseline than subjects in the control group.

Table 2 Exposure to submicrometer sized airborne particles < 700 nm during 4,5 h of the work shift at 5 different locations

Location	Duration (in hours)	AM particle concentration (n/cm^3)	Median particle size (nm)	Mean particle size (nm)	Dominating Mode (nm)
A1	3.5	3.57×10^5	54.7	67.2	56.6
A2	3.5	5.31×10^5	62.3	72.8	63.3
B1	3.5	4.66×10^5	58.8	70.1	60.1
B2	3.5	5.93×10^5	60.3	70.3	64.5
B3	4	5.39×10^5	62.1	72.3	65.8
C	3.5	4.28×10^5	62.8	75.4	63.4
D	3.5	7.58×10^5	78.1	89.2	83.3
E	2	3.34×10^5	98.2	109.8	101.0

A-E: different locations, at location A and B the measurements were repeated on 2 and 3 study days, respectively, in parallel to the medical examinations
AM arithmetic mean

Spirometry

- At baseline

Baseline spirometry values significantly differed between the exposed and non-exposed subjects. Baseline vital capacity (VC) values in control subjects were lower than the baseline VC values in exposed subjects (5.01 ± 0.93 [SD] L vs. 5.45 ± 0.97 [SD] L, respectively, $p = 0.0165$) as shown in Table 1. In the exposed shooting instructors a significant reduction of the FEV_1 lung function parameter (for 0.23 L on average $p = 0.0104$) was found only in the 24 h after exposure spirometry when compared to baseline values. No reduction in MEF_{50} or in MEF_{25} was found at any time point (Tables 3 and 4) in exposed subjects. In the control group no significant difference between time point 0^{con} and time point 1^{con} in FEV_1 ($p = 0.5517$), MEF_{50} ($p = 0.7302$) and MEF_{25} ($p = 0.6537$) was found.

- After 4 h of UFP exposure and 24 h after exposure

No significant differences in lung function parameters were found after 4 h of UFP exposure between exposed and control subjects when adjusted for baseline value, age and package years. Since measurements after 24 h have only been available for the exposed group we performed a pairwise comparison within the group of exposed subjects. No significant changes were found in lung function parameters, except for the mentioned FEV_1 decrease 24 h after exposure when compared to baseline FEV_1.

Blood cell count and serum parameters

- At baseline

Table 3 Lung function in shooting instructors occupationally exposed to UFPs (3 study points)

	Timepoint 0	Timepoint 1	Timepoint 2
VC (L)	5.5 ± 1.0	5.3 ± 0.9	5.4 ± 0.7
VC (%)	95.6 ± 15.5	93.2 ± 16.2	94.6 ± 13.5
FEV_1 (L)	4.6 ± 0.7	4.5 ± 0.7	4.3 ± 0.6
FEV_1 (%)	96.8 ± 13.2	95.0 ± 11.2	92.5 ± 10.5
MEF_{50} (L/s)	2.8 ± 0.8	2.8 ± 0.8	2.6 ± 0.7
MEF_{50} (%)	94.7 ± 25.7	95.8 ± 25. 7	89.6 ± 23.0
MEF_{25} (L/s)	1.9 ± 0.3	2.0 ± 0.2	2.0 ± 0.2
MEF_{25} (%)	85.7 ± 34.8	82.2 ± 32.9	77.2 ± 27.2

Data expressed in mean ± standard deviation
VC, vital capacity; FEV_1, forced expiratory volume in one second; MEF_{50}, maximum expiratory flow at 50% of forced VC; MEF_{25}, maximum expiratory flow at 25% of forced VC

Table 4 Lung function of control participants (2 study points)

	Timepoint 0	Timepoint 1
VC (L)	5.0 ± 0.9	5.1 ± 0.8
VC (%)	90.1 ± 13.4	92.6 ± 12.8
FEV_1 (L)	4.2 ± 0.8	4.1 ± 0.5
FEV_1 (%)	92.8 ± 17.0	91.15 ± 10.1
MEF_{50} (L/s)	2.4 ± 0.7	2.4 ± 0.7
MEF_{50} (%)	90.0 ± 11.9	87.1 ± 29.2
MEF_{25} (L/s)	1.7 ± 0.3	1.7 ± 0.3
MEF_{25} (%)	72.3 ± 36.8	69.2 ± 26.8

Data expressed in mean ± standard deviation
VC vital capacity, *FEV_1* forced expiratory volume in one second, *MEF_{50}* maximum expiratory flow at 50% of forced VC, *MEF_{25}* maximum expiratory flow at 25% of forced VC

Table 6 Biochemical serum parameters of control participants at 2 study points

	Timepoint 0	Timepoint 1	*p* value
HDL	50.2 ± 8.9	53.0 ± 9.5	n.s.
LDL	137.3 ± 35.0	139.7 ± 32.5	n.s.
Cholesterol	220.0 ± 38.3	225.5 ± 38.0	n.s.
Albumin	45.1 ± 1.9	44.8 ± 1.8	n.s.
IgG	1085.1 ± 203.0	1099.5 ± 208.4	n.s.
FVII	110.5 ± 20.2	115.0 ± 18.8	n.s.
Fibrinogen	2.6 ± 0.4	2.7 ± 0.4	n.s.

Data expressed in mean ± standard deviation
HDL high-density lipoprotein, *LDL* low-density lipoprotein, *IgG* immunoglobulin G, *FVII* factor VII, *n.s.* non significant

Exposed subjects had higher albumin values at baseline ($p = 0.004$). Apart from that no significant difference between exposed and control subjects was found in complete and differential blood cell count, biochemical parameters, haemostasis factors, immunoglobulins (IgA, IgG, IgE) and in acute phase proteins (C-reactive protein [CRP] and fibrinogen).

- After 4 h of UFP exposure and 24 h after exposure

No difference in measured serum parameters was found after 4 h of UFP exposure in the exposure group and at the second time point in the control group (see Tables 5 and 6) compared to baseline values. 24 h after UFP exposure a slight decrease within exposed subjects was observed for albumin (mean difference: 0.96, $p = 0.0093$), IgG (mean difference 45.3, $p = 0.0001$), coagulation factor VII (mean difference: 4.87; p = 0.009) and fibrinogen (mean difference: 0.8; $p = 0.003$) compared to baseline.

Cytokine levels in serum

- At baseline

There was no significant difference in cytokine levels in serum (IL-2, IL-4, IL-5, IL-6, IL-8, IFN-γ and GM-CSF) between exposed subjects and controls at baseline (see Tables 7 and 8).

- After 4 h of UFP exposure and 24 h after exposure

No significant changes were found after 4 h of exposure to UFPs except for a significant increase in IFN-γ serum concentration (1.5-fold increase in exposed subjects) ($p = 0.022$, Tables 7 and 8). No significant changes in cytokine levels were found 24 h after UFP exposure.

Blood metal concentration

A higher blood lead concentration ($p = 0.0008$) was found in shooting instructors than in controls (109.33 ± 103.63 (SD) μg/L vs. 36.24 ± 20.42 μg/L, respectively) at baseline. No significant change in blood lead and other metal concentrations was found following UFP exposure and 24 h after exposure compared to baseline in the exposed group and at both time points in the control group.

Table 5 Biochemical serum parameters in shooting instructors occupationally exposed to UFPs (3 study points)

	Timepoint 0	Timepoint 1	Timepoint 2	*p* value
HDL	51.0 ± 11.6	49.2 ± 11.1	50.6 ± 11.2	n.s.
LDL	121.3 ± 39.8	111.0 ± 33.9	114.0 ± 41.4	n.s.
Cholesterol	201.3 ± 46.3	189.4 ± 44.0	196.2 ± 44.3	n.s.
Albumin	46.8 ± 2.4	46.5 ± 3.2	45.8 ± 2.7	0.0093
IgG	1066.7 ± 180.5	1042.0 ± 183.1	1021.4 ± 170.7	0.0001
FVII	101.9 ± 31.0	99.0 ± 41.7	97.0 ± 33.1	0.009
Fibrinogen	2.5 ± 0.5	2.1 ± 0.9	2.0 ± 0.7	0.003

Data expressed in mean ± standard deviation
HDL high-density lipoprotein, *LDL* low-density lipoprotein, *IgG* immunoglobulin G, *FVII* factor VII, *n.s.* non significant

Table 7 Cytokines in sera from shooting instructors occupationally exposed to UFPs ($N = 30$)

Cytokines	Timepoint 0	Timepoint 1	Timepoint 2
IL-2 ng/ml	4.4 (0–29.9)	4.0 (0–21.8)	5.8 (0–51.8)
IL-4 ng/ml	0.2 (0–3.2)	0.5 (0–2.7)	0.1 (0–1.0)
IL-5 ng/ml	2.2 (0–28.6)	2.7 (0–26.5)	1.4 (0–39.4)
IL-6 ng/ml	0.4 (0–3.1)	0.9 (0–4.3)	0.3 (0–1.7)
IL-8 ng/ml	16.0 (0–73.8)	28.8 (0–244.2)	25.7 (0–172.6)
IFN-γ	9.6 (0–87.3)	25.1 (0–153.2)	10.7 (0–75.1)
GM-CSF	0.6 (0–4.1)	1.0 (0–6.3)	0.8 (0–8.4)

Data expressed in mean (range)
IL interleukin, *IFN-γ* interferon gamma, *GM-CSF* granulocyte macrophage colony-stimulating factor

Table 8 Cytokines in sera of control participants ($N = 30$)

Cytokines	Timepoint 0	Timepoint 1
IL-2 ng/ml	3.0 (0–33.4)	2.6 (0–34.5)
IL-4 ng/ml	0.02 (0–0.7)	0.5 (0–13.8)
IL-5 ng/ml	7.5 (0–101.9)	4.5 (0–43.4)
IL-6 ng/ml	0.3 (0–3.0)	1.3 (0–26.3)
IL-8 ng/ml	9.6 (0–24.0)	14.0 (0–87.0)
IFN-γ	11.5 (0–89.1)	10.6 (0–53.6)
GM-CSF	0.3 (0–1.9)	0.2 (0–3.4)

Data expressed in mean (range)
IL interleukin, *IFN-γ* interferon gamma, *GM-CSF* granulocyte macrophage colony-stimulating factor

Discussion

Contrary to our expectations, occupational exposure to high doses of submicrometer (< 700 nm) particles, with predominant concentrations in the UFP range, did not cause complaints or significant respiratory effects, neither acutely (after 4 h hours of exposure) nor belatedly (24 h after exposure) in our study subjects working as instructors at shooting ranges.

These findings are remarkable because the amount of UFPs at the presented occupational setting (shooting ranges) reached approximately twice the level of episodic peak environmental concentration of UFPs (up to 300,000/cm^3 with approximately 50 μg/m^3 of mass) and belongs to the highest known occupational exposures. UFPs are known to be generally much more biologically aggressive than larger environmental particles, due to their physical properties and their ability to readily cross the alveolo-vascular barrier [23, 37, 38]. The results of our "real life exposure" setting are in concordance with results from controlled laboratory exposures to 500 μg/m^3 of fine (1.9×10^5 FP/cm^3, median diameter 291.2 ± 20.2 nm) and UF zinc oxide particles (4.6×10^6 UFPs/cm^3, median diameter 40.4 ± 2.7 nm) [39].

A possible explanation for the lack of significant pathological observations after exposure to UFPs could be the characteristics of our examined study population, which were predominantly healthy, young and well trained men. Like in other potentially health-adverse occupational environments, the possibility of a "healthy worker effect" could be considered. According to information obtained from the study subjects themselves, however, ex-collaborators who left this particular working environment rarely did so for health related reasons. In currently available scientific literature, the majority of previously documented harmful effects of UFPs in human subjects were shown in susceptible subjects or in patient groups. Those epidemiologic studies have shown that increased particulate air pollution (PM10 and PM2.5) is significantly associated with increased respiratory and cardiovascular morbidity, worsening of asthma, intensified medication, higher hospital admissions and mortality [1–3, 7]. Furthermore another study found associations even between ambient UFPs and mortality. Our study group mainly consisted of healthy and physically fit young men, as mentioned above [4].

Although we found a statistically significant late onset impairment (24 h after exposure) of FEV_1 air flow, we doubt that it is caused by the exposure to UFPs. Firstly, small airways, which are the target for deposition of fine and ultrafine particles, would be the first to show obstruction in air flow. A matching impairment of MEF_{50} and MEF_{25} which reflect the function of the small airways was not found in our subjects. Secondly, FEV_1 is, equally to other lung function parameter, influenced by subjects' motivation and effort; thus a decline in readiness for collaboration cannot be excluded at the final measurement. The interpretation of our results is in accordance with several studies [36, 40, 41] who all failed to show a reduction in lung function parameters after exposure to UFPs. Even in asthmatics and patients with chronic pulmonary disease (COPD) no decrease in lung function after exposure to UFPs could be demonstrated [42–44].

Although UFPs readily cross the alveolo-capillary barrier the chosen circulating inflammatory markers (serum cytokine levels and haemostatic factors, as well as biochemical parameters), did not indicate any systemic reaction neither after 4 h of exposure nor 24 h after occupational UFP exposure [23, 45, 46], except for an increase in circulating IFN-γ levels 4 h after UFP exposure compared to baseline values. IFN-γ is involved in first line innate immune responses to potential pathogens by activation of macrophages [47] and can be released from several cell types, e.g. T cells, natural killer cells and epithelial cells. Immediate increase in IFN-γ levels after UFP exposure has not been previously reported in vivo, however, Huang et al. found that ultrafine carbon particle inhalation in healthy individuals induced inflammation related pathways, e.g. T cell receptor and natural killer cell signalling, which might be an associated mechanism for preformed IFN-γ release [48]. Notably, a significant decrease of serum albumin, immunoglobulin G (IgG), coagulation factor VII, and fibrinogen was measured 24 h after UFP exposure. Albumin, IgG and fibrinogen have been shown to bind to ultrafine particles in the bloodstream and are most likely associated with physiological clearance processes [49]. Most available literature showed either no change in IgG levels or a slight increase. These studies were, however, done in sensitized experimental animal models, therefore more research on human participants will be necessary in order to provide a basis for a clinical significance of this finding [50, 51].

A clinical significance of these findings is arguable. In terms of haemostasis, Gilmour et al. [52] previously examined but could not find effects of ultrafine and fine carbon black particle exposure using similar UFP concentrations as measured in our study. Recent data indicates an association between exposure to UFPs (and larger particles) and both, acute-phase proteins and pro-coagulation parameters, in the same time span considered in our study, which was described as a possible link between air pollution and cardiovascular events [53–56]. Negative correlations between environmental particulate air pollution (PM_{10}) and haemoglobin concentration, packed cell volume, red blood count ($p < 0.001$), platelets and factor VII levels ($p < 0.05$), were reported [57] previously, but did not match our results. Data on systemic effects of UFP exposure is in fact controversial in literature, probably depending on the study design, studied population, particle type, model used and questions asked.

The content of lead in blood was significantly higher in the exposed subjects than in the control group (109.33 ± 103.63 (SD) µg/L vs. 36.24 ± 20.42 µg/L; $p = 0.0008$), which not only shows that metal particles were indeed incorporated but also that the incorporation exceeded the recommended doses (in Austria maximum blood lead concentrations should be below 90 µg/L in male workers), putting them at higher risk for adverse health effects associated with higher blood lead levels [58].

In occupational settings the concentration and size of UFPs depends not only on the (technological) process, but also on the efficacy of the exhaust system. Efficient exhaust systems predominantly reduce large particle load of the breathing air. Unexpectedly, at two other typical occupational settings with high burdens of UFPs, welding and laser beam application on a glass coating, Riediger and Möhlman [59] have demonstrated that by switching the local exhaust system on, the number of UFPs is reduced for 1 to 1,5 orders of magnitude. In our study, we did not measure the number and size of particles when the exhaust system was turned off because of ethical considerations.

Study limitations

There are some limitations to our study. Firstly, we initially measured submicrometer sized particles (< 700 nm), but since we did not find adverse respiratory effects and monodispersed particles ranged between 58.85 ± 16.94 and 98.19 ± 22.83 nm in our measurements, we did not calculate the exact concentrations of UFP (< 100 nm). Secondly, a possible limitation for the lack of adverse effects found in our study could be the absence of reactive metals, since it has been shown before, that oxidative stress induced by UFPs depends on the content of reactive metals. Thirdly, gender differences could not be assessed in this study due to the lack of exposed female subjects, but men may be more resistant to UFPs related adverse health effects than women. Further there were only three time points of air flow measurements: before, 4 h and 24 h after exposure. Thus, short-term changes following exposure to UFPs might have been missed. Finally, the young age of our subjects, as well as their overall good health and relatively short continuous exposure to UFPs at the workplace (4.7 years on average) might have been limiting study factors.

Conclusions

We could not detect consistent indications for adverse respiratory or inflammatory effects directly following exposure and 24 h after exposure to high levels of submicrometer and UFPs in our study group. These findings imply that high levels of submicrometer sized airborne particle concentrations, with a predominant fraction of UFPs, do not induce significant airway inflammation in healthy male subjects. The value of this study is the assessment of the short-term exposure effects to UFPs at a genuine occupational setting, which might is relevant when a risk assessment of high level occupational exposures to UFPs is considered. The implication, furthermore is, that our study supports the theory of a threshold value under which no observed effects level (NOEL) could be found by conventional diagnostic measures in otherwise healthy workers. Long-term prospective studies evaluating the effects of occupational UFPs exposure on human health are however required for the development of reasonable safety measures and preventive work-place related medical surveillance methods.

Acknowledgements

The authors thank Mr. Karl Mayr and his colleagues from Federal Ministry of Internal Affairs for their contribution and support of this work. We also thank Magdalena Kirnbauer for her valuable technical assistance.

Funding

This study was funded by the Austrian General Insurance Board (AUVA).

Authors' contributions

IG and GJ interpreted the data and wrote the text of the article. EV and JGC wrote the study protocol. KES, AGr, AS, KHS, CO and OS recruited the patients and did the laboratory analyses. AGo did the statystical analysis. All the authors read and agreed on the final version of the manuscript.

Competing interests

The authors declare that they have no competing interests.

Author details
[1]University Department of Physical Medicine, Rehabilitation and Occupational Medicine, Medical University of Vienna, Waehringer Guertel 18-20, A-1090 Vienna, Austria. [2]Department of Social and Preventive Medicine, Centre for Public Health, Medical University of Vienna, Kinderspitalgasse 15/1, A-1090 Vienna, Austria. [3]Austrian Worker's Compensation Board (AUVA), HUB, Adalbert-Stifter-Straße 6, 1200 Vienna, Austria. [4]University Clinic of Internal Medicine II, Institute of Occupational Medicine, Medical University of Vienna, Waehringer Guertel 18-20, A-1090 Vienna, Austria. [5]Austrian Dust-Silicosis Control Center (ÖSBS), Einödmayergasse 12, 8700 Leoben, Austria. [6]Department of Pathophysiology and Allergy Research, Medical University of Vienna, Waehringer Guertel 18-20, A-1090 Vienna, Austria. [7]Section of Medical Statistics, Core Unit for Medical Statistics and Informatics, Medical University of Vienna, Waehringer Guertel 18-20, A-1090 Vienna, Austria.

References

1. Dockery DW, Schwartz J, Spengler JD. Air pollution and daily mortality: associations with particulates and acid aerosols. Environ Res. 1992;59:362–73.
2. Dockery DW, Pope CA 3rd, Xu X, et al. An association between air pollution and mortality in six U.S. cities. N Engl J Med. 1993;329:1753–9.
3. Dockery DW. Epidemiologic evidence of cardiovascular effects of particulate air pollution. Environ Health Perspect. 2001;109(Suppl 4):483–6.
4. Ibald-Mulli A, Wichmann HE, Kreyling W, Peters A. Epidemiological evidence on health effects of ultrafine particles. J Aerosol Med. 2002;15:189–201.
5. Buonanno G, Marks GB, Morawska L. Health effects of daily airborne particle dose in children: direct association between personal dose and respiratory health effects. Environ Pollut. 2013;180:246–50.
6. Pope CA 3rd, Dockery DW. Health effects of fine particulate air pollution: lines that connect. J Air Waste Manag Assoc. 2006;56:709–42.
7. Donaldson K, Stone V, Clouter A, Renwick L, MacNee W. Ultrafine particles. Occup Environ Med. 2001;58:211–6. 199.
8. Utell MJ, Frampton MW. Acute health effects of ambient air pollution: the ultrafine particle hypothesis. J Aerosol Med. 2000;13:355–9.
9. Donaldson K, Tran L, Jimenez LA, et al. Combustion-derived nanoparticles: a review of their toxicology following inhalation exposure. Part Fibre Toxicol. 2005;2:10.
10. MacNee W, Donaldson K. Mechanism of lung injury caused by PM10 and ultrafine particles with special reference to COPD. Eur Respir J Suppl. 2003; 40:47s–51s.
11. Oberdorster G, Oberdorster E, Oberdorster J. Nanotoxicology: an emerging discipline evolving from studies of ultrafine particles. Environ Health Perspect. 2005;113:823–39.
12. Borm PJ, Robbins D, Haubold S, et al. The potential risks of nanomaterials: a review carried out for ECETOC. Part Fibre Toxicol. 2006;3:11.
13. Oberdorster G. Pulmonary effects of inhaled ultrafine particles. Int Arch Occup Environ Health. 2001;74:1–8.
14. Salvi SS, Nordenhall C, Blomberg A, et al. Acute exposure to diesel exhaust increases IL-8 and GRO-alpha production in healthy human airways. Am J Respir Crit Care Med. 2000;161:550–7.
15. Totlandsdal AI, Cassee FR, Schwarze P, Refsnes M, Lag M. Diesel exhaust particles induce CYP1A1 and pro-inflammatory responses via differential pathways in human bronchial epithelial cells. Part Fibre Toxicol. 2010;7:41.
16. Donaldson K, Brown D, Clouter A, et al. The pulmonary toxicology of ultrafine particles. J Aerosol Med. 2002;15:213–20.
17. Reibman J, Hsu Y, Chen LC, et al. Size fractions of ambient particulate matter induce granulocyte macrophage colony-stimulating factor in human bronchial epithelial cells by mitogen-activated protein kinase pathways. Am J Respir Cell Mol Biol. 2002;27:455–62.
18. Hohr D, Steinfartz Y, Schins RP, et al. The surface area rather than the surface coating determines the acute inflammatory response after instillation of fine and ultrafine TiO2 in the rat. Int J Hyg Environ Health. 2002;205:239–44.
19. Riedl M, Diaz-Sanchez D. Biology of diesel exhaust effects on respiratory function. J Allergy Clin Immunol. 2005;115:221–8. quiz 9.
20. Diaz-Sanchez D, Tsien A, Fleming J, Saxon A. Combined diesel exhaust particulate and ragweed allergen challenge markedly enhances human in vivo nasal ragweed-specific IgE and skews cytokine production to a T helper cell 2-type pattern. J Immunol. 1997;158:2406–13.
21. Diaz-Sanchez D, Tsien A, Casillas A, Dotson AR, Saxon A. Enhanced nasal cytokine production in human beings after in vivo challenge with diesel exhaust particles. J Allergy Clin Immunol. 1996;98:114–23.
22. Jantzen K, Roursgaard M, Desler C, Loft S, Rasmussen LJ, Moller P. Oxidative damage to DNA by diesel exhaust particle exposure in co-cultures of human lung epithelial cells and macrophages. Mutagenesis. 2012;27:693–701.
23. Nemmar A, Hoet PH, Vanquickenborne B, et al. Passage of inhaled particles into the blood circulation in humans. Circulation. 2002;105:411–4.
24. Frampton MW. Systemic and cardiovascular effects of airway injury and inflammation: ultrafine particle exposure in humans. Environ Health Perspect. 2001;109(Suppl 4):529–32.
25. Oberdorster G, Utell MJ. Ultrafine particles in the urban air: to the respiratory tract–and beyond? Environ Health Perspect. 2002;110:A440–1.
26. Stewart JC, Chalupa DC, Devlin RB, et al. Vascular effects of ultrafine particles in persons with type 2 diabetes. Environ Health Perspect. 2010;118:1692–8.
27. Vattanasit U, Navasumrit P, Khadka MB, et al. Oxidative DNA damage and inflammatory responses in cultured human cells and in humans exposed to traffic-related particles. Int J Hyg Environ Health. 2014;217:23–33.
28. Nemmar A, Hoylaerts MF, Hoet PH, et al. Ultrafine particles affect experimental thrombosis in an in vivo hamster model. Am J Respir Crit Care Med. 2002;166:998–1004.
29. Mills NL, Donaldson K, Hadoke PW, et al. Adverse cardiovascular effects of air pollution. Nat Clin Pract Cardiovasc Med. 2009;6:36–44.
30. Wurster U. Nanomaterialien: Arbeitsschutzpakete. In: LUBW Landesanstalt für Umwelt MuNB-W, ed. wwwlubwbadem-wuertembergde. Postfach 10 01 63, 76231 Karlsruhe: LUBW Landesanstalt für Umwelt, Messungen und Naturschutz Baden-Württemberg; 2009.
31. Melo G, Martiny A, Pinto AL. Nano characterization of gunshot residues from Brazilian ammunition. Forensic Sci Int. 2014;240:69–79.
32. Airports Council International. Ultrafine Particles at Airports. Discussion and Assessment of Ultrafine Particles (UFP) in Aviation and ant Airports in 2012. Available at: https://www.cph.dk/contentassets/04a9b35237a547d1a924ea3c9df25c31/aci-europe-study-on-ultrafine-particles-at-airports.pdf. Accessed 11 Sept 2017.
33. Landesanstalt für Umwelt, Messungen und Naturschutz Baden-Württemberg. Umweltforschung Journal 2006. Available at: https://www4.lubw.baden-wuerttemberg.de/servlet/is/19970/umweltforschung_journal_2006.pdf?command=downloadContent&filename=umweltforschung_journal_2006.pdf. Accessed 10 Sept 2017.
34. Viana M, Fonseca AS, Alastuey A, Querol X, Rodriguez A. Exposure to nanoparticle emissions inside firing ranges. Available at: http://www.isiaq.org/docs/Papers/Paper427.pdf. Accessed 10 Sept 2017.
35. Campagna M, Marcias G, Angius N, et al. 0277 Environmental exposure to nanoparticles in Sardinia, Italy: a pilot study of residential exposure nearby an industrial area and a military shooting range. Occup Environ Med. 2014;71:A99.
36. Quanjer PH, Tammeling GJ, Cotes JE, Pedersen OF, Peslin R, Yernault JC. Lung volumes and forced ventilatory flows. Report working party standardization of lung function tests, European Community for steel and coal. Official statement of the European Respiratory Society. Eur Respir J Suppl. 1993;16:5–40.
37. Brown DM, Wilson MR, MacNee W, Stone V, Donaldson K. Size-dependent proinflammatory effects of ultrafine polystyrene particles: a role for surface area and oxidative stress in the enhanced activity of ultrafines. Toxicol Appl Pharmacol. 2001;175:191–9.
38. Li N, Sioutas C, Cho A, et al. Ultrafine particulate pollutants induce oxidative stress and mitochondrial damage. Environ Health Perspect. 2003;111:455–60.
39. Beckett WS, Chalupa DF, Pauly-Brown A, et al. Comparing inhaled ultrafine versus fine zinc oxide particles in healthy adults: a human inhalation study. Am J Respir Crit Care Med. 2005;171:1129–35.
40. Oberdorster G, Gelein RM, Ferin J, Weiss B. Association of particulate air pollution and acute mortality: involvement of ultrafine particles? Inhal Toxicol. 1995;7:111–24.
41. Li XY, Brown D, Smith S, MacNee W, Donaldson K. Short-term inflammatory responses following intratracheal instillation of fine and ultrafine carbon black in rats. Inhal Toxicol. 1999;11:709–31.

42. Gong H Jr, Sioutas C, Linn WS. Controlled exposures of healthy and asthmatic volunteers to concentrated ambient particles in metropolitan Los Angeles. Res Rep Health Eff Inst. 2003;(118):1-36. discussion 37-47.
43. Frampton MW, Utell MJ, Zareba W, et al. Effects of exposure to ultrafine carbon particles in healthy subjects and subjects with asthma. Res Rep Health Eff Inst. 2004;(126):1-47. discussion 49-63.
44. de Hartog JJ, Ayres JG, Karakatsani A, et al. Lung function and indicators of exposure to indoor and outdoor particulate matter among asthma and COPD patients. Occup Environ Med. 2010;67:2–10.
45. Geiser M, Kreyling WG. Deposition and biokinetics of inhaled nanoparticles. Part Fibre Toxicol. 2010;7:2.
46. Elder A, Oberdorster G. Translocation and effects of ultrafine particles outside of the lung. Clin Occup Environ Med. 2006;5:785–96.
47. Schroder K, Hertzog PJ, Ravasi T, Hume DA. Interferon-γ: an overview of signals, mechanisms and functions. J Leukoc Biol. 2003;75(2):163–89.
48. Beck-Speier I, Karg E, Behrendt H, Stoeger T, Alessandrini F. Ultrafine particles affect the balance of endogenous pro- and anti-inflammatory lipid mediators in the lung: in-vitro and in-vivo studies. Part Fibre Toxicol. 2012 Jul 18;9:27.
49. Aggarwal P, Hall JB, McLeland CB, Dobrovolskaia MA, McNeil SE. Nanoparticle interaction with plasma proteins as it relates to particle biodistribution, biocompatibility and therapeutic efficacy. Adv Drug Deliv Re. 2009;61(6):428–37.
50. Barrett EG, Rudolph K, Bowen LE, Muggenburg BA, Bice DE. Effect of inhaled ultrafine carbon particles on the allergic airway response in ragweed-sensitized dogs. Inhal Toxicol. 2003;15:151–65.
51. Kleinman MT, Hamade A, Meacher D, et al. Inhalation of concentrated ambient particulate matter near a heavily trafficked road stimulates antigen-induced airway responses in mice. J Air Waste Manag Assoc. 2005;55:1277–88.
52. Gilmour PS, Ziesenis A, Morrison ER, et al. Pulmonary and systemic effects of short-term inhalation exposure to ultrafine carbon black particles. Toxicol Appl Pharmacol. 2004;195:35–44.
53. Ruckerl R, Greven S, Ljungman P, et al. Air pollution and inflammation (interleukin-6, C-reactive protein, fibrinogen) in myocardial infarction survivors. Environ Health Perspect. 2007;115:1072–80.
54. Tsai DH, Amyai N, Marques-Vidal P, et al. Effects of particulate matter on inflammatory markers in the general adult population. Part Fibre Toxicol. 2012;9:24.
55. Miller KA, Siscovick DS, Sheppard L, et al. Long-term exposure to air pollution and incidence of cardiovascular events in women. N Engl J Med. 2007;356:447–58.
56. Ruckerl R, Phipps RP, Schneider A, et al. Ultrafine particles and platelet activation in patients with coronary heart disease–results from a prospective panel study. Part Fibre Toxicol. 2007;4:1.
57. Seaton A, MacNee W, Donaldson K, Godden D. Particulate air pollution and acute health effects. Lancet. 1995;345:176–8.
58. Wilhelm M, Heinzow B, Angerer J, Schulz C. Reassessment of critical lead effects by the German human biomonitoring commission results in suspension of the human biomonitoring values (HBM I and HBM II) for lead in blood of children and adults. Int J Hyg Environ Health. 2010;213:265–9.
59. Riediger G, Möhlmann C. Ultrafeine Aerosole an Arbeitsplätzen. Konventionen und Beispiele aus der Praxis Gefahrenstoffe Reinhalt Luft. 2001;61:42.

20

Validating the Demand Control Support Questionnaire among white-collar employees

Daniel Mauss[1*], Raphael M. Herr[1], Töres Theorell[2], Peter Angerer[3] and Jian Li[3]

Abstract

Background: The Demand Control Support Questionnaire (DCSQ) is an established self-reported tool to measure a stressful work environment. Validated German and English versions are however currently missing. The aim of this study was therefore to evaluate the psychometric properties of German and English versions of the DCSQ among white-collar employees in Switzerland and the US.

Methods: This cross-sectional study was carried out on 499 employees in Switzerland and 411 in the US, respectively. The 17-item DCSQ with three scales assessed psychosocial stress at work (psychological demands, decision latitude, and social support at work). Depressive symptoms were measured by the 2-item Patient Health Questionnaire. Cronbach's α and item-total correlations tested the scale reliability (internal consistency). Construct validity of the questionnaire was examined using exploratory factor analysis (EFA). Logistic regressions estimated associations of each scale and job strain with depressive symptoms (criterion validity).

Results: In both samples, all DCSQ scales presented satisfactory internal consistency (Cronbach's $\alpha \geq 0.72$; item-total correlations ≥ 0.33), and EFA showed the 17 items loading on three factors, which is in line with the theoretically assumed structure of the DCSQ construct. Moreover, all three scales as well as high job strain were significantly associated with depressive symptoms. The associations were stronger in the US sample.

Conclusions: The German and the English versions of the DCSQ seem to be reliable and valid instruments to measure psychosocial stress based on the job demand-control-support model in the workplace of white-collar employees in Switzerland and the US.

Keywords: Demand-control-support model, Depressive symptoms, Job strain, Psychosocial stress, Validation

Background

The job demand-control model proposed by Karasek [1] is one of the best evaluated models of stress at work [2]. It has been associated with the onset of major diseases such as depression [3] and cardiovascular disease [4, 5]. Furthermore, a reduction of this work-related stress can improve work ability, well-being and productivity of employees [6–8]. The job demand-control model takes psychological demands (e.g. workload and time pressure) and decision latitude (also called job control including decision authority and skill discretion) into consideration. High job strain usually leads to negative bodily responses (stress) and is defined as a mismatch of high demands and low decision latitude, whereas low strain is theoretically defined as low job demands with high decision latitude; meanwhile active job and passive job refer to both high job demands and decision latitude or both low, respectively. In 1988, the additional component of social support by peers and supervisors was added to the model as a possible resource to buffer the impact of job strain on health [9].

* Correspondence: dmousetrap@googlemail.com
[1]Mannheim Institute of Public Health, Social and Preventive Medicine, Medical Faculty Mannheim, Heidelberg University, Ludolf-Krehl-Str. 7-11, D-68167 Mannheim, Germany
Full list of author information is available at the end of the article

To operationalize the job demand-control-support model, two questionnaires were developed. The job content questionnaire (JCQ), which contains of 49 items in five scales such as decision latitude, psychological demands and mental workload, social support, physical demands, and job insecurity [10], has been validated in various languages and job profiles. The other instrument, the Demand Control Support Questionnaire (DCSQ), is an economical 17-item short form of the JCQ [11]. It comprises three scales of psychological demands (work fast, work intensely, work effort, overtime work, and conflicting demands), decision latitude divided in skill discretion (learning new things, skill level, being creative, variety of work), and decision authority (how to do the work, what to do at work), and social support at work (pleasant atmosphere, spirit of unity, colleagues support, helpful colleagues, relationship with superiors, relationship with colleagues). Thus, the DCSQ does not assess physical demands and is therefore much shorter and not that time-consuming compared to the JCQ.

Although the DCSQ has been validated in various languages like Brazilian-Portuguese [12, 13], Swedish [14], Norwegian [15], Turkish [16], and Japanese [17], no validated German or English version exists so far. Therefore, the aim of this study was to investigate the psychometric properties of the German version as well as the English version of the DCSQ among white-collar employees from Switzerland and the US. Firstly, the internal consistency reliability and construct validity of the questionnaires and its scales were analyzed. Secondly, we selected depressive symptoms as a criterion to test its associations of DCSQ scales and the job strain categories in order for criterion validity. In the past years, substantial evidence has been gained to establish a causal relation between job strain measured by the demand-control model and depressive symptoms [3, 18]. For instance, a recent review and meta-analysis showed that decision latitude (158,251 subjects in 19 studies) and job strain (197,682 subject in 14 studies) exerted the largest effects: an odds ratio for job strain was 1.74 to develop depressive symptoms, while high decision latitude protected against depressive symptoms with an odds ratio of 0.73 [3].

Methods

Study sample

A voluntary online questionnaire was offered to 1944 white-collar employees (48.4% female, 40.2 years) of a large multi-national insurance company in either German (944 employees in Switzerland) or English (1000 employees in the US). Employees in Switzerland were based in Zurich where German is the main language. Employees in the US were based in Minnesota. The study sample included various jobs of in-house staff, but no call center and sales activities. In total, 970 employees (537 from Switzerland and 433 from the US) answered the questionnaire (overall response rate = 49.9%). Participants with missing values were excluded from further analysis. The final sample comprised of 910 employees presenting a full data set with 499 participants from Switzerland and 411 from the US.

Procedure

The survey was conducted in December 2014 during official office hours, and participation was anonymous. Sociodemographic characteristics included age (≤ 34, 35-49, ≥ 50 years), gender, job position (employee, employee with management responsibility), and tenure (< 5, 5-9, ≥ 10 years). Managers (employees with management responsibility) were defined as having a leadership role. Informed consent was given by each participant. Data collection and study procedure was approved by the corporate data protection officers and by the Ethical Committee of the Bavarian State Chamber of Physicians in Munich as the study was designed there at the headquarters of the company.

Measurements

Demand Control Support Questionnaire (DCSQ)

The 17-item DCSQ includes the three scales of psychological demands (five items), decision latitude (six items), and social support at work (six items) [14]. In our present study, all the 17 items were expressed as statements and the respondents were asked to report their levels of agreement or disagreement on a four-point Likert scale, with higher values indicating higher psychological demands (range 5–20), higher decision latitude (range 6–24), and higher social support at work (range 6–24). All scale scores were calculated by summing up the respective unweighted item scores after appropriate reverse scoring of item 4 (overtime work) and item 9 (variety of work). As an English translated but not validated version of the DCSQ items already existed, there was no translational process from the original Swedish version into English needed. After reviewing national databases on literature of prior use of a German version, one of the authors (P.A.) translated the English DCSQ version into German supported by an English-speaking German translator. This first version was also reviewed and modified by the other German-speaking authors separately to rule out translational problems. All versions were returned to P.A. and consolidated for a consensual version. Finally, this version was approved by Prof. Theorell. Furthermore, a median split of the scale values of the samples were used to calculate low and high levels of psychological demands and decision latitude, and four groups of low strain, active, passive, and high strain were categorized accordingly.

Patient Health Questionnaire (PHQ-2)

Depressive symptoms were measured by the two-item Patient Health Questionnaire [19] using a four-point Likert scale (from "0 = not at all" to "3 = nearly every day"). Unweighted sum scores ranging 0-6 were calculated with scores ≥ 3 indicating a high risk for depressive symptoms. Cronbach's α was 0.75 for the Swiss sample and 0.85 for the US sample.

Statistical analysis

Based on the quality criteria of evaluating health-related questionnaires [20], three established psychometric properties were tested in our study: internal consistency reliability, construct validity, and criterion validity.

Consistency reliability

Internal consistency reliability refers to the overall consistency of a measure meaning that similar results are produced if conditions are consistent [20]. Internal consistency was evaluated by Cronbach's α and item-total correlations. Values > 0.7 for Cronbach's α and > 0.3 for item-total correlation were considered to be acceptable [21].

Construct and criterion validity

The validity of a measurement tool is the degree to which the tool measures what it claims to measure, including construct validity (i.e., extent to which a theoretical construct is measured) and criterion validity (i.e., comparison of the tool with other measures or outcomes) [20]. Construct validity was assessed by exploratory factor analysis (EFA) using principal axis extraction and varimax rotation. A factor loading ≥ 0.35 was considered satisfactory [22]. All the 17 items of the DCSQ were included in the EFA. Criterion validity was tested using multivariate logistic regression analyses to assess associations between the three DCSQ scales and depressive symptoms, adjusting for age, gender, job position, and tenure as these variables are known to influence the association of stress with depressive symptoms [18, 23, 24]. Results are shown as standardized odds ratios (ORs), defined as ORs per standard deviation change, with 95% confidence intervals (CIs). Furthermore, multivariate logistic regression models explored associations of the four stress groups (i.e., low strain, active, passive, and high strain) with depressive symptoms in both countries. A p-value < .05 was considered as statistically significant. SAS 9.4 (SAS Institute Inc., North Carolina, US) was used for all statistical analyses.

Results

Study population

Characteristics of both study samples including age, gender, job position, and tenure as well as depressive symptoms were comparable (see Table 1).

Consistency reliability

Mean values with standard deviations (SDs) of the three scales are presented in Table 2. Compared to the Swiss sample, demands and control were slightly higher whereas social support was slightly lower in the US sample. Cronbach's α indicated satisfactory internal consistency for all three scales (psychological demands, decision latitude, and social support) of the German (0.72, 0.77, and 0.83, respectively) and the English version (0.78, 0.78, and 0.84, respectively). Values for item-total correlations varied between 0.33 and 0.69 for the German version, and between 0.38 and 0.73 for the English version indicating satisfactory internal consistency.

In addition, we observed significant differences according to gender (female employees had lower decision latitude, in the Swiss sample only), age (decision latitude increased with higher age in both samples), and position (managers had higher psychological demands and decision latitude in both samples), suggesting good discriminant validity (data not shown).

Construct validity

Results of the explanatory factor analysis are presented in Table 3. In accordance with the criterion of Kaiser's eigenvalue > 1 and the scree plot analysis, a three-factorial solution was applied. In both the Swiss and the US sample, the factor patterns were similar and the hypothesized factorial structure was well identified. All items of a respective scale were loaded onto one of the three factors with factor loadings between 0.38 and 0.77.

Criterion validity

In multivariate logistic regression analysis, for every SD increase in psychological demands a significantly ($p < .001$) elevated standardized OR of 1.86 for depressive symptoms was observed in the Swiss sample. For every SD increase in decision latitude and social support a decreased standardized OR of 0.52 and 0.40 respectively was observed for depressive symptoms. Notably, the magnitude of associations with depressive symptoms was relatively larger in the US sample (Table 4). Compared to low strain, high strain showed a standardized OR of 5.91 ($p < .001$) in Switzerland and 12.22 ($p < .001$) in the US after adjusting for age, gender, job position, and tenure.

Discussion

The aim of the present study was to validate the German and English versions of the DCSQ in white-collar employees in Switzerland and the US. Our results demonstrate a good internal consistency, construct validity, and criterion validity across both samples.

The properties of the German and English DCSQ versions are in line with findings from validation studies in other languages. Cronbach's alpha coefficients explored

Table 1 Characteristics of study subjects ($N = 910$), N (%)

Variables		Switzerland ($N = 499$)	United States ($N = 411$)
Age	≤ 34 years	175 (35.07%)	119 (28.95%)
	35-49 years	201 (40.28%)	178 (43.31%)
	≥ 50 years	123 (24.65%)	114 (27.74%)
Gender	Men	264 (52.91%)	171 (41.61%)
	Women	235 (47.09%)	240 (58.39%)
Job position	Manager	78 (15.63%)	96 (23.36%)
	Employee	421 (84.37%)	315 (76.64%)
Tenure	< 5 years	225 (45.09%)	133 (32.36%)
	5-9 years	90 (18.04%)	111 (27.01%)
	≥ 10 years	184 (36.87%)	167 (40.63%)
Depressive symptoms		63 (12.62%)	54 (13.14%)

in our samples are similar to DCSQ versions validated in Brazil [12, 13], Sweden [14], Norway [15], Turkey [16], and Japan [17]. As supported by these studies, social support showed the highest internal consistency in both samples of our study. However, our results indicated lower sum scores for psychological demands and decision latitude compared to other DCSQ validation studies [14, 17]. Regarding discriminant validity we observed significant differences according to age, gender, and position, which are consistent with previous studies, showing that women have lower decision latitude [25], decision latitude increases with age [26], and managers having higher psychological demands and decision latitude [27]. The DCSQ factorial patterns in the two samples from Switzerland and the US reflected well the theoretical structure and the three-factor solution of this questionnaire. Explanatory factor analysis in Norwegian workers [15] and Japanese nurses [17] confirmed this structure as well. On the other hand, a recent longitudinal study using confirmatory factor analysis found a

Table 2 Mean, standard deviation (SD), item-total correlation and Cronbach's alpha coefficients of the scales of the DCSQ

Items	Switzerland			United States		
	Mean (SD)	Item-total correlations	Alpha of scale	Mean (SD)	Item-total correlations	Alpha of scale
Psychological demands (scale range: 5-20)	12.59 (2.44)		0.72	13.27 (2.43)		0.78
Item 1: work fast		0.59			0.58	
Item 2: work intensively		0.50			0.57	
Item 3: work effort		0.48			0.54	
Item 4: overtime work		0.51			0.55	
Item 5: conflicting demands		0.33			0.54	
Decision latitude (scale range: 6-24)	16.60 (3.00)		0.77	17.31 (2.84)		0.78
Item 6: learning new things		0.45			0.54	
Item 7: skill level		0.48			0.38	
Item 8: being creative		0.64			0.62	
Item 9: variety of work		0.45			0.49	
Item 10: how to do the work		0.57			0.60	
Item 11: what to do at work		0.50			0.57	
Social support at work (scale range: 6-24)	18.88 (2.82)		0.83	18.34 (2.68)		0.84
Item 12: pleasant atmosphere		0.62			0.52	
Item 13: spirit of unity		0.68			0.73	
Item 14: colleagues support		0.69			0.69	
Item 15: helpful colleagues		0.53			0.52	
Item 16: relationship with superiors		0.49			0.65	
Item 17: relationship with colleagues		0.66			0.59	

Table 3 Exploratory factor analysis of the 17-item DCSQ using principal axis extraction and varimax rotation

Scales	Items	Switzerland			United States		
		F1	F2	F3	F1	F2	F3
Psychological demands	Item 1: work fast			0.72		0.66	
	Item 2: work intensively			0.67		0.66	
	Item 3: work effort			0.51		0.59	
	Item 4: overtime work			0.60		0.61	
	Item 5: conflicting demands			0.38		0.60	
Decision latitude	Item 6: learning new things		0.47				0.54
	Item 7: skill level		0.55				0.45
	Item 8: being creative		0.71				0.67
	Item 9: variety of work		0.52				0.55
	Item 10: how to do the work		0.66				0.65
	Item 11: what to do at work		0.60				0.61
Social support at work	Item 12: pleasant atmosphere	0.68			0.44		
	Item 13: spirit of unity	0.72			0.70		
	Item 14: colleagues support	0.77			0.77		
	Item 15: helpful colleagues	0.57			0.48		
	Item 16: relationship with superiors	0.52			0.66		
	Item 17: relationship with colleagues	0.73			0.73		
Variance explained (%)		17.73	13.19	11.52	16.18	15.93	13.96

Only items with factor loading ≥ 0.35 are shown

four-factor structure, dividing decision latitude into the two subscales of skill discretion and decision authority [14]. We conducted supplementary EFA among the six items of the decision latitude scale, two distinct factorial loadings representing skill discretion and decision authority were also observed (data not shown).

Although internal consistency and construct validity were similar between the Swiss and the US sample, criterion validity is somewhat different. It seems like the associations of psychosocial stress in the workplace with depressive symptoms were stronger in the US sample than in the Swiss sample. It might be the case that protective labor and social policies modify the strength of these associations. A study assessing depressive symptoms among 14,236 older employees experiencing higher levels of psychosocial stress at work found higher risk estimation in the US (OR = 2.28) compared to Europe (OR = 1.97) and Japan (OR = 1.64) in cross-sectional data, while longitudinal analysis indicated somewhat smaller but still significant associations [28]. To explain these results, Lunau and colleagues longitudinally explored the impact of national labor and social policies on this association in European countries and the US. They used six macro indicators defined by the Organization for Economic Co-operation and Development (OECD) including active labor market policy expenditures,

Table 4 Associations of the scales of the DCSQ with depressive symptoms (standardized odds ratios (ORs) and 95% confidence intervals (CIs))

		Switzerland	United States
Psychological demands	Increase per SD	1.86 (1.40, 2.47) ***	2.20 (1.57, 3.08) ***
Decision latitude	Increase per SD	0.52 (0.39, 0.71) ***	0.41 (0.30, 0.57) ***
Social support at work	Increase per SD	0.40 (0.29, 0.54) ***	0.47 (0.34, 0.66) ***
Low strain		1.00	1.00
Active		2.58 (0.96, 6.96)	3.55 (1.06, 11.91) *
Passive		3.55 (1.33, 9.47) **	4.01 (1.19, 13.50) **
High strain		5.91 (2.28, 15.30) ***	12.22 (4.06, 36.83) ***

Multivariate logistic regression, * $p < .05$, ** $p < .01$, *** $p < .001$
Adjusted for age, gender, job position, and tenure

investments in rehabilitation services, participation of older employees in learning offerings, support for unemployed people, degree of union density, and income inequalities. Switzerland scored better for every one of these six indicators than the US with the Scandinavian countries having the best scores. It was suggested these macro indicators modified the effect of work-related stress on depressive symptoms across countries [29]. As for our present study, given the consideration that national labor and social policies in Switzerland are generally more protective than those in the US, the effect of work stress might be less health threatening if stress is experienced in a protective society. Interestingly, an active job which is defined as combination of high job demands with high decision latitude is usually assumed to be health-promoting [10]. In contradiction to that, in our sample an active job was associated with higher poor mental health compared to a low strain job, although this finding was not significant in the Swiss sample and slightly significant in the US sample. A similar result was described by Madsen in a recent meta-analysis [18].

Limitations and strengths

Our study has some limitations to address. First, the analysis is based on cross-sectional data. That did not allow us to test for longitudinal stability and test-retest reliability. Second, we could not rule out the healthy worker effect, i.e., employees with reduced health status have been sick at home or had already left the company and therefore did not participate in this study. Third, the study sample was comprised of employees of a multi-national insurance company based in Switzerland and the US. Generalization to other industries in both countries as well as to other languages within Switzerland (French, Italian, Swiss-German, Rhaeto-Romanic) cannot be made. As Swiss people are usually very familiar with German, especially in Zurich, we do not think that using a German questionnaire may have biased the results due to any dialectical misunderstandings. Additionally, the fact that all variables had been measured by a self-rated questionnaire could lead to common method variance bias. Fourth, although the PHQ-2 is a validated instrument to screen depressive symptoms, it is based on two cardinal symptoms only ("little interest" and "feeling down"). Therefore, it must be distinct from clinically diagnosed depression [30]. Nevertheless, these limitations are balanced by several strengths. Compared to some of the other DCSQ validation studies [13, 16, 17] the sample size of our study was somewhat bigger providing good statistical power and allowing us to test the categorized job strain model (low strain, active job, passive job, high strain). Furthermore, our study is the first to validate the psychometric properties of the German and English versions of the DCSQ. This validation of the 17-item parsimonious and economical instrument would provide more option for studies on psychosocial working conditions and health outcomes in German and English speaking countries.

Conclusions

Both the German and the English versions of the DCSQ seem to be reliable and valid instruments to measure psychosocial stress in the workplace, based on the job demand-control-support model, in white-collar employees in Switzerland and the US.

Abbreviations

DCSQ: Demand control support questionnaire; EFA: Exploratory factor analysis; JCQ: Job content questionnaire; OECD: Organization for economic co-operation and development; OR: Odds ratio; PHQ-2: Patient health questionnaire; SD: Standard deviation; US: United States of America

Acknowledgements

Not applicable

Funding

All authors declare that they had no external funding for the study.

Authors' contributions

All authors agreed to be accountable for all aspects of the work ensuring accuracy and integrity. DM conceived this study and drafted the manuscript assisted by RMH and JL who additionally performed all analyses. PA and TT provided scientific advice, supported in the interpretation of the data and editing the manuscript. All authors read and approved the final manuscript.

Competing interests

The authors declare that they have no competing interests.

Author details

[1]Mannheim Institute of Public Health, Social and Preventive Medicine, Medical Faculty Mannheim, Heidelberg University, Ludolf-Krehl-Str. 7-11, D-68167 Mannheim, Germany. [2]Institute for Stress Research, Stockholm University, Stockholm, Sweden. [3]Institute of Occupational, Social and Environmental Medicine, Centre for Health and Society, Faculty of Medicine, University of Düsseldorf, Düsseldorf, Germany.

References

1. Karasek RA. Job demands, job decision latitude, and mental strain: implications for job redesign. Adm Sci Q. 1979;24:285–308.
2. Tabanelli MC, Depolo M, Cooke RMT, Sarchielli G, Bonfiglioli R, Mattioli S, et al. Available instruments for measurement of psychosocial factors in the work environment. Int Arch Occup Environ Health. 2008;82:1–12.
3. Theorell T, Hammarstrom A, Aronsson G, Traskman Bendz L, Grape T, Hogstedt C, et al. A systematic review including meta-analysis of work environment and depressive symptoms. BMC Public Health. 2015;15:738.
4. Theorell T, Jood K, Jarvholm LS, Vingard E, Perk J, Ostergren PO, et al. A systematic review of studies in the contributions of the work environment to ischaemic heart disease development. Eur J Pub Health. 2016;26:470–7.
5. Schnall PL, Dobson M, Landsbergis P. Globalization, work, and cardiovascular disease. Int J Health Serv. 2016;46:656–92.

6. Schulte P, Vainio H. Well-being at work–overview and perspective. Scand J Work Environ Health. 2010;36:422–9.
7. Lamontagne AD, Keegel T, Louie AM, Ostry A, Landsbergis PA. A systematic review of the job-stress intervention evaluation literature, 1990-2005. Int J Occup Environ Health. 2007;13:268–80.
8. Joyce S, Modini M, Christensen H, Mykletun A, Bryant R, Mitchell PB, et al. Workplace interventions for common mental disorders: a systematic meta-review. Psychol Med. 2016;46:683–97.
9. Johnson JV, Hall EM. Job strain, work place social support, and cardiovascular disease: a cross-sectional study of a random sample of the Swedish working population. Am J Public Health. 1988;78:1336–42.
10. Karasek R, Brisson C, Kawakami N, Houtman I, Bongers P, Amick B. The job content questionnaire (JCQ): an instrument for internationally comparative assessments of psychosocial job characteristics. J Occup Health Psychol. 1998;3:322–55.
11. Theorell T, Perski A, Akerstedt T, Sigala F, Ahlberg-Hulten G, Svensson J, et al. Changes in job strain in relation to changes in physiological state. A longitudinal study. Scand J Work Environ Health. 1988;14:189–96.
12. MGDM A, Chor D, Faerstein E, CDS L, Werneck GL. Short version of the "job stress scale": a Portuguese-language adaptation. Rev Saude Publica. 2004;38:164–71.
13. Hokerberg YHM, Aguiar OB, Reichenheim M, Faerstein E, Valente JG, MDJ F, et al. Dimensional structure of the demand control support questionnaire: a Brazilian context. Int Arch Occup Environ Health. 2010;83:407–16.
14. Chungkham HS, Ingre M, Karasek R, Westerlund H, Theorell T. Factor structure and longitudinal measurement invariance of the demand control support model: an evidence from the Swedish longitudinal occupational survey of health (SLOSH). PLoS One. 2013;8:e70541.
15. Sanne B, Torp S, Mykletun A, Dahl AA. The Swedish demand-control-support questionnaire (DCSQ): factor structure, item analyses, and internal consistency in a large population. Scand J Public Health. 2005;33:166–74.
16. Demiral Y, Ünal B, Kılıç B, Soysal A, Bilgin AC, Reyhan U, et al. Validity and reliability of job stress questionnaire in Izmir-Konak municipality workers [in Turkish]. Toplum Hekimligi Bülteni. 2007;26:11–8.
17. Mase J, Ota A, Inoue K, Iida T, Tsutsumi A, Yatsuya H, et al. Reliability and validity of the Japanese translated version of the Swedish demand-control-support questionnaire. Ind Health. 2012;50:467–75.
18. Madsen IEH, Nyberg ST, Magnusson Hanson LL, Ferrie JE, Ahola K, Alfredsson L, et al. Job strain as a risk factor for clinical depression: systematic review and meta-analysis with additional individual participant data. Psychol Med. 2017;47:1342–56.
19. Kroenke K, Spitzer RL, Williams JBW. The patient health questionnaire-2: validity of a two-item depression screener. Med Care. 2003;41:1284–92.
20. Terwee CB, Bot SDM, de Boer MR, van der Windt DAWM, Knol DL, Dekker J, et al. Quality criteria were proposed for measurement properties of health status questionnaires. J Clin Epidemiol. 2007;60:34–42.
21. Schmitt N. Uses and abuses of coefficient alpha. Psychol Assess. 1996;8:350–3.
22. Tabachnick BG, Fidell LS. Using multivariate statistics. New York: Allyn and Bacon. 2007.
23. Stansfeld SA, Shipley MJ, Head J, Fuhrer R. Repeated job strain and the risk of depression: longitudinal analyses from the Whitehall II study. Am J Public Health. 2011;102:2360–6.
24. Chaney BH, Torres E. Covariates of identified stress and depression among seasonal farmworkers. Int J Environ Res Public Health. 2017;14:1–12.
25. Braun S, Hollander RB. Work and depression among women in the Federal Republic of Germany. Women Health. 1988;14:3–26.
26. Vanagas G, Bihari-Axelsson S. Interaction among general practitioners age and patient load in the prediction of job strain, decision latitude and perception of job demands a cross-sectional study. BMC Public Health. 2004;4:59.
27. Bernin P, Theorell T. Demand–control–support among female and male managers in eight Swedish companies. Stress Health. 2001;17:231–43.
28. Siegrist J, Lunau T, Wahrendorf M, Dragano N. Depressive symptoms and psychosocial stress at work among older employees in three continents. Glob Health. 2012;8:27.
29. Lunau T, Wahrendorf M, Dragano N, Siegrist J. Work stress and depressive symptoms in older employees: impact of national labour and social policies. BMC Public Health. 2013;13:1086.
30. Solomon A, Haaga DA, Arnow BA. Is clinical depression distinct from subthreshold depressive symptoms? A review of the continuity issue in depression research. J Nerv Ment Dis. 2001;189:498–506.

Association of plasma PCB levels and HbA1c concentration in Iran

Sahar Eftekhari[2], Omid Aminian[3], Zeinab Moinfar[4], Thomas Schettgen[1], Andrea Kaifie[1], Michael Felten[1], Thomas Kraus[1] and André Esser[1*]

Abstract

Background: The rapid increase in prevalence of diabetes mellitus over the last decades warrants more attention to the effects of environmental and occupational exposures on glucose metabolism. Our study aimed to assess the association between the plasma levels of various congeners of polychlorinated biphenyls (PCBs) and the serum concentration of glycated haemoglobin (HbA1c).

Methods: Our study population consisted of 140 Iranian adults from seven different occupational groups and a group of non-occupationally exposed female participants. The plasma concentration of PCBs were determined at the laboratory of occupational toxicology at RWTH Aachen University, Germany. We considered an HbA1c concentration of 5.7% and more as indicating a disturbed glucose metabolism. Logistic regression was used to assess the association between quartiles of concentrations of PCB congeners and serum HbA1c.

Results: Participants with an increased HbA1c value had higher plasma levels of PCB 138, 153, 180 and the PCB sum, although this association was statistically not significant. There was no significant difference between the levels of PCB 138, 153, 180, the sum of these congeners, and PCB 118 in their quartiles when comparing with HbA1c concentrations.

Conclusions: For our cohort, we could not demonstrate a significant association between PCB and HbA1c concentrations indicating a disturbance of glucose metabolism.

Keywords: PCB, HbA1c, Glucose disturbance polychlorinated biphenyls; diabetes mellitus

Background

Diabetes mellitus (DM) is a common non-communicable disease and a leading cause of death worldwide with more than one million casualties in 2010 [1]. According to the International Diabetes Federation (IDF), in 2011 366 million cases of diabetes (8.3% adults) were reported worldwide. In Iran the prevalence of the disease was 11.4% of the total population in 2011, representing an increase of about 35% since 2005 [2]. A further mean increase of 194,000 DM patients per year among the Iranian adult population aged 20–79 years is projected [3]. In addition to patients suffering from clinically manifest DM there is an unknown number of individuals with glycated haemoglobin (HbA1c) values between 5.7 and 6.4% indicating the status of pre-diabetes which is known to significantly increase the risk of developing type 2 diabetes mellitus (T2DM) and cardiovascular complications [4]. The rapidly increasing incidence of T2DM around the world calls for a better understanding of the role of environmental and occupational pollutants such as the ubiquitous polychlorinated biphenyls (PCB) as potential additional risk factors, along with known factors such as obesity, sedentary life style, genetic predisposition and smoking [5–8].

PCBs are a form of halogenated organic compounds that had been widely used as additives in hydraulic fluids, industrial capacitors, transformers, and as plasticizers for expansion joints until approximately three decades ago [9]. Due to the long half-lives of certain PCB congeners, exposure to these compounds continues through food chains, indoor air pollution and at certain industrial plants and workplaces. In addition, occupational contact with PCB is still

* Correspondence: anesser@ukaachen.de
[1]Institute for Occupational, Social and Environmental Medicine, University Hospital Aachen, RWTH University Aachen, Pauwelsstr 30, D-52074 Aachen, Germany
Full list of author information is available at the end of the article

common during maintenance and de-installation of electrical equipment manufactured in the past [10–12].

Recently, numerous studies assessed the association between PCB exposure and the development of diabetes and pre-diabetes, which was confirmed with some results particularly for dioxin-like PCB congeners [12–16]. There were also reports of a positive association between increased blood glucose levels and the contamination with non-dioxin-like higher-chlorinated PCB congeners [17–20]. Other studies found no such association between serum PCB and diabetes development [21]. However, results of experimental studies suggested possible mechanisms linking glucose metabolism disorders and PCB exposure. They found that certain PCB congeners may act as endocrine disrupters [22], exacerbate insulin resistance [23] and cause depletion of beta cells [24]. Our study presented here aimed to analyse the association between the serum concentration of PCB and increased levels of blood glucose indicated by the HbA1c level.

Methods

The participants of the study were recruited among the employees of six companies in the Tehran region, each representing an industry with an assumedly high or low exposure level of PCB. The employees of the companies and the group of non-occupationally exposed housewives had been selected according to their willingness to participate and good accessibility for setting up the collection of samples. High exposure industries were represented by an electrical power distribution company and manufacturers of paint and pesticides, whereas turning and casting operations, polymer plastic manufacturing and professional driving and office work were considered as low exposure occupations for PCB. „After introducing the study to the company management and their agreement to cooperate, all employees were informed verbally and by notice board on the project, and invited to participate voluntarily. As the allocation to the different professional groups was done only afterwards on the basis of the interviews, a systematic bias by filtering the participants was largely avoided. After excluding missing data for HbA1c or cases with missing biomonitoring (6 samples were damaged during transport to Germany), 140 cases remained. The distribution among the groups is shown in Fig. 1.

A single interviewer collected all data on demographic status, diet habits and occupational history, and measured the participants' height and weight using calibrated standard devices. All serum samples, obtained from approximately five ml venous blood, were analysed in the same laboratory in Tehran for HbA1c concentrations and lipid profiles. Plasma samples were shipped by commercial mailing service to the occupational toxicology laboratory of the Institute of Occupational, Social and Environmental Medicine at RWTH Aachen University, Germany for determining nine non-dioxin-like (28, 52, 66, 74, 99, 101, 138, 153, 180) and 12 dioxin-like (77, 81, 105, 114, 118, 123, 126, 156, 157, 167, 169, 189) PCB congeners by using gas chromatography coupled with mass spectrometry (GC/MS). For a detailed description of the method we refer to Schettgen et al. [25, 26].

Congeners concentrations of less than 10% above the lower limit of detection (LOD) were excluded from statistical analysis. Therefore, the further analyses have been carried out for PCB 138, 153, 180 and 118. In this study we used a LOD of 0.01 μg/l. All results below this threshold were set to 0.005 μg/l. The plasma concentration of PCBs were categorized using their quartile values. The first quartile (25%) was used as the reference category. If more than 25% of the values of congeners were below LOD, all these values were added to the first quartile. The remaining values were divided into three equal groups forming the quartiles two to four [9]. Following current recommendations by the American Diabetes Association, we used the serum concentration of HbA1c (5.7% or more) for the diagnosis of diabetes or pre-diabetes. Using the HbA1c concentration had several advantages compared with other laboratory parameters, such as fasting plasma glucose or the oral glucose tolerance test, including greater convenience as pre-test fasting was not required, a better pre-analytical stability, and less day-to-day perturbations during stress and illness [27].

We categorized the participants metabolic disorders status according to the HbA1c level, as it is more reliable while some of them might not adhere to the restrict recommended fasting period despite prior rigorous advice.

Statistical tests

For statistical analysis we used the IBM SPSS Statistics 22 package. Comparing variable distributions with normal distribution curve was done by using the *Kolmogorov–Smirnov test.* A *P*-value of less than 0.05 was considered significant for all statistical tests. Logistic regression modelling was used to evaluate the association between diabetes, pre-diabetes and serum concentrations of PCB congeners, as well as the other considered covariates (age, gender, BMI and total lipid concentration). Adjusted odds ratios (ORs) for these covariates and their corresponding 95% confidence intervals (CIs) are reported. Total serum lipid was calculated using the short formula proposed by Phillips: Total lipids (mg/dL) = 2.27*Total cholesterol + TG (triglycerides) + 0.623 [28]. A generalized maximum likelihood Wald X^2 test was used on dummy variables of four quartiles to evaluate the differences of the average proportion of diabetic cases across the quartiles [29].

Ethical considerations

All participants of the study gave written informed consent beforehand. Participation in the study was voluntary.

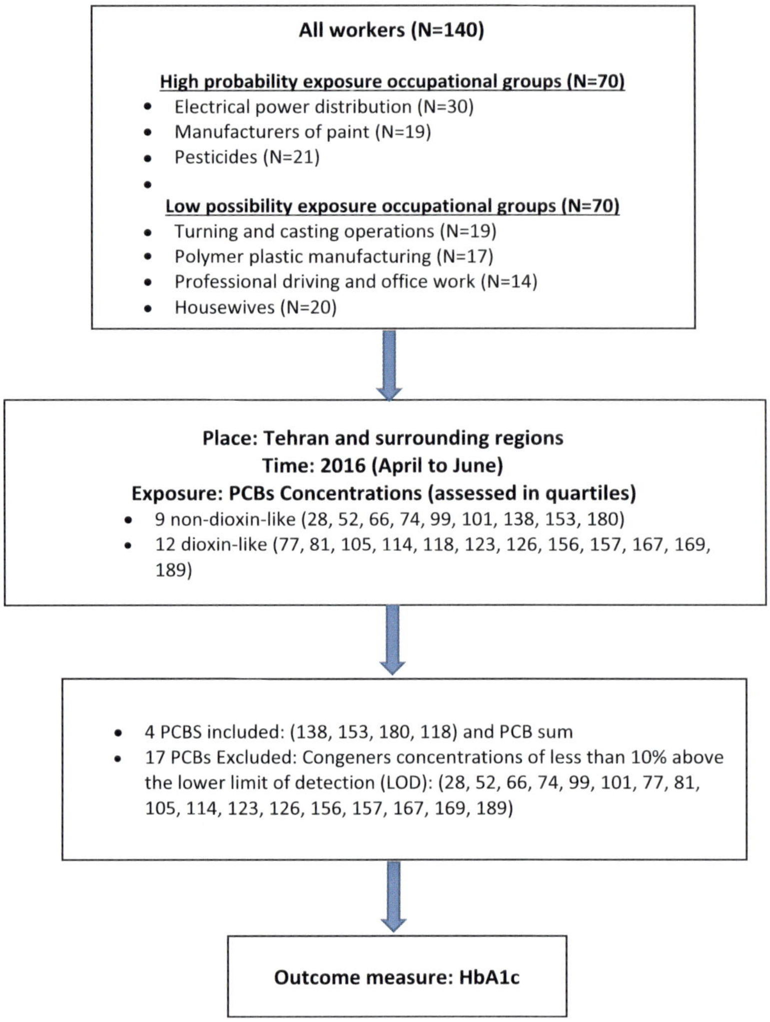

Fig. 1 Project outline

Confidentiality was guaranteed through anonymous data gathering. The study was approved by the Ethics Committee at the Research Division of the Ministry of Health in Tehran (Project number: 93–03–103-26,804-144,653).

Results

Table 1 shows the demographic characteristics and metabolic key values of the 140 examined participants, of which 83% were males. The age range lay between 20 and 71 years (mean 38.6, SD ± 10.38 years). Mean and median BMI were 26.41 and 26.34 kg/m^2 respectively and thus falling into the "overweight" category (BMI between 25 and 30 kg/m^2) [30]. Of the 140 participants, 77 (55%) were classified as being diabetic or pre-diabetic, and were also older than the participants with normal HbA1c values ($P = 0.002$). In addition, they had higher values of PCB 138, 153, 180 and the PCB sum, although this was not statistically significant.

The mean plasma concentrations of PCB 138, 153, 180, 118 and the PCB sum, as well as their 25th, 50th and 75th percentiles, subdivided in two groups (HbA1c ≥ 5.7% and < 5.7%) are shown in Table 2.

The relationship between the concentrations of PCB 138, 153, 180, the PCB sum, and PCB 118 in different quartiles and according to blood glucose status is shown in Table 3. The first quartile was used as the reference group. The third quartiles of the values for PCB 138 and 153 were significantly increased ($P = 0.01$) compared to the reference group. Regarding the relationship in other quartiles, only PCB 153 in the second quartile and PCB 180 in the fourth quartile showed statistically significant differences in both glucose status groups ($P = 0.03$ and 0.01 respectively). The highest ORs were found for the third quartiles of PCB153 and PCB138 (OR = 3.51 and 3.44, respectively). As there was no difference of the categorized HbA1c levels among the PCB 118 quartiles, and a large number of participants fell into the first quartile, the same analysis with dichotomous PCB 118

Table 1 Demographic and metabolic characteristics of the two blood glucose status groups, as determined by HbA1c level

		Total ($N = 140$)	Metabolic disorder (HbA1C ≥ 5.7) ($N = 77$)	Without Metabolic disorder (HbA1C < 5.7) ($N = 63$)	*P* value
Gender	N (%)				
	Male	116 (82.9)	62 (53.4)	54 (46.6)	0.42
	Female	24 (17.1)	15 (62.5)	9 (37.5)	
Age	[Year] Mean (Sd)	38.61 (10.38)	41.04 (11.04)	35.63 (8.7)	0.002*
BMI Mean	[Kg/M^2] (Sd)	26.41 (3.76)	26.52 (3.62)	26.26 (3.96)	0.69
HbA1c Mean	[%] (Sd)	5.86 (1.12)	6.28 (1.35)	5.34 (0.27)	< 0.001*
FBS Mean	[Mg/Dl] (Sd)	99.90 (37.02)	106.31 (47.89)	92.27 (13.52)	0.03*
Total Lipid Mean	[Mg/Dl] (Sd)	577.09 (162.91)	583.70 (151.26)	569.09 (176.90)	0.30

BMI Body Mass Index, *HbA1c* glycated hemoglobin, *FBG* Fasting Blood Glucose
*Statistically significant relation (*P* value < 0.05)

values (LOD 0.005 as cut off) was performed. This analysis showed that 20 (55.6%) participants with a PCB 118 level above LOD had also an increased HbA1c level of 5.7% or more, compared to 57 (54.8%) in the other group with no detected PCB 118 ($P = 0.94$, OR = 1.03 CI 95%: 0.48–2.21).

The relationship between PCB levels and indications of a disturbed of blood glucose is shown in Table 4. In the logistic regression, adjusted for age, gender, BMI and total lipid concentrations, none of the pairwise differences between the first quartile and the remaining 2nd, 3rd and 4th quartiles reached statistical significance.

Discussion

In this study we investigated 140 participants categorized in two groups according to their HbA1c level, either indicating a disturbed glucose metabolism or showing normal values of less than 5.7%. For our cohort we could not find a significant association between plasma PCB levels and HbA1c values. As expected, age as one of the other tested co-variables, had the strongest effect on HbA1c. We have also found that the PCB-burden of our study population was lower in comparison with similar study groups [31].

The high number of male participants in this study was due to the fact that the study population originated from an occupational health investigation among workers from industrial workplaces. In Iran the majority of the working population particularly in the manufacturing and power industry is male. In view of the overall low PCB burden, however, an influence of gender on the results can be denied, especially since the regression has been adjusted for gender. Published results of a study among the American native population suggested that the strongest association with diabetes was due to the lower-chlorinated PCB congeners, which are less persistent in the human body [32]. In our study group, for none of the low chlorinated PCB congeners more than 10% of the measured plasma values lay above the LOD. Therefore we had to exclude the results for these congeners, which had probably the strongest effect on glucose metabolism, from further analysis. This together with the small sample size and the limited overall PCB

Table 2 Distribution of PCB 138, 153, 180, sum, and 118 in two blood glucose status groups, determined by HbA1c level

	Total (N = 140)					Metabolic disorder (HbA1C ≥ 5.7) (N = 77)					Without Metabolic disorder (HbA1C < 5.7) (N = 63)				
	PCB 138 [μg/l]	PCB 153 [μg/l]	PCB 180 [μg/l]	PCB sum [μg/l]	PCB 118 [μg/l]	PCB 138 [μg/l]	PCB 153 [μg/l]	PCB 180 [μg/l]	PCB sum [μg/l]	PCB 118 [μg/l]	PCB 138 [μg/l]	PCB 153 [μg/l]	PCB 180 [μg/l]	PCB sum [μg/l]	PCB 118 [μg/l]
Mean	0.026	0.038	0.027	0.107	0.009	0.029	0.043	0.032	0.120	0.009	0.023	0.032	0.020	0.090	0.010
SD	0.03	0.03	0.03	0.08	0.01	0.03	0.04	0.03	0.10	0.01	0.02	0.03	0.02	0.07	0.01
Minimum	0.005	0.005	0.005	0.030	0.005	0.005	0.005	0.005	0.030	0.005	0.005	0.005	0.005	0.030	0.005
Percentile 25	0.005	0.016	0.005	0.050	0.005	0.008	0.020	0.005	0.058	0.005	0.005	0.014	0.005	0.039	0.005
Median	0.020	0.032	0.017	0.082	0.005	0.023	0.034	0.021	0.09	0.005	0.014	0.027	0.014	0.070	0.005
Percentile 75	0.036	0.053	0.039	0.140	0.009	0.037	0.053	0.047	0.156	0.011	0.033	0.051	0.033	0.132	0.006
Maximum	0.171	0.170	0.173	0.450	0.109	0.171	0.170	0.173	0.450	0.068	0.154	0.151	0.069	0.393	0.109

There was no statistically significant difference of the PCB congener levels between the two groups

Table 3 The relationship between level of PCB 138, 153, 180, sum, and 118 in different quartiles and blood glucose status (divided into 2 groups considering HBA1c = 5.7% as cut-off), considering the first quartile as the reference group (unadjusted ORs)

Variables	Quartile 1	Quartile 2	Quartile 3	Quartile 4
PCB138 N (HbA1c ≥ 5.7%)	47 (19)	31 (18)	30 (21)	32 (19)
OR (CI)	1.0 (Ref)	2.04 (0.81–5.12)	3.44 (1.30–9.11)	2.15 (0.86–5.38)
P value	–	0.13	0.01*	0.10
PCB153 N (HbA1c ≥ 5.7%)	34 (12)	36 (22)	35 (23)	35 (20)
OR (CI)	1.0 (Ref)	2.88 (1.09–7.61)	3.51 (1.30–9.46)	2.44 (0.93–6.45)
P value	–	0.03*	0.01*	0.07
PCB180 N (HbA1c ≥ 5.7%)	51 (23)	30 (18)	29 (14)	30 (22)
OR (CI)	1.0 (Ref)	1.83 (0.73–4.56)	1.14 (0.46–2.83)	3.35 (1.26–8.91)
P value	–	0.19	0.78	0.01*
PCB sum[a] N (HbA1c ≥ 5.7%)	36 (15)	34 (20)	35 (20)	35 (22)
OR (CI)	1.0 (Ref)	2 (0.77–5.18)	1.87 (0.73–4.79)	2.37 (0.91–6.15)
P value	–	0.15	0.19	0.07
PCB118 N (HbA1c ≥ 5.7%)	104 (57)	12 (6)	12 (7)	12 (7)
OR (CI)	1.0 (Ref)	0.82 (0.25–2.73)	1.15 (0.34–3.87)	1.15 (0.34–3.87)
P value	–	0.75	0.82	0.82

[a]Calculated as sum of PCB 28 + 52 + 101 + 138 + 153 + 180 according to the German PCB-guideline [37, 38]
*Statistically significant relation (*P* value < 0.05)

burden may explain the discrepancy between our results and other cross sectional studies showing a strong dose-response relationship between serum concentrations of PCB 153 and diabetes [17, 31]. We can still say that these findings are not contradicting our results, although the dose response relationship lost statistical significance after adjustment for the co-variables age, gender, BMI and serum total lipid in the regression model. Considering the strong influence of age on the plasma levels of higher chlorinated PCBs [25], the reduced observed relationship in the statistical model may be contributed primarily to the effect of age.

In 2010, Lee et al. showed a non-linear U-shaped relation between high chlorinated PCBs and diabetes risk [16]. Their separate analysis of the different PCB congeners indicated that the blood concentrations of PCB 74, 118 and 126 (dioxin like PCBs) as well as PCB 138, 153, 170, 180 and 187 (non-dioxin like PCBs) were associated with signs of the metabolic syndrome. This association was much stronger between lower concentrations than higher background concentrations [16], which was explained by the role of PCB as an endocrine disrupter. High-dose exposure may lead to down-regulation of receptors as the dose further increases [33]. This finding

Table 4 Logistic regression, model adjusted for sex, age, BMI, total lipid assessing the relationship between level of PCB 138, 153, 180, sum, and 118 in different quartiles and blood glucose status (divided into 2 groups considering HBA1c = 5.7% as cut-off), considering the first quartile as the reference group

Variables		Quartile 1	Quartile 2	Quartile 3	Quartile 4	Wald χ2 *p*-value
PCB138	Exp (B)	1.0	1.52	2.44	1.12	0.34
	P Value	–	0.44	0.09	0.85	
PCB153	Exp (B)	1.0	2.45	2.55	1.00	0.12
	P Value	–	0.09	0.08	1	
PCB180	Exp (B)	1.0	1.23	0.72	1.66	0.53
	P Value	–	0.69	0.53	0.39	
PCB sum[a]	Exp (B)	1.0	1.38	1.25	0.93	0.87
	P Value	–	0.54	0.68	0.91	
PCB118	Exp (B)	1.0	0.62	0.87	0.47	0.73
	P Value	–	0.48	0.82	0.32	

[a]Calculated as sum of PCB 28 + 52 + 101 + 138 + 153 + 180 according to the German PCB-guideline [37, 38]

may warrant the conclusion that exposure to low doses of PCB can be at least as harmful as to higher doses [34, 35]. However, in the present study, we could not investigate low chlorinated congeners, such as PCB 74 and 126, since less than 10% of the studied population had serum concentrations above the LOD. Although the analysis of PCB 138 and 153 showed some effect on the glucose metabolism in the second and third quartiles, this association did not reach a statistically significant level.

The results of our study did not demonstrate any association between the serum values of PCB 118 and the PCB sum on the one hand and the risk of developing a disturbed glucose metabolism on the other, which is inconsistent with previous studies [16, 36]. A large Japanese study demonstrated a significantly higher prevalence of DM at the third and fourth quartiles of dioxin like PCBs [13]. That may be due to the fact that PCBs plasma levels of the Iranian population are generally low. We must however also keep in mind that we could not analyse the association of all dioxin like PCBs as mentioned formerly.

This study's major strength was the use of HbA1c rather than e.g. fasting blood glucose as an indicator of an unbalanced glucose metabolism or manifest diabetes. The assessment of a specific additional effect of raised PCB levels on the glucose metabolism was further validated in our participants by controlling for other important risk factors. Another important strength was the inclusion of different occupational groups with a wide range of assumed PCB-exposure risks, together with the housewives as a non-occupationally exposed reference group and possibly indicating the background exposure of a typical urban population. This was an advantage over previous studies on PCB only assessing subjects with known high exposures to various pollutants in occupational settings, and thus avoiding a selection bias.

Due to the cross sectional design of our study and the anonymity of all participants, only one contact could be made to collect blood samples and record demographic data. Therefore it was not possible to assess incidence and changes over time in exposed and non-exposed subgroups. The low overall levels of dioxin-like PCBs, except for PCB 118, made it impossible to assess their association with increased glucose levels and diabetes. Our attempt to consider the effect of each PCB congener separately, rather than building groups of similar types, hampered significant results.

Conclusion

For our study cohort of male industrial workers and not-occupationally exposed housewives we could not demonstrate a significant effect of different PCB congeners on the concentration of HbA1c.

Abbreviations

ADA: American Diabetes Association; CI: Confidence interval; DM: Diabetes mellitus; FPG: Fasting plasma glucose; HbA1c: % of glycosylated haemoglobin; IDF: International Diabetes Federation; LOD: Limit of detection; OGTT: Oral glucose tolerance test; ORs: Adjusted odds ratios; PCB: Polychlorinated biphenyls; POPs: Persistent organic pollutants; RWTH: Rheinisch-Westfaelische Technische Hochschule / rhenish-westphalian technical University; T2DM: Type 2 diabetes mellitus

Authors' contributions

SE managed communications and collaboration with German colleagues and was involved in the design of the study, literature search, data acquisition from study population, manuscript preparation and manuscript editing. OA was involved in the design of the study, definition of intellectual content and manuscript review. ZM was involved in literature search, data analysis, statistical analysis, and manuscript editing. TS was responsible for conduction and evaluation of biomonitoring. T.S. was involved in the study design, manuscript editing and review and interpretation of the results. AK was involved in data analysis, interpretation of results and manuscript review. MF was involved in in the design of the study, definition of intellectual content, manuscript review, and interpretation of the results. TK was involved in in the design of the study, definition of intellectual content, manuscript review, and interpretation of the results. AE managed communications and collaboration with Iranian partners, logistical procedures of blood samples and material shipment. A.E. was involved in the design of the study, definition of intellectual content, data analysis and statistical analysis, manuscript review and interpretation of the results. All authors read and approved the final manuscript.

Competing interests

The authors declare that they have no competing interests.

Author details

[1]Institute for Occupational, Social and Environmental Medicine, University Hospital Aachen, RWTH University Aachen, Pauwelsstr 30, D-52074 Aachen, Germany. [2]School of Medicine- International Campus, Tehran University of Medical Sciences (TUMS), Tehran, Iran. [3]Center for Research on Occupational Diseases, Tehran University of Medical Sciences (TUMS), Tehran, Iran. [4]Community and Preventive Medicine Department, Tehran University of Medical Sciences (TUMS), Tehran, Iran.

References

1. Lozano R, Naghavi M, Foreman K, Lim S, Shibuya K, Aboyans V, et al. Global and regional mortality from 235 causes of death for 20 age groups in 1990 and 2010: a systematic analysis for the global burden of disease study 2010. Lancet. 2013;380(9859):2095–128.
2. Esteghamati A, Etemad K, Koohpayehzadeh J, Abbasi M, Meysamie A, Noshad S, et al. Trends in the prevalence of diabetes and impaired fasting glucose in association with obesity in Iran: 2005–2011. Diabetes Res Clin Pract. 2014;103(2):319–27.
3. Whiting DR, Guariguata L, Weil C, Shaw J. IDF diabetes atlas: global estimates of the prevalence of diabetes for 2011 and 2030. Diabetes Res Clin Pract. 2011;94(3):311–21.
4. Kim C-H, Kim H-K, Kim E-H, Bae S-J, Choe J, Park J-Y. Risk of progression to diabetes from prediabetes defined by HbA1c or fasting plasma glucose criteria in Koreans. Diabetes Res Clin Pract. 2016;118:105–11.
5. Kriska AM, Saremi A, Hanson RL, Bennett PH, Kobes S, Williams DE, et al. Physical activity, obesity, and the incidence of type 2 diabetes in a high-risk population. Am J Epidemiol. 2003;158(7):669–75.
6. Hu FB, Manson JE, Stampfer MJ, Colditz G, Liu S, Solomon CG, et al. Diet, lifestyle, and the risk of type 2 diabetes mellitus in women. N Engl J Med. 2001;345(11):790–7.
7. Rimm EB, Chan J, Stampfer MJ, Colditz GA, Willett WC. Prospective study of cigarette smoking, alcohol use, and the risk of diabetes in men. BMJ. 1995; 310(6979):555–9.

8. Will JC, Galuska DA, Ford ES, Mokdad A, Calle EE. Cigarette smoking and diabetes mellitus: evidence of a positive association from a large prospective cohort study. Int J Epidemiol. 2001;30(3):540–6.
9. Esser A, Schettgen T, Gube M, Koch A, Kraus T. Association between polychlorinated biphenyls and diabetes mellitus in the German HELPcB cohort. Int J Hyg Environ Health. 2016;219(6):557–65.
10. La Rocca C, Mantovani A. From environment to food: the case of PCB. Annali-Istituto Superiore di Sanita 2006;42(4):410.
11. Kohler M, Zennegg M, Waeber R. Coplanar polychlorinated biphenyls (PCB) in indoor air. Environmental science & technology. 2002;36(22):4735–40.
12. Persky V, Piorkowski J, Turyk M, Freels S, Chatterton R, Dimos J, et al. Polychlorinated biphenyl exposure, diabetes and endogenous hormones: a cross-sectional study in men previously employed at a capacitor manufacturing plant. Environ Health. 2012;11(1):57.
13. Uemura H, Arisawa K, Hiyoshi M, Satoh H, Sumiyoshi Y, Morinaga K, et al. Associations of environmental exposure to dioxins with prevalent diabetes among general inhabitants in Japan. Environ Res. 2008;108(1):63–8.
14. Everett CJ, Frithsen IL, Diaz VA, Koopman RJ, Simpson WM, Mainous AG. Association of a polychlorinated dibenzo-p-dioxin, a polychlorinated biphenyl, and DDT with diabetes in the 1999–2002 National Health and nutrition examination survey. Environ Res. 2007;103(3):413–8.
15. Lee D-H, Lee I-K, Porta M, Steffes M, Jacobs D. Relationship between serum concentrations of persistent organic pollutants and the prevalence of metabolic syndrome among non-diabetic adults: results from the National Health and nutrition examination survey 1999–2002. Diabetologia. 2007;50(9):1841–51.
16. Lee D-H, Steffes MW, Sjödin A, Jones RS, Needham LL, Jacobs Jr DR. Low dose of some persistent organic pollutants predicts type 2 diabetes: a nested case-control study. Environ Health Perspect. 2010; 118(9):1235.
17. Lee D-H, Lee I-K, Song K, Steffes M, Toscano W, Baker BA, et al. A strong dose-response relation between serum concentrations of persistent organic pollutants and diabetes. Diabetes Care. 2006;29(7):1638–44.
18. Philibert A, Schwartz H, Mergler D. An exploratory study of diabetes in a first nation community with respect to serum concentrations of p, p'-DDE and PCBs and fish consumption. Int J Environ Res Public Health. 2009;6(12): 3179–89.
19. Tanaka T, Morita A, Kato M, Hirai T, Mizoue T, Terauchi Y, et al. Congener-specific polychlorinated biphenyls and the prevalence of diabetes in the Saku control obesity program (SCOP). Endocr J. 2011; 58(7):589–96.
20. Gasull M, Pumarega J, Téllez-Plaza M, Castell C, Tresserras R, Lee DH, et al. Blood concentrations of persistent organic pollutants and prediabetes and diabetes in the general population of Catalonia. Environmental science & technology. 2012;46(14):7799–810.
21. Wu H, Bertrand KA, Choi AL, Hu FB, Laden F, Grandjean P, et al. Plasma levels of persistent organic pollutants and risk of type 2 diabetes: a prospective analysis in the nurses' health study and meta-analysis. 2013.
22. Casals-Casas C, Desvergne B. Endocrine disruptors: from endocrine to metabolic disruption. Annu Rev Physiol. 2011;73:135–62.
23. Gray SL, Shaw AC, Gagne AX, Chan HM. Chronic exposure to PCBs (Aroclor 1254) exacerbates obesity-induced insulin resistance and hyperinsulinemia in mice. J Toxic Environ Health A. 2013;76(12):701–15.
24. Fischer LJ, Zhou H-R, Wagner MA. Polychlorinated biphenyls release insulin from RINm5F cells. Life Sci. 1996;59(24):2041–9.
25. Schettgen T, Gube M, Alt A, Fromme H, Kraus T. Pilot study on the exposure of the German general population to non-dioxin-like and dioxin-like PCBs. Int J Hyg Environ Health. 2011;214(4):319–25.
26. Schettgen T, Alt A, Esser A, Kraus T. Current data on the background burden to the persistent organochlorine pollutants HCB, p, p'-DDE as well as PCB 138, PCB 153 and PCB 180 in plasma of the general population in Germany. Int J Hyg Environ Health. 2015;218(4):380–5.
27. Association AD. Diagnosis and classification of diabetes mellitus. Diabetes Care. 2014;37(Supplement 1):S81–90.
28. Bernert JT, Turner WE, Patterson Jr DG, Needham LL. Calculation of serum "total lipid" concentrations for the adjustment of persistent organohalogen toxicant measurements in human samples. Chemosphere. 2007;68(5):824–31.
29. Myers RH, Montgomery DC, Vining GG. Robinson TJ. In: Generalized linear models: with applications in engineering and the sciences. Hoboken: Wiley; 2012. https://onlinelibrary.wiley.com/doi/pdf/10.1002/9780470556986.
30. Flegal KM, Carroll MD, Kuczmarski RJ, Johnson CL. Overweight and obesity in the United States: prevalence and trends, 1960–1994. Int J Obes. 1998; 22(1):39–47.
31. Codru N, Schymura MJ, Negoita S, Rej R, Carpenter DO. Environment ATFot. Diabetes in relation to serum levels of polychlorinated biphenyls and chlorinated pesticides in adult native Americans. Environ Health Perspect. 2007;115(10):1442.
32. Aminov Z, Haase R, Rej R, Schymura MJ, Santiago-Rivera A, Morse G, et al. Diabetes prevalence in relation to serum concentrations of polychlorinated biphenyl (PCB) congener groups and three chlorinated pesticides in a native American population. Environ Health Perspect. 2016;124(9):1376.
33. Medlock KL, Lyttle CR, Kelepouris N, Newman ED, Sheehan DM. Estradiol down-regulation of the rat uterine estrogen receptor. Exp Biol Med. 1991; 196(3):293–300.
34. Welshons WV, Thayer KA, Judy BM, Taylor JA, Curran EM, Vom Saal FS. Large effects from small exposures. I. Mechanisms for endocrine-disrupting chemicals with estrogenic activity. Environ Health Perspect. 2003;111(8):994.
35. Hennig B, Meerarani P, Slim R, Toborek M, Daugherty A, Silverstone AE, et al. Proinflammatory properties of coplanar PCBs: in vitro and in vivo evidence. Toxicol Appl Pharmacol. 2002;181(3):174–83.
36. Turyk M, Anderson H, Knobeloch L, Imm P, Persky V. Organochlorine exposure and incidence of diabetes in a cohort of Great Lakes sport fish consumers. Environ Health Perspect. 2009;117(7):1076.
37. Knipschildt F, Kommune K. Miljøforvaltningen T-o. Sundhedsmæssig vurdering af PCB-holdige bygningsfuger.
38. Wang RY, Jain RB, Wolkin AF, Rubin CH, Needham LL. Serum concentrations of selected persistent organic pollutants in a sample of pregnant females and changes in their concentrations during gestation. Environ Health Perspect. 2009;117(8):1244.

Oxygen Consumption (V'O2) and physical Strainas measured by the occupational activity of cleaning personnel

M. J. Fröhlich[1*], R. F. Kroidl[2] and T. Welte[1]

Abstract

Background: The aim of the study was to determine the physical effort and energy expenditure needed over a working period of 45–60 min, specifically for the occupational activity of cleaning. The effort was demonstrated in absolute terms (V'O2), in relation to the involved person's maximum physical capacity (peak V'O2) and in relation to the individual aerobic-anaerobic threshold (V'O2 at VT1, the point when lactate starts to accumulate but can be cleared). In addition to this, the aim was to verify the suitability of portable ergospirometry in determining the occupational workload in a real-life setting.

Methods: Thirty-five cleaners performed a bicycle ergospirometry to determine their maximum physical capacity (peak V'O2 = L/min) and their aerobic-anaerobic threshold (V'O2 at the Ventilatory Threshold 1 [VT1]). This was followed by portable ergospirometry lasting 45–60 min while pursuing regular cleaning activities.

Results: Performance V'O2 (the average oxygen consumption over 45–60 min of work- time) was 1.06 L/min or 4.4 METs. This was scarcely lower than the individual V'O2 at VT1 and approached 45% of the maximum physical capacity (peak V'O2). In addition, there was positive feedback regarding the wearability of the portable device. The dropout rate was low.

Conclusion: The occupational activity of cleaning was defined as a "committed activity", performed close to the upper limit of the continuous physical capacity (approaching V'O2 at VT1). The positive feedback and a low dropout rate proved good acceptance of portable ergospirometry in this field of work over a 45–60 min period.

Keywords: Occupational workload, Real-life setting, Ergospirometry, Cardiopulmonary exercise testing, Disability

Background

A frequent medical task involves the evaluation of an individual's physical capacity with regard to his or her work demands. According to the recommendations of the WHO and its ICF-classification [1] such a judgment should include the total bio-psycho-social context of the individual. As part of the bio-psycho-social context the clinician needs to assess the physical capability of the person to perform his occupational activity. The performance demand (load) should be reflected against the performance ability (capacity), leading to the concept of "load to capacity". Two questions must be answered:

- How great are the physical demands caused by the work?
- How high is this person's physical capacity? It should be kept in mind that usual conditions and not peak performances are involved.

In Germany, physical workload is estimated according to the REFA-classification (REFA: Reichsausschuß für Arbeitszeitermittlung, now known as Verband für Arbeitsgestaltung, Betriebsorganisation und Unternehmensentwicklung e. V.). It has four gradings: "light", "light to moderate", "moderate" and "hard" [2]. This classification dates back to the 1920s and 1930s and primarily relates to carrying and holding work with emphasis placed on different physical positions.

* Correspondence: michaeljoachimfroehlich@yahoo.com
[1]Department of Respiratory Medicine, Medizinische Hochschule Hannover, Carl-Neuberg Str. 1, 30625 Hannover, Germany
Full list of author information is available at the end of the article

In order to gain better and more concrete information as well as numeric values for performance demands, studies on energy consumption in diverse professional sectors were carried out in the 1950s and 1960s [3–6]. Oxygen uptake (V'O2 in L/min) was determined as the central measured parameter, providing energy consumption (in kcal) via the caloric equivalent. The measurements did not exclusively monitor conditions at the actual workplace (i.e. field tests) but were mostly carried out in standardised settings.

Energy expenditure is also the basis of the compendium of physical activities as compiled by Ainsworth et al. [7, 8]. This compendium takes the metabolic rate obtained during quiet sitting down (resting period) as the standard metabolic rate. It is assigned a valued with 1 MET (4184 kJ/kg body weight/h). The compendium lists 605 specific activities. The activities are classified according to the number of MET needed to perform them and classifies activities in terms of light, moderate or vigorous intensity activities. For example, "interior cleaning" is valued 3,01 MET. The compendium was compiled to standardize and classify the physical intensity of activities in previously done research. It is based on data acquired before the 1990's, before the use of portable ergospirometry. It does not take individual variation (for example: fitness levels or medical disabilities) into account.

According to pertinent literature and widely accepted consent in occupational medicine, a person can be declared "fit for work" if the continuous workload does not exceed 40% of the individual's peak V'O2. The aerobic-anaerobic threshold is regarded as the upper limit of the continuous physical performance capacity [9–14].

Given the possibilities of portable ergospirometry, we have a new and precise way to ascertain physical workload under authentic working conditions. It is important to demonstrate the workload in relation to the maximal capacity ("load to capacity"). Portable ergospirometry has been used in the field of occupational medicine. Among other fields it has been used in research pertaining to firefighters, in forestry and in the military [15–18]. Most of the common occupations have however not been investigated and not all studies were done in real-life settings (i.e. how does marching on an indoor treadmill relate to a field march in battle, or do firefighters experience the same amount of stress when performing a pre-trainer practise routine in comparison with a real firefight). In one recent study concerning municipal refuse collectors the "load to capacity" was evaluated by use of portable ergospirometry in a real-life setting [19]. The implementation of portable ergospirometry in daily practice remains an area of interest that needs to be evaluated further. Its use is not yet standard in determining the workload of an individual.

Study goal

The goal of this study was firstly to determine in a group of cleaning personnel how great the physical performance needs to be to carry out cleaning work and how this activity is related to the actual maximum performance capacity and the aerobic-anaerobic threshold.

Secondly, our study focussed on determining if portable ergospirometry is suited for displaying the actual workload in a workplace related field test.

Methods

Participants and study design

Employees were recruited from the cleaning departments of rehabilitation centres on the island of Borkum as well as employees from several hotels and guest houses. All participants were of good health and gave informed consent before study entry. The study was presented to and approved by the ethical committee of the "Medizinische Hochschule Hannover". Included were persons ranging in age from 18 to 65 years.

Measurements

At first the maximum physical capacity (peak V'O2) was determined by an exhaustive bicycle ergospirometry. This was done in the facilities of the "Knappschaft-Bahn-See" rehabilitation centre. A Ganshorn Power Cube LF8, 5F paired with an Ergoline Ergometrics 900 ergometer in a semi-recumbent position was used. A Radiometer Copenhagen ABL700 was used to conduct capillary blood gas analyses.

The exhaustive bicycle ergospirometries were carried out according to current clinical practise [20–22]. They were scheduled either early in the morning or early in the afternoon. The following test protocol was used: After 3 min of rest and 3 min of unloaded pedalling at 60 rpm, the workload was started at 25 watts. The workload was increased gradually in intervals of one minute. The increases were estimated according to the person's prevailing physical abilities and with the help of tables, formulas and clinical experience in order to reach exhaustion after about 10 [8–15] min. Every subject had an individual testing protocol. Physical exhaustion was determined by clinical judgement, by use of the Borg Scale and by passing the aerobe-anaerobe threshold, V'O2 at VT1 (Ventilatory Threshold 1) [21], the point when lactate starts to accumulate but can be cleared. Capillary blood gas analyses were conducted at rest and close to exhaustion. The results were compiled in tables and depicted in the 9-panel plot according to Wasserman [20, 21]. The individual aerobic-anaerobic threshold was assessed predominantly with the use of panels 5, 6 and 9. As reference values, we used data from Wasserman and Jones [20]. All results were reviewed and validated by the second investigator. (Fig. 1).

At a later stage, the tests were continued by using portable ergospirometry while the cleaners carried out their cleaning work, the "field test". The cleaners were accompanied to their actual workplace and were monitored during their usual, daily work routine. After applying the portable ergospirometry device and measuring for 2–5 min at rest, the cleaners resumed their regular work. The cleaners were asked to continue the work that they were doing at their usual pace. The specific tasks were not standardized. The aim was to measure the workload in a real-life setting. The work consisted mostly of mopping and vacuuming floors, making beds and cleaning bedrooms as well as bathrooms. The aim was to record a period of between 45 and 60 min. The recording time variation was caused by work requirements. For example, recording continued until a subject had finished cleaning a specific section. (Fig. 2).

The Metamax 3B device® by Cortex, Leipzig, was used along with a pulsar pulse belt by Pulsar®. The Metamax 3B device® consists of two approximately 10 cm × 8 cm × 5 cm size parts which are connected by a cable. The cable is hung around the neck and the parts are attached with a harness to the front of the chest. The device itself weighs about 500 g. A mask, made of soft silicone, is placed with an elastic belt system over the face. A sensor piece fits onto the mask and connects to the chest device. The collected data can be stored in the device and/or sent wirelessly to a normal PC. The field test was only performed on persons who had previously undergone stationary ergospirometry without complications.

Statistical analysis

We compiled and analysed the data with the use of Microsoft Excel 2013 (v15.0) and its statistical calculators (Microsoft Redmond campus, Redmond, Washington, United States). Categorical variables are shown as numbers (n) and percentages (%). Continuous variables are shown as mean ± SD, unless indicated otherwise. For comparisons a two-sided paired t-test was used as appropriate. All reported *p*-values are two-sided unless indicated otherwise; p-values < 0.05 were considered statistically significant.

Results

Altogether 44 persons were recruited. Due to 9 dropouts (20%) a total of 35 subjects, 4 men (11%) and 31 women (89%) made up the test group. No prioritising in terms of sex was made. The mean age was 37.4 years (Standard Deviation, SD = 9.6) the median 37 years (Interquartile Range, IQR = 31–45). The mean height was 169 cm (SD 7.8), the median 168 cm (IQR = 163–172.5). The mean weight was 66 kg (SD = 18.3), the median 69 kg (IQR = 64–83). The mean BMI was 23.1 kg/m^2 (SD = 5.8), the median 25.8 kg/m^2 (IQR = 23.2–27.95). The mean recorded

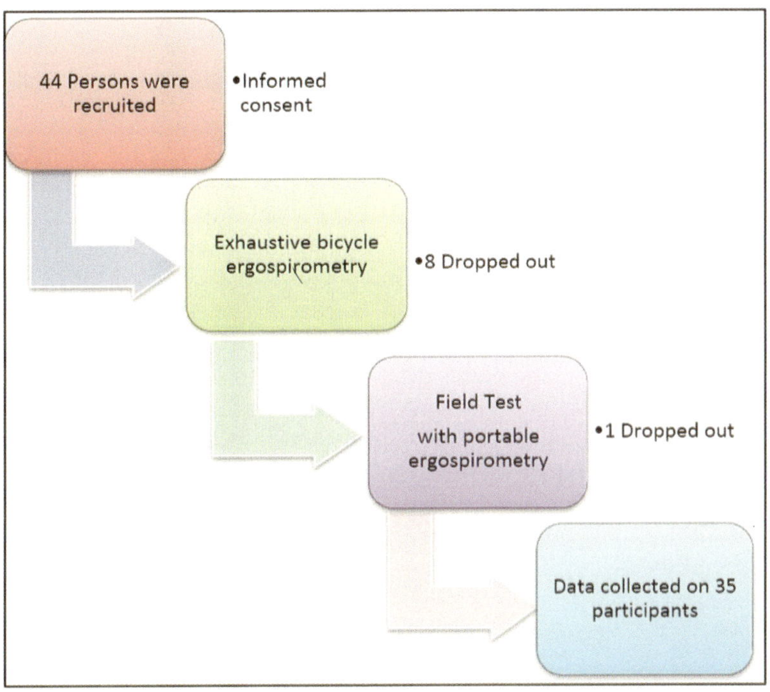

Fig. 1 The Procedural Path

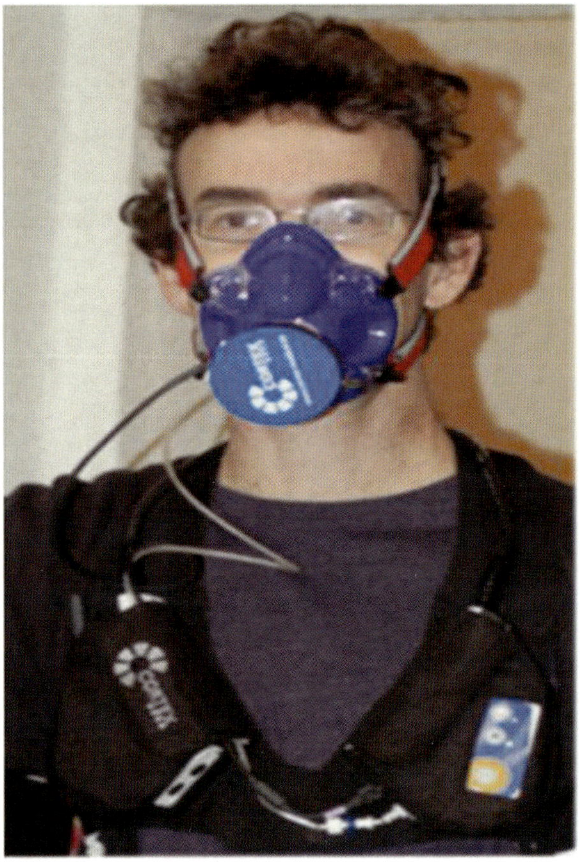

Fig. 2 Test person wearing the portable ergospirometry device. Source: Own image library, reproduction with subjects' permission

time in the field test was 52 min (SD 10.7), the median 50 min (IQR = 48–55).

It is noteworthy that the method of portable ergospirometry was well tolerated and accepted. Minor complaints such as increased sweating and oral dryness were reported in half of the cases. Work mobility was only slightly impaired. Altogether (stationary and portable ergospirometry combined) nine participants opted out. Reasons given were claustrophobia (four participants), the participant relocated (one), restriction of free movement during work (two participants) and revocation of consent without reason (two participants). The acceptance of these investigations by the working environment resulted in mixed responses: the appearance of an employee wearing a mask was (understandably) unusual and sometimes a cause for concern among bystanders. These concerns were, however, dealt with easily by the attending investigator.

The results showed that the resting V′O2 obtained during the bicycle ergospirometry compared well with the resting V′O2 measured before the field test.

- Bicycle ergospirometry: mean resting V′O2 0.38 L/min (SD = 0.11), median 0.35 L/min (IQR = 0.31–0.41)
- Portable ergospirometry: mean resting V′O2 0.38 L/min (SD = 0,12), median 0.41 L/min (IQR = 0.32–046)

A paired t-test revealed $p = 0.19$, stating no statistically relevant difference.

The mean peak V'O2 gained from bicycle ergospirometry was 2.06 L/min (SD = 0.54) or 28 ml/kg/min (SD = 7.4). The median peak V'O2 was 1.9 L/min (IQR = 1.78–2.16) or 26 ml/kg/min (IQR = 23–28). It corresponds to approximately 9 MET.

The mean V'O2 at VT1 (gained from bicycle ergospirometry) was 1.28 L/min (SD 0.34). Median V'O2 at VT1 was 1.25 L/min (IQR = 1–1.48).

To qualify the data, we introduced two terms:

- **Performance V'O2:** Total oxygen consumption while carrying out the work.
  This value includes the oxygen consumption at rest in addition to V'O2 allocated to the specific workload. The mean performance V'O2 was 1.06 L/min (SD = 0.24), the median performance V'O2 was 1.02 L/min (IQR = 0.92–1.19). This corresponds to approximately 4.5 MET.
- **Work V'O2:** Additional oxygen consumption needed to perform work, not including the oxygen consumption needed for basal metabolism. The mean work V'O2 was 0.68 L/min (SD = 0.19), the median work V'O2 was 0.65 L/min (IQR = 0.6–0.79). Therefore, the mean work-specific energy demand was calculated at $(0.68 \times 4.82) \approx 3.3$ kcal/min [21]. This is the energy expenditure needed for this specific professional activity.

Stationary semi-recumbent bicycle ergospirometry is not entirely suitable for determining the maximum physical capacity in relation to the measurements gained with a portable device. This is due to peak V'O2 being higher when weight-bearing activities are performed as opposed to non-weight-bearing activities [23–25]. We increased the peak V'O2 value as determined with the bicycle ergospirometry (non-weight-bearing activity) by 15% to 2.37 L/min in order to compare it with the "field test" of cleaning work (weight-bearing activity). The cleaner's workload amounted to 45% of the maximum available physical capacity. Performance V'O2 reached 90% of the V'O2 at VT1.

A t-test between performance V'O2 and V'O2 at VT1 revealed $p = 0.0015$, confirming a statistically relevant difference. (Fig. 3).

Discussion

The physical workload of cleaning work, especially how this activity relates to the individual's actual maximum

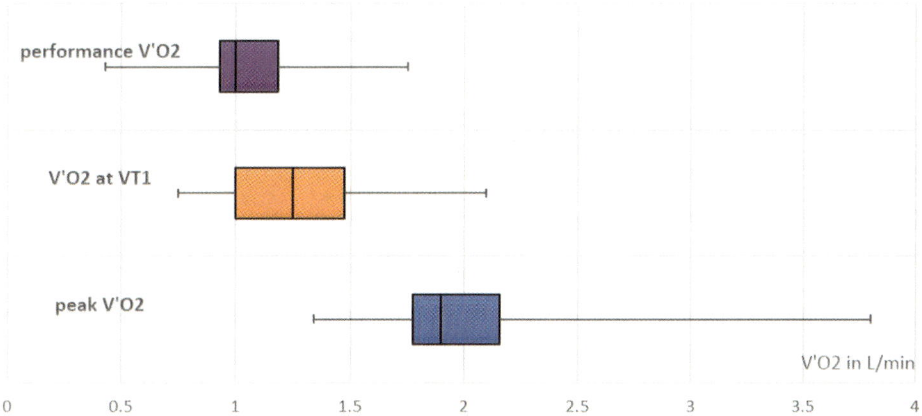

Fig. 3 Comparison of performance V'O2, V'O2 at VT1 and the peak V'O2

performance capacity and the aerobic-anaerobic threshold was noticeably higher than expected. The performance V'O2 almost reached 45% of the peak V'O2 and 90% of the V'O2 at VT1. According to pertinent literature and widely accepted consent in occupational medicine, a continuous permanent workload of around 40% of peak V'O2 is seen as the upper limit of continuous physical performance capacity [9–14]. Cleaning work exceeded this value, but not by a large margin. The work was done just within the boundary of predominantly aerobic metabolism.

If we use the criteria of the Compendium of Physical Activities by Ainsworth et al. [7, 8], our study showed that cleaning work could be classified as a moderate activity (3–6 MET) as it accounts for approximately 4.5 MET. Our study also showed the energy expenditure to be considerably higher than the assigned value of 3.01 MET (interior cleaning, 7, 8).

Work V'O2 is defined as the additional oxygen consumption needed to perform work, not including the oxygen consumption needed for the basal metabolism. This corresponds to a work-specific energy demand of approximately 3.3 kcal/min. This is relevant because if our results are compared with the studies completed during the 1950's and 1960's (Max Planck Institute, Dortmund) [3–6], we find that the results are very similar. With the technical possibilities available at that time, they measured the average energy consumption for cleaning work to be approximately 4 kcal/min.

Portable ergospirometry was suited for displaying the actual workload in field tests. The handling of the portable ergospirometry device turned out to be simple and intuitive. The measured values were plausible and the resting V'O2 compared well with that of the bicycle ergospirometry. The measurements were obtained without any complications. Mobility during the operation was marginally limited but restrictions were generally well tolerated. Claustrophobia seldom arose and portable ergospirometry was indeed practical in this setting. It is, however, important to mention that portable testing was only carried out on persons who had already tolerated face masks during earlier bicycle ergospirometry. Furthermore, not all occupations allow this type of testing, e.g. a salesperson or a telephone operator in a call centre cannot be tested. Also, it was noted that a cleaner wearing the portable ergospirometry device did (at times) elicit quite a bit of curiosity amongst bystanders. These factors could prove to be restricting in terms of the utilisation of portable ergospirometry testing in occupational medicine. Wearing the portable ergospirometry device (the mask) is not comfortable (sweating, dry mouth) and testing over longer periods of an entire shift, e.g. 4–6 or 8 h, is therefore not feasible.

The stationary bicycle ergospirometry in semi-recumbent position is not completely suitable for determining the maximum physical capacity in relation to the measurement done with the portable device. This is due to the difference in peak V'02 between weight-bearing and non-weight-bearing activities. Literature showed that a weight-bearing activity produces a higher peak V'O2 value of about 15% in comparison to a non-weight-bearing activity [23–25]. Having done the capacity measurements with an ergometer in semi-recumbent position, we corrected the peak V'O2 measurement obtained by means of bicycle ergospirometry through increasing it with 15% in order to compare it to the field test. The peak V'O2 measurement obtained by means of a bicycle ergospirometry as a surrogate for maximum V'O2 remains, however, a noteworthy limitation of our study.

Conclusion

These real-life measurements showed that the performance requirements for professional cleaning work are higher than expected. The REFA-classification as traditionally used in Germany today would classify cleaning workload as "light work". Our study shows that cleaning work reached the upper limit of continuous physical capacity. Thus, we do not classify cleaning as "light" work.

We propose the introduction of an extended classification system that would compare the prevailing physical capacity of a person with the real-life demands of the occupation, based on the concept of "load to capacity". Our study showed that with the current increasing availability of stationary and portable ergospirometry the amount of physical effort needed to perform work and the physical capacity involved can be assessed, compared and studied further [26, 27]. In order to increase the accuracy we advise the use of a treadmill ergospirometry to obtain the maximal physical capacity.

In our opinion the present classifications do not provide an adequate representation for the workload of professional cleaning and therefore we suggest that a new term "committed activity" could be used to describe the work that was carried out at the upper limit of continuous physical capacity.

Abbreviations

IQR: Interquartile Range; MET: Metabolic Equivalent of Task; Peak V'O2: The highest oxygen consumption achieved in a ergospirometry; Performance V'O2: Total oxygen consumption while performing the work; REFA: Reichsausschuss für Arbeitsstudien, currently: Verband für Arbeitsgestaltung, Betriebsorganisation und Unternehmensentwicklung e. V.; RER: Respiratory Exchange Rate; Resting V'O2: Oxygen consumption needed for the basal metabolism; SD: Standard deviation; V'O2 at the VT1: Ventilatory Threshold 1. The point where lactate starts to accumulate but can be cleared; V'O2: Oxygen consumption; Work V'O2: Additional oxygen consumption needed to perform work, not including the oxygen consumption needed for the basal metabolism

Acknowledgements

We thank the following institutions and persons for their respective contributions:
The Knappschaft-Bahn-See Klinik, Borkum for the use of their facilities.
Cortex, Leipzig, for the use of the Metamax 3B device®.
Jan Fuge, BREATH - Member of the German Center for Lung Research (DZL) Medizinische Hochschule Hannover, for his help with the statistics.
Susanne Lindemann for her help in sourcing the reference material from the 1950's and 1960's (Max Planck Institute, Dortmund).

Funding

We received financial support from the "Norddeutsche Gesellschaft für Pneumologie (NdGP)" and "Niedersächsischer Verein zur Bekämpfung der Tuberkulose e.V".

Authors' contributions

The examinations were mainly performed and interpreted by the corresponding author. All results were reviewed and validated by a second investigator, Rolf Kroidl. All authors contributed to writing the manuscript. All authors read and approved the final manuscript.

Competing interests

The authors declare that they have no competing interests.

Author details

[1]Department of Respiratory Medicine, Medizinische Hochschule Hannover, Carl-Neuberg Str. 1, 30625 Hannover, Germany. [2]Stade, Germany.

References

1. 54th World Health Assembly (WHA 54.21), 2001. International classification of functioning, disability and health.
2. Die REFA-Klassifikation, Verband für Arbeitsgestaltung, Betriebsorganisation und Unternehmensentwicklung e. V. Der ärztliche Reha- Entlassungsbericht: Deutsche Rentenversicherung; 2015. http://www.deutsche-rentenversicherung.de/cae/servlet/contentblob/215334/publicationFile/2078/download_leitfaden_einheitl_e_bericht.pdf. Accessed 15 Jan 2018.
3. Lehmann G, Müller EA, Spitzer H. Der Calorienbedarf bei gewerblicher Arbeit. Arbeitsphysiologie. 1950;14:166–235.
4. Lehmann G, Kwilecki CG. Untersuchung zur Frage des maximal zumutbaren Energieverbrauches arbeitender Frauen. Arbeitsphysiologie. 1959;17:438–51.
5. Müller EA. Werkzeug, Leistung und Energieverbrauch beim Schraubenziehen. Arbeitsphysiologie. 1952;14:477–88.
6. Hettinger T, Wirths W. Der Energieverbrauch beim Hand und Motorpflügen. Arbeitsphysiologie. 1953;15:41–6.
7. Ainsworth BE, et al. Compendium of physical activities: an update of activity codes and MET intensities. Med Sci Sports Exerc. 2000;32:498–516.
8. Ainsworth BE, Haskell WL, Leon AS. Compendium of physical activities: classification of energy costs of human physical activities. Med Sci Sports Exerc. 1993;25(1):71–80.
9. Ortega F, Montemayor T, Sanchez A, Cabello F, Castillo J. Role of cardiopulmonary exercise testing and the criteria used to determine disability in patients with severe COPD. Am J Respir Crit Care Med. 1994;150:747–51.
10. American Thoracic Society. Evaluation of impairment/disability secondary to respiratory disease. American Review Respiratory Disease. 1982;126:945–51.
11. American Thoracic Society. Evaluation of impairment/disability secondary to respiratory disorders. American Review Respiratory Disease. 1986;133:1205–9.
12. Killian KJ, Summers E, Jones NL, Campbell EJM. Exercise capacity and Ventilatory, circulatory and symptom limitations in patient with chronic airflow limitation. American Review Respiratory Disease. 1990;1992:935–40.
13. Medical Section of the American Lung Association. Guidelines for the Evaluation of Impairment/Disability in Patients with Asthma. Am Rev Respir Dis. 147(4):1056–61.
14. González CM, Barcala FJG, Ramírez JB, Ros IG, Michavila IM, Martínez CO, Rodríguez-Moro JMG, Portal JAR, Álvareza RF. Recommendations for fitness for work medical evaluations in chronic respiratory patients. Arch Bronchopneumol. 2013;49(11):480–90.
15. Harvey DG, Kraemer JL, Sharratt MT, Hughson RL. Respiratory gas exchange and physiological demands during a fire fighter evaluation circuit in men and women. Eur J Appl Physiol. 2008;103(1):89–98.
16. Williams-Bell FM, Villar R, Sharratt MT, Hughson RL. Physiological demands of the firefighter candidate physical ability test. Med Sci Sports Exerc. 2009; 41(3):653–62.
17. Christie CJ. A field investigation of physical workloads imposed on harvesters in south African forestryDissertation. Submitted in fulfillment of the requirements for the Degree Doctor of Philosophy. Grahamstown: Department of Human Kinetics and Ergonomics, Rhodes University; 2006.
18. Christie CJ, Scott PA. Metabolic responses of south African soldiers during simulated marching with sixteen combinations of speed and backpack load. Mil Med. 2005;170(7):69–76.
19. Preisser A, Zhou L, Velasco Garrido M, Harth V. Measured by the oxygen uptake in the field, the work of refuse collectors is particularly hard work: are the limit values for physical endurance workload too low? Int Arch Occup Environ Health. 2016;89(2):211–20. Epub 2015 Jun 19.
20. Wasserman K, Hansen JE, Sue DY, Stringer WW, Whipp BJ. Principles of exercise testing and interpretation: including Pathophysiology and clinical applications. 4th ed: Lippincott, Williams & Wilkins Publisher; 2005.

21. Kroidl RF, Schwarz S, Lehnigk B, Fritsch J. Kursbuch Spiroergometrie. 3rd ed: Thieme Publisher; 2015.
22. McArdle WD, Katch FI, Katch VL. Sports and exercise nutrition. 3rd ed: Wolters Kluwer/Lippincott Williams & Wilkins Publisher; 2007.
23. Venkata Ramana Y, Surya Kumari MV, Sudhakar RS, Balakrishna N. Comparison of training loads and physiological responses in athletes: consideration of body weight implication. N JEP online. 2004;7(3):134–9.
24. McArdle WD, Katch FI, Pechar GS. Comparison of continuous and discontinuous treadmill and bicycle test for V'O2 max. Medicine and science in sports. 1973;5(3):156–60.
25. Myers J, Buchanan N, Walsh D, Kraemer M, McAuley P, Hamilton-Wessler M, Froelicher VFJ. Comparison of the ramp versus standard exercise protocols. Am Coll Cardiol. 1991;17(6):1334–42.
26. Baur X, Clasen M, Fissler-Eckhoff A, et al. Diagnostisch und Begutachtung asbestbedingter Berufskrankheiten. Interdisziplinäre S 2-Leitlinie der Deutschen Gesellschaft für Pneumologie und Beatmungsmedizin und der Deutschen Gesellschaft für Arbeitsmedizin und Umweltmedizin. Pneumologie. 2011;65:e1–e47.
27. Reichenhaller, Empfehlung 2012: Deutsche Gesetzliche Unfallversicherung (DGUV). Empfehlung für die Begutachtung der Berufskrankheiten der Nummern 1315 (ohne Alveolitis), 4301 und 4302 der Anlage zur Berufskrankheiten-Verordnung (BKV). Berlin: DGUV; 2012.

23

Prevalence of hidden carbon monoxide poisoning in auto service workers

Oğuzhan Bol[1*], Serhat Koyuncu[2] and Nurullah Günay[3]

Abstract

Background: Carbon monoxide (CO) is formed as a result of the incomplete burning of hydrocarbon-containing fuels such as natural gas, coal, liquid petroleum gas, and wood. CO is a colorless, odorless, and poisonous gas that produces various acute and chronic effects in CO-exposed people. In this study, we aimed to measure CO levels in auto care repairmen with chronic CO-related illnesses using a serial, non-invasive method.
A prospective cohort study.

Methods: A total of 99 people from six different auto-repair services were included in the study. Carboxyhemoglobin (COHb) levels were measured at four different times with 2-hour intervals starting at 08:00 AM. Data concerning employees' ages, working hours, smoking statuses, and types of home heating fuel were collected. A control group of 100 cases was created based on this data. The measurements were done on the control group in the morning with a Masimo Rad-57 CO-oximeter.

Results: The highest mean (± SD) COHb value was 7.04% ± 3.32% after the third measurement. The mean value for the control group was 1.61% ± 1.43%. A statistically significant difference between the groups was found for each value.

Discussion: We determined that the risk of being affected by CO is high in buildings in which the auto services were located. The effects of chronic or prolonged exposure to low amounts of CO were found to be ambiguous. However, in some studies, it was found that low-grade CO exposure could lead to coronary artery disease and some neurological complications. Therefore, it is necessary to be careful about the health of employees who have been exposed to CO.

Conclusions: We concluded that there is a need for more detailed studies concerning chronic CO poisoning. Also, in workplaces in which there is high exposure to CO, proper workplace safety measures should be taken to reduce this gas's harmful effects to employees.

Objectives

Carbon monoxide (CO) is a colorless and odorless toxic gas [1, 2] that is produced mainly as a result of incomplete combustion of hydrocarbon fuels such as natural gas, coal, liquefied petroleum gas, and wood [1, 3, 4]. In people's daily lives, environmental CO exposure is typically < 0.001% or 10 ppm (ppm) [1, 2, 5]. While an adult cigarette smoker is exposed to an estimated 400 to 500 ppm of CO during active smoking, automobile exhaust may contain around 100,000 ppm CO as measured inside a closed garage [1, 4, 6]. Based on these values, the Air Quality Guidelines for Europe (Second Edition), which were published by the World Health Organisation, stated that a COHb level of 2.5% should not be exceeded depending on the CO levels in the environment and duration of exposure. Ambient CO values that are required to reach this maximal acceptable value of serum COHb are presented in Table 1 in units of mg/m^3 and ppm [5].

Reports on the acute phase of CO gas exposure are prevalent, whereas chronic exposure has rarely been reported. Chronic CO exposure is considered to be more prevalent and much more closely associated with increased morbidity and mortality than previously accepted or assumed [1, 2]. Chronic exposure is defined as prolonged

* Correspondence: mariachiozi@gmail.com
[1]Health Science University Kayseri Training and Research Hospital Emergency Medicine Department, Kayseri, Turkey
Full list of author information is available at the end of the article

Table 1 Air Quality Guidelines for Europe, Second Edition published by the World Health Organisation (WHO) state that a carboxyhemoglobin (COHb) level of 2.5% should not be exceeded as determined in ambient carbon monoxide (CO) concentrations after a given exposure period

CO concentration (mg/m^3)	CO concentration (ppm)	Exposure Time (Minute)
100	90	15
60	50	30
30	25	60
10	10	480

exposure to low amounts of CO [7]. Chronic exposure can be an underlying cause of nonspecific complaints such as headaches, nausea, vomiting, and asthenia and dizziness in addition to clinical manifestations, including cerebellar dysfunction and acute coronary syndrome [1, 2].

CO poisoning is quite common among the population but there are certain occupational groups who carry a greater risk of exposure to this gas due to their occupation [8]. These occupational groups include auto service maintenance personnel, exhaust pipe repairmen, chefs using ovens or grills in which charcoal is used, gasoline pumpers, and traffic policemen. Although chronic exposure of these people to CO gas has been reported previously, insufficient scientific data exist concerning possible chronic daytime CO exposure of these individuals, particularly the ones who work in auto service centers [9]. Therefore, autoworkers were selected as the target occupational group for this study.

Study design

A prospective cohort study was conducted.

Methods

This study was conducted between 10.12.2012 and 10.01.2013 after obtaining approval from the local and ethics committees (Erciyes University Ethics Committee approval date: 04.12.2012 and the Decision Number: 2012/701). A total of 99 male employees working at six different car service centers in Kayseri were included. For each participant, a total of four serial daytime CO measurements were made, and COHb levels were recorded on the same day starting at 08:00 AM (beginning of office hours) followed by measurements at 10.00 AM, 12.00 PM and 14.00 PM. The measurements were done at the workplace and were performed in a noninvasive manner with Masimo Rad-57 Oximeter (Masimo Corporation, Irvine), which has an accuracy of 3% according to the manufacturer. The device has the same format as the commonly known finger pulse oximeter. Additionally, workers were asked questions such as whether they smoked, what kind of fuel they used to heat their home, how long they had been working, and whether they had recently complained of a headache, weakness, nausea, insomnia, and/or confusion (delay in understanding what has been said). In order to be eligible for this study, the car service had to be a closed area and heated without using an energy source that potentially emits CO (such as charcoal/ wood or similar fuels). Inclusion criteria for autoworkers included a minimum of 1 month of work experience at their current auto service, > 18 years of age, and working in the auto service's mechanic division.

A control group of 100 subjects who were matched with the study group with regard to age, gender, and the use of a stove or natural gas for heating was included. The control group consisted of the relatives of patients who were admitted to the emergency department triage unit between 08:00 AM and 10:00 AM. As with the study group, the ones with a chronic illness were excluded by evaluating them with routine histories and physical examinations. Also, initial COHb values of the study group were compared with those of control group.

The following protocol was applied for autoworkers with regard to the measurement of COHb levels: The threshold COHb value was determined as 10% in smokers and 5% in non-smokers, and any value exceeding this was considered an indication of CO poisoning. Threshold levels of COHb poisoning were determined with reference to previous studies [10–12]. Workers with symptoms of acute poisoning were admitted to our emergency department and managed by emergency medicine physicians. An additional blood sample was obtained from these individuals, and patients were treated if toxicity was detected.

Data from patient and control groups were recorded into the licensed SPSS (IBM, ver21, United State) software package. Categorical variables were compared using the chi-square exact test. Normal distribution of numerical variables was checked using the Shapiro-Wilk test. Comparisons between measurements were performed by one-way repeated variance analysis (ANOVA) and multiple comparisons were performed using the Bonferroni test. Two independent sample t- and one-way ANOVA tests were used for intergroup comparisons. The relationship between numerical variables was evaluated by Pearson's correlation analysis. A p-value < 0.05 was considered statistically significant.

Results

Of 14 auto service centers with a certificate of authorization for operating in the city of Kayseri, six were included in the study. In this study group of 99 workers, duration of work experience in the field of occupation ranged between 3 months and 25 years with a mean ± SD of 15.16 ± 9.9 years. Their ages ranged from 18 to 45 years (mean ± SD, 31.59 ± 8.98). For the control group, ages ranged between 19 and 45 years (mean ± SD, 30.4 ± 7.4).

COHb values of the groups, smoking statuses, and types of heating are shown in Fig. 1. In the study group, the highest and lowest COHb values were 18 and 0%, respectively. In the control group, the corresponding COHb values were 4 and 0%, respectively.

In our study, 10 smokers (18%) with a COHb value of $\geq$ 10% and 33 non-smokers (73%) with a COHb value $\geq$ 5% were detected at any time of measurement.

When we analyzed the results individually, the highest COHb values of 15, 15, 18, 13, 11 and 15% were obtained from six different auto service centers after four measurements. The total number of workers who had at least one measurement exceeding the pre-specified threshold exposure level of 5 or 10% based on smoking status were nine, five, 10, five, six, and eight, and a total of 43 workers were found to have threshold levels that exceeded this level.

Among workers, the highest mean (± SD) COHb value of 7.040 ± 3.32% was obtained during the third measurement. The mean (± SD) value was 1.61 ± 1.43% in the control group. Other values are shown in Table 2.

Differences between four measurements and the relationship of the values obtained with smoking and the type of heating were also analyzed for the study group. Values obtained from the control group were statistically analyzed together with the initial values of the study group.

Within the study group, there was a significant difference in COHb levels from all four measurements.

This difference between measurements was also significant when each sub-group in the control and test subject groups was compared: smokers ($p < 0.001$), nonsmokers ($p = 0.004$), charcoal users ($P = 0.004$), and natural gas users ($p < 0.001$) employees.

For the study group, a statistically significant difference in mean COHb was obtained at the third measurement at 12:00 PM was detected between smoking and non-smoking employees ($p = 0.021$). Other measurements did not show a statistically significant difference; $p = 0.28$ at 08:00 AM, $p = 0.10$ at 10:00 AM, and $p = 0.33$ at 02:00 PM (Fig. 2).

For the study group, a statistically significant difference was not found when workers using natural gas for heating were compared with workers using charcoal.

A statistically significant difference was observed between all measurements of study group and control group ($p < 0.001$).

When we analyzed smokers in the study and control groups, a statistical difference was not found between COHb values. Nonsmokers in study and control groups did not show significant differences regarding the measured COHb values either. (Table 3).

There was no statistically significant difference in measured COHb values between study and control groups regarding those who used natural gas for heating. Similarly, a significant difference was not observed in measured

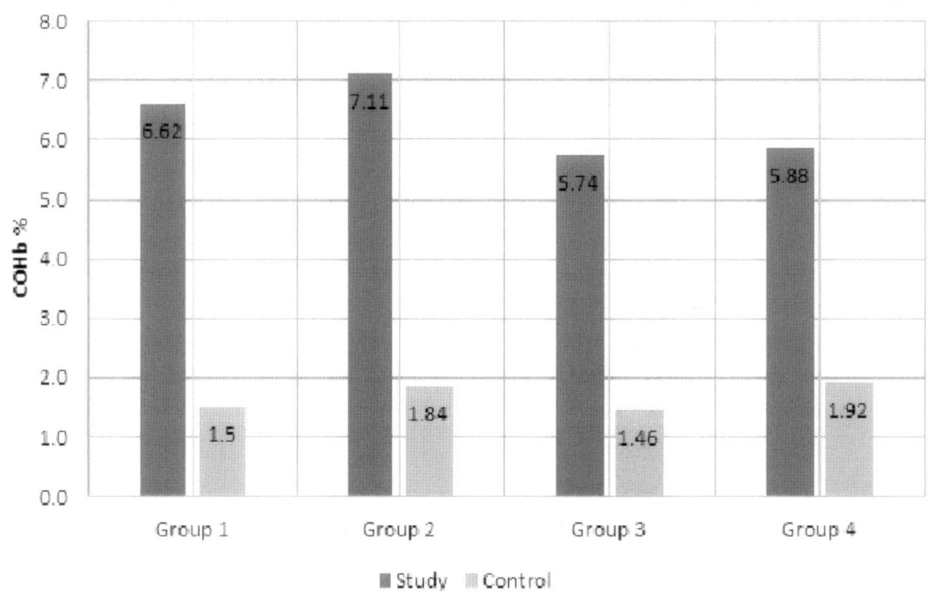

Fig. 1 Carboxyhemoglobin values in workers and controls, stratified by smoking status and home heating system. **Group 1:** Smokers who use natural gas for heating (study; n:35, control; n:36, min-max value worker and control group; 0–18 and 0–4, 95% CI of study group 5.68% to 7.55%). **Group 2**: Smokers who use charcoal for heating (study; n:19, control; n:19) (study; n:19, control; n:19, min-max value worker and control group; 1–15 and 0–4, 95% CI of study group 5.84% to 8.38%). **Group 3:** Non-smokers who use natural gas for heating (study; n:32, control; n:32, min-max worker value and control group; 0–13 and 0–4, 95% CI of study group 4.76% to 6.72%). **Group 4**: Non-smokers who use charcoal for heating (study; n:13, control; n:13, min-max value worker and control group; 0–14 and 0–4, 95% CI of study group 4.34% to 7.42%)

Table 2 Mean carboxyhemoglobin [%] in the control and study groups at different time points

	08:00	10:00	12:00	14:00
Study Group	5.21 ± 3.23	6.44 ± 3.34	7.04 ± 3.32	6.64 ± 3.28
Control Group	1.61 ± 1.43	–	–	–

COHb values between study and control groups for those who used charcoal for heating.

Discussion

We believe that CO poisoning cases other than acute poisoning are even more remarkable because of the difficulty of detecting such cases and the impossibility of finding them without definitive proof. Diagnosis of chronic CO poisoning in patients admitted to emergency services is still not easy as the presence of similar clinical presentations cannot be excluded. CO gas may harm any cell in the body which is dependent on oxygen regardless of its amount, causing a range of conditions from acute coronary syndrome to detectable damages in the brain [1]. Based on this knowledge, we planned to conduct a study with autoworkers due to their involvement in an occupational group that is known to be associated with risk factors for CO-related chronic poisoning and because of the inability to diagnose such cases in the emergency room.

Even the highest and lowest COHb values (18 and 0%, respectively) that are found in members of an occupational group who had a risk factor for chronic CO exposure alone supported our hypothesis that chronic and even acute effects of CO poisoning can be seen in autoworkers. That is to say, breathing CO of 18% itself calls for suspicion of an acute poisoning that requires urgent treatment. However, we believe that the aforementioned complaints are often overlooked and not verbally expressed in daily life and/or thought of as signs of other ailments. Another possibility is that even if employees are chronically exposed to CO, they might spontaneously recover from its effects before they decide to seek medical attention, which would preclude a proper diagnosis at the time of presentation. Our research may be valuable for demonstrating the possible effects of CO exposure in the sense that measurements should be performed right after exposure and at the site of exposure. On the other hand, detection of a

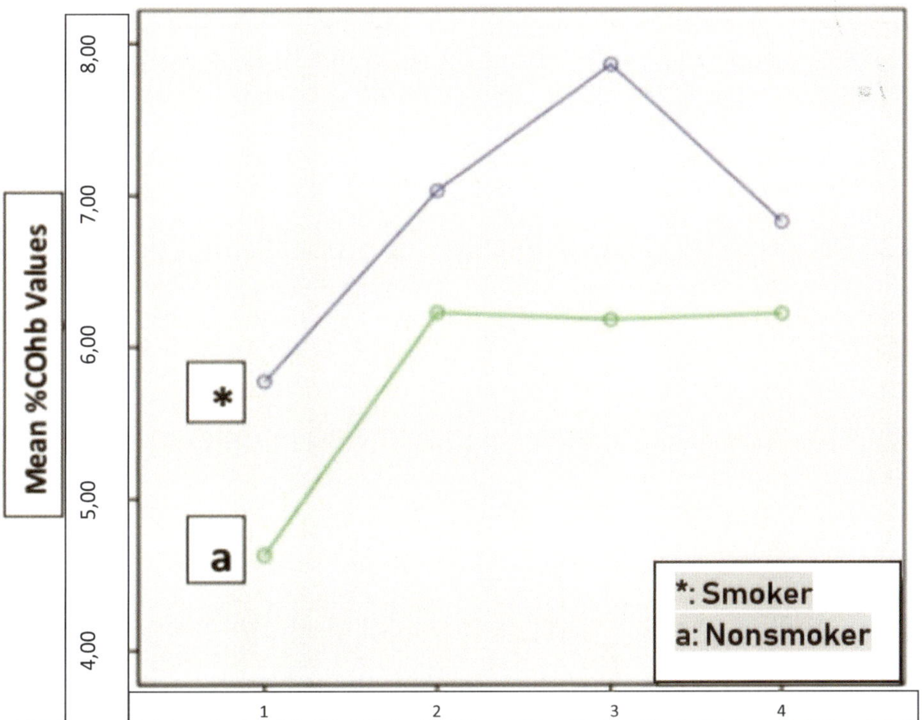

Hours:	08:00	10:00	12:00	14:00
P values:	p:0.28	p:0.10	p:0.021	p:0.33
5th-95th% Smoker	4.85-6.68	6.09-7.96	6.93-8.78	5.88-7.75
Nonsmoker	3.57-5.68	5.14-7.30	5.10-7.24	5.14-7.29

Fig. 2 Statistical difference in mean carboxyhemoglobin between the 4 different measurements times in the study group

Table 3 CoHb values in smokers and non-smokers in the study and control groups

	95% Confidence Interval for Mean Lower Bound/Upper Bound	Mean, Min-Max
CoHb values in smokers (n:109)	2,9566/ 4,2361	3,5963, 0–17
CoHb values in non-smokers (n:90)	2,6048/ 3,7285	3,1667, 0–10

COHb value of 0% was interpreted as a lack of absolute homogeneity in a given auto service and accordingly, autoworkers may be exposed to CO at different levels depending on their location and the work they perform in the auto service.

By examining the number of workers with values exceeding the threshold, one might assume that these workers are chronically affected by CO gas and beyond that, they are actually on the brink of acute poisoning. Since elevated COHb values were detected in 43 workers in the study group, all of them were invited to be examined in our emergency department because of the possibility of acute poisoning. Among these workers, 33 accepted the invitation and came to the emergency department after work followed by diagnostic testing and treatment. During this time, invasive COHb measurements were conducted to confirm exposure to CO gas, and 26 workers who were found to have serum COHb values exceeding the pre-determined threshold were administered normobaric oxygen treatment at a flow rate of 2 to 4 L/min for nearly 1 h. The absence of complaints at the time of ER admission in the other workers with normal serum COHb values, which were detected by invasive measurements, suggested that workers might have experienced clinical relief as a result of being away from the CO source and cleared the CO gas during the time period after leaving the workplace until admission to the emergency department. Workers were discharged after evaluation of both laboratory parameters and symptoms (if there were any) as observed by pre- and post-treatment monitoring, and they were considered to be affected by CO gas. Despite the presence of a control group, baseline COHb value of the workers was also determined using their initial measurements. Even when the control group was not considered, readings in the study group obtained at 10:00 AM, 12:00 PM, and 02:00 PM were found to be significantly elevated compared to their baseline values. Thus, during the day, workers continued to be incrementally affected by CO gas at 2-h interval beginning from the time (08:00 AM) they started working. As a study objective, smoking habits and types of home heating were also examined in detail in order to demonstrate the presence of an occupational risk factor for chronic CO exposure after taking these parameters into account.

Employees usually do their job in a closed area and remain continuously close to a CO source, especially in the presence of running motor vehicles. In our study, a possible CO source was considered to be the auto service center itself. Although there were smokers among the employees, we observed that they avoided smoking in closed areas of all areas of the car services. Thus, the car service was considered to be the CO source among nonsmokers.

While subsequent COHb readings were elevated compared to baseline, a statistically significant increase that was found at the third measurement of smokers was not due to smoking alone. This elevated third reading was considered to be associated with increased admission of more motor vehicles during that time period to the car service. Another interesting point was that the third reading roughly coincided with the time of the employees' lunch break. During this break, smokers were observed to smoke cigarettes more frequently.

A comprehensive study similar to ours was conducted by Kelman et al. who measured the serum COHb values of 61 employees working at 35 Leicestershire garages. A single sample was obtained in that study, which found elevated COHb values in 20% of smokers and 43.8% of non-smokers. Their threshold values were the same as ours ($\geq$ 10% for smokers and 5% for nonsmokers); however, the authors did not take the difference between invasive and non-invasive measurements into account (11). As an interesting finding in our study, elevated COHb values were obtained among non-smokers in contrast to that study. Smokers are exposed to a certain amount of CO on a daily basis as a result of to their habit, but nonsmokers are only exposed to CO at their workplaces. Persistently high CO exposure among nonsmokers and continuous near-threshold CO exposure among smokers puts these individuals at a higher risk for chronic CO poisoning. Also, our study used serial measurements instead of a single reading. Since CO exposure was monitored among both smokers and nonsmokers throughout the day, we believe that our study demonstrates the danger of chronic exposure more accurately.

In a study by C. M. Castleden et al., COHb values obtained from smoking and non-smoking employees working in different occupations were analyzed. Smokers were found to have a significantly higher mean COHb value (5.8%) in comparison to that of nonsmokers (1.3%) [13]. In the present study, smoking and non-smoking employees differed only with regard to the values of the third measurement.

We conducted a literature scan in order to identify the studies that focused on a link between CO exposure and the type of home heating used by employees and could not find one. When we analyzed CO values according to the type of household heating, a statistically significant association was not found. Before initiating the study, we expected to see different results among employees who used charcoal for home heating. We also considered that a possible CO elevation cannot be identified among employees based on these data during the time period between leaving the house and starting of jobs.

We obtained a statistically significant difference between the data that were obtained from the study and control groups. This major difference that we observed between control group consisting of individuals who left their living environment and were admitted to hospital in the early hours and the study group might actually indicate the risks that the study group encounters on a daily basis. Workers in the study group are exposed to a considerable amount of CO not only for a short-term but also throughout their office hours and even for the majority of their lifetime. Moreover, we believe that these individuals might experience a diminished quality of life over long-term, especially after considering their smoking habits.

In one study, G. Kocasoyet al. compared CO and COHb before and after working values obtained from 72 employees and those of a control group (smoking and non-smoking), who worked at the Istanbul Bosphorus Bridge tolls. In comparison to the control group, CO and COHb values showed a statistically significant difference between smoking and non-smoking employees. A significant difference was found between smoking and non-smoking employees with regard to CO and COHb values before and after working hours [14]. In the present study, the opposite results were obtained. There was a statistically significant difference between our study and control groups with regard to CO values; the study group had a significantly elevated CO exposure. However, we did not find a statistically significant difference between the study and control groups when we examined smoking and non-smoking employees separately.

In a study by M. Abdollahi et al., bus drivers working in the city center were found to have significantly higher blood COHb values (4.19% ± 0.65%) compared to those of control group (1.09% ± 0.27%) [15]. These findings are similar to ours.

S. Nizaet al. conducted a study with employees working in toll bridges and offices in the surrounding area and found higher COHb levels among toll bridge workers than office employees. They observed an increase in the COHb levels, especially during the rush hour when the traffic intensity increased [16]. These findings are consistent with ours.

What these three studies have in common is the presence of elevated COHb values among employees who are exposed to intense exhaust gas at their workplaces. These results are also consistent with ours. In this study, COHb levels of the study group were significantly higher than the control group. These data show that individuals working in garages are persistently exposed to the effects of CO when compared to people living under normal environmental conditions.

To this date, studies have investigated the effects of chronic CO exposure in different occupational groups. However, no studies using serial measurements have been conducted that have explored possible chronic CO exposure among auto service workers. As a result of the data presented in this study, it can be concluded that auto workers were chronically exposed to a substantial amount of CO gas during their working hours irrespective of their smoking habits and from the carbon-based fuels they use for heating their homes. At this point, as researchers, we are left in the dark regarding long-term clinical manifestations that may occur in the participating auto workers. A study of the long-term clinical manifestations might be an interesting starting point for enthusiastic researchers who wish to conduct further extensive studies about this matter.

Limitations

The most important limitation of this study was the lack of air sampling from the environment around the study or the control group.

Authors' contributions

This article is the thesis of the OB. OB and NG developed the project and selected the variables. NG coordinated the project and OB collected, interpreted and drafted all the data. SK was involved in the composition at the organizational level of the control group data collection. All writers contributed to the discussion. All authors gave their final approval of the version to be published and agreed to be responsible for all aspects of the work to ensure that questions about the integrity or completeness of any part of the work were appropriately researched and resolved.

Consent for publication

Not applicable

Competing interests

The authors declare that they have no competing interests.

Author details

[1]Health Science University Kayseri Training and Research Hospital Emergency Medicine Department, Kayseri, Turkey. [2]Gaziosmanpasa University Emergency Medicine, Tokat, Turkey. [3]Erciyes University Emergency Medicine, Kayseri, Turkey.

References

1. Kao LW, Nañagas KA. Carbon monoxide poisoning. Med Clin North Am. 2005;89:1161–94.
2. Tintinalli JE, Kelen GD, Stapczynski JS. Tintinalli's emergency medicine a comprehensive study guide. 7th ed; 2011.
3. Blumenthal I. Carbon monoxide poisoning. J R Soc Med. 2001;94:270–2.
4. Abelsohn A, Sanborn MD, Jessiman BJ, Weir E. Identifying and managing adverse environmental health effects: 6. Carbon monoxide poisoning. Can Med Assoc J. 2002;166(13):1685–90.
5. WHO Air Quality Guidelines. 2000. Available from: http://www.euro.who.int/__data/assets/pdf_file/0005/74732/E71922.pdf.
6. Federal-Provincial Advisory Committee On Environmental And Occupational Health (Canada). Exposure guidelines for residential indoor air quality: a report of the federal-provincial advisory committee on environmental and occupational health. Rev Ed Otta.
7. Townsend CL, Maynard RL. Effects on health of prolonged exposure to low concentrations of carbon monoxide. Occup Environ Med. 2002;59(10):708–11.
8. Brvar M, Luzar B, Finderle Z, Šuput D, Bunc M. The time-dependent protective effect of hyperbaric oxygen on neuronal cell apoptosis in carbon monoxide poisoning. Inhal Toxicol. 2010;22(12):1026–31.
9. Güvendik G, Yılmaz A. Egzos kirliliğine maruz kalan kişilerde kan karboksihemoglobin düzeyi. Adli Tıp Bülteni. 2001;6(2).
10. O'donnell P, Buxton PJ, Pitkin A, Jarvis LJ. The magnetic resonance imaging appearances of the brain in acute carbon monoxide poisoning. Clin Radiol. 2000;55(4):273–80.
11. Kelman GR, Davies TJ. Carboxyhaemoglobin levels in workers in Leicestershire garages. Br J Ind Med. 1979;36(3):238–41.
12. Heliövaara M, Karvonen MJ, Vilhunen R, Punsar S. Smoking, carbon monoxide, and atherosclerotic diseases. Br Med J. 1978;1(6108):268.
13. Castleden CM, Cole PV. Carboxyhaemoglobin levels of smokers and non-smokers working in the City of London. Br J Ind Med. 1975;32(2):115–8.
14. Kocasoy G, Yalin H. Determination of carboxyhemoglobin levels and health effects on officers working at the Istanbul Bosphorus bridge. J Environ Sci Heal Part A. 2004;39(4):1129–39.
15. Abdollahi M, Zadparvar L, Ayatollahi B, Baradaran M, Nikfar S, Hastaie P. Hazard from carbon monoxide poisoning for bus drivers in Tehran, Iran. Bull Environ Contam Toxicol 1998;61(2):210–215.
16. Niza S, Jamal HH. Carbon monoxide exposure assessment among toll operators in Klang Valley, Kuala Lumpur, Malaysia. Int J Environ Health Res Nisan. 2007;17(2):95–103.

24

Hepatitis C in healthcare personnel: secondary data analysis of therapies with direct-acting antiviral agents

Claudia Westermann[1*], Dana Wendeler[2] and Albert Nienhaus[1,2]

Abstract

Background: Hepatitis C Virus (HCV) infections are blood-borne, generally chronic and are associated with increased morbidity and mortality. The aim of this study is to describe the results of therapies with direct-acting antiviral agents (DAAs) in healthcare personnel.

Methods: Secondary data analysis using data from the Statutory Accident Insurance of the Health and Welfare Service. The study surveyed DAA therapies administered to insured parties (healthcare personnel with an HCV infection recognised as an occupational disease) in Germany between 01/01/2014 and 30/11/2016. The end points were results of monitorings carried out twelve weeks after the end of treatment (SVR12), side effects and the results of the assessment of reduced work ability after treatment. Multivariate logistic regression models were constructed to model SVR12.

Results: The study population (n = 180) comprised 74% women, 90% of the participants had an HCV genotype 1 infection. Two-thirds had fibrosis or cirrhosis and were treatment experienced. The most common combined therapy was ledipasvir and sofosbuvir (49%). A DAA therapy with ribavirin was administered in 20% of cases, with (pegylated) interferon and ribavirin used in 2% of cases. The majority of therapies were completed without any side effects. The overall SVR12 rate was 94%. Significant independent predictor of decrease odds of SVR12 was liver cirrhosis. Positive effects on the healthcare personnel's work ability were observed after successful therapy.

Conclusion: High SVR12 rates were achieved in the sample population, with positive effects on their work ability. Early HCV therapy seems reasonable due to the increased chance of successful treatment of the infection.

Keywords: Hepatitis C virus, Occupational exposure, Blood-borne infections, Healthcare personnel, Direct-acting antiviral agents

Background

The hepatitis C virus (HCV) is one of the most common infectious diseases in the world and develops into a chronic infection in up to 85% of cases. According to data from the World Health Organisation (WHO), approx. 71 million people globally have a chronic hepatitis C (CHC) infection [1, 2]. CHC is associated with higher morbidity and higher mortality [2, 3]. The use of direct-acting antiviral agents (DAAs) is currently leading to a major shift in the management of chronic HCV infections. DAAs open up the possibility for efficient oral therapy regimens with fewer side effects for patients with or without treatment experience. As recent studies have shown, interferon-free DAA treatments have achieved substantial sustained virological response rates (SVRs) of over 90% [4, 5]. For CHC infections, treatment success is achieved when the HCV virus's RNA can no longer be detected in the blood (SVR), generally twelve weeks after the end of treatment [6, 7]. SVRs are associated with lowering morbidity and mortality caused by CHC [8, 9].

* Correspondence: c.westermann@uke.de
[1]Competence Centre for Epidemiology and Health Services Research for Healthcare Professionals (CVcare), Institute for Health Services Research in Dermatology and Nursing (IVDP), University Medical Centre Hamburg-Eppendorf (UKE), Martinistr. 52, 20146 Hamburg, Germany
Full list of author information is available at the end of the article

Healthcare personnel (HP) have contact with infected patients as part of their work. Injuries caused by sharp or pointed objects are some of the most commonly reported workplace accidents [10]. In Germany, reports detailing a reasonable suspicion of occupational illness are submitted to the statutory accident insurance carriers. Despite being on the decrease, Hepatitis C is still one of the most common infections leading to the recognition of an occupational illness among German HP. It is also the most common reason for newly approved retirement on the grounds of occupational disease [11]. Data analysis of an accident insurer shows that despite the number of cases has declined, the costs of HCV infection as an occupational disease (OD) have been significantly increasing over the past 15 years. These costs are the result of the increase in compensation payments for retirement on the grounds of OD and, since 2012, as a result of an increase in the cost of the drugs used to treat the infection [12]. The high costs of DAA therapies are offset by the potentially considerable benefits. The aim of this study is to investigate the treatment results of the DAA therapies in HP.

Methods

Analysis of the DAA therapies using data from the Statutory Accident Insurance of the Health and Welfare Service (Berufsgenossenschaft für Gesundheitsdienst und Wohlfahrtspflege, BGW). This analysis was carried out in line with the Consensus German Reporting Standard for Secondary Data Analyses (STROSA) [13]. When applying for DAA therapy for a HP with an occupational CHC infection, the BGW collects data (using a standardised input mask (Excel table)) about the course of treatment for the purposes of conducting an analysis. For quality assurance purposes, this process was discussed and aided by the BGW's Occupational Diseases working group. Following data was anonymised extracted from doctors' letters and test results in the insured party's medical files: genotype, reduced work ability (RWA) grading, treatments used, treatment status (naive/experienced), cirrhosis (yes/no), start and end of treatment (duration), treatment result (RNA evidence), side effects, and assessment of the RWA after DAA therapy. The analysis included data from insured individuals who completed DAA therapy between 01/01/2014 and 30/11/2016 and for whom treatment results were available twelve weeks after the end of therapy. In cases of treatment failure directly following the end of therapy, if there was no data available at twelve weeks after the end of treatment, it was also assumed that treatment had failed. Evidence of virus RNA twelve weeks after the end of treatment following previous ETR (end-of-treatment sustained virological response) was considered a relapse. The end points investigated were treatment success twelve weeks after the end of treatment (SVR12), side effects and the results of assessment of the RWA after the conclusion of DAA therapy.

Determination of RWA in occupational disease procedures

Statutory accident insurance is one of the pillars of German social insurance. On the basis of the 7th German Social Security Code (Siebtes Buch, Sozialgesetzbuch, SGB VII), every employer is legally obliged to insure employees against accidents at work. The sponsorship of statutory accident insurance, the group of insured persons and the procedure in the event of a claim as well as the benefits in the event of an insured event are regulated in this code of law. The essential benefit for insured persons who get injured at the workplace following an accident or who suffer an occupational disease is the entitlement to compensation if their performance and thus their ability to work cannot be fully restored. This entitlement for the injured person's pension is dependent on the assessment of the RWA and the extent to which the reduction in the physical and mental capacity of an insured person restricts their work opportunities. In the event of a complete loss of working ability (100%), a full pension is paid, which amounts to two thirds of the annual earnings before the occupational disease. In the case of a partial RWA, a partial pension corresponding to the degree of RWA is paid. The entitlement starts with a RWA of at least 20%. For claimants suffering HCV, the RWA is determined by the fibrosis stage and the degree of inflammatory activity of the disease. The initial assessment requires a detailed anamnesis, the clinical status and an abdominal sonography as well as a sufficient laboratory program with clinical-chemical, virological and immunoserological parameters. A reliable differential diagnostic and functional assessment of the liver situation needs to be ensured. Further assessment criteria are the probable duration and the course of the disease and the associated statement on the prognosis. A RWA of 20% should be granted when the CHC infection is accompanied with an increased concentration of the liver enzymes but not with a fibrosis of the liver, whereas a RWA of 50 to 100% should be granted when a cirrhosis is present. However, the grading is performed individually and personal circumstances like fatigue or depression should also be considered. The grading is performed by the case manager of the insurance with the support of a physician. The RWA determines the amount of the pension to be paid, even over the period of working life.

Statistical analysis

Univariate comparisons were made to describe the correlations between treatment success (SVR12) and the categorical variables treatment status (naive/experienced), cirrhosis (yes/no), RWA (≤50%/> 50%) and gender. The significance of the correlations was tested using the Fisher's exact test. Pearson's correlation coefficient was calculated to measure the statistical association between age and RWA. Multivariate logistic regression models were constructed to model SVR12. Models included cirrhosis, prior treatment, gender, and age (as a continuous variable). Nagelkerke's R-squared was calculated and used to derive Cohen's effect size [14]. Using the measure according to Cohen, an *f*-value of 0.10 equates to a small effect, an *f*-value of 0.25 to a medium effect and an *f*-value of 0.40 to a large effect. For all comparisons, a *p*-Value < 0.05 was considered statistically significant. Data analysis was done using IBM SPSS Statistics version 23.

Results

During the analysis period, a DAA therapy was administered to 180 HP and the SVR was determined twelve weeks after the end of treatment.

Description of the sample (Table 1)

The mean age of the insured individuals was 62 years. For the period under analysis, 60% were under the statutory retirement age of 65 years. The sample population comprised 74% women. The most common type of infection among the sample was HCV genotype 1 (91%), with individual cases caused by viruses of genotypes 2, 3 or 4. No co-morbidities with Hepatitis B or HIV infections were documented. There were histological indications in 76% of the participants (fibrosis 43%; compensated or decompensated cirrhosis 24 and 9%, respectively) before the DAA therapy started and 72% had already experienced a prior treatment. More than 90% of the insured individuals had a RWA, approximately a third had a RWA of more than 50%.

Table 1 Baseline characteristics (n = 180)

Characteristic (missing values n/%)	Valid values n	%
Gender		
Women	133	74
Men	47	26
Age		
Mean (SD)	62 (10)	
Median/Minimum/Maximum	62/21/88	
Age group		
30–39	4	2
40–49	12	7
50–59	50	28
60–64	42	23
≥ 65[a]	72	40
Genotype (11/6)		
1 sub-type not recognised	15	9
1a	50	29
1b	88	52
2	6	4
3	7	4
3a	2	1
4	1	< 1
RWA % (5/3)		
0 < 20	12	7
20	59	34
30–40	46	26
50–60	35	20
70–80	11	6
90–100	12	7
Stage of liver disease (28/16)		
No findings	37	24
Fibrosis	65	43
Compensated cirrhosis	37	24
Decompensated cirrhosis	13	9
Therapy status (21/12)		
Naive	45	28
Experienced	114	72

[a]statutory retirement age; *RWA* reduced work ability, *SD* standard deviation

DAA-regimens and side effects (Table 2)

The most common treatment was a combination therapy of ledipasvir (LDV) and sofosbuvir (SOF) (n = 88/49%). A DAA therapy with ribavirin (RBV) was administered in 36 cases (20%), and (pegylated) interferon (PEG-IFN) and RBV were used in four cases (2%). Treatment duration was between eight and 24 weeks, with the majority lasting twelve weeks (71%). For 67% of insured individuals, the treatment was not associated with any side effects. The most common side effect was a combination of mild symptoms such as headaches, nausea and sleep disorders and/or fatigue (26%). 4% of the sample population suffered from skin reactions (pruritus to generalised skin rash, phototoxic reactions), and there were individual cases of decrease in haemoglobin, feelings of anxiety or depression and isolated gastrointestinal disorders. Side effects not linked to the DAA therapy, but seen as symptoms of an advanced CHC infection were summarised as other side effects (bleeding of the oesophageal varices, incipient hepatorenal syndrome). The observed side effects of a decrease in haemoglobin (n = 2) occurred in DAA therapy (LDV/SOF) combined with RBV in priory treated patients with liver cirrhosis. These therapies were conducted for twelve or 24 weeks and led to SVR12 in the insured individuals. Anxiety and depression were observed in

Table 2 DAA treatment regimens and results ($n = 180$)

Characteristic (missing values n/%)	Valid values	
	n	%
Therapies total (2/1)	178	
LDV, SOF	88	49
SOF, DCV	29	16
LDV, SOF, RBV	17	10
SOF, SMV	11	6
DSV, OBV, PTV, RTV, RBV	11	6
DSV, OBV, PTV, RTV	9	5
SOF, RBV	7	4
SOF, RBV, PEG-IFN	3	2
DCV, SOF, RBV	1	< 1
SOF, SMV, RBV	1	< 1
PEG-IFN, TVR, RBV	1	< 1
Therapy result		
Directly after therapy (1/< 1)	179	
ETR	173	97
Remission	6	3
Twelve weeks after therapy	180	
SVR12	170	94
Remission/viral load unchanged	6	> 2
Relapse	4	> 3
Side effects (13/7)	167	
None	110	66
Headaches, nausea, sleep disorder	43	26
Skin reactions	6	4
Anaemia	2	> 1
Depression, anxiety	2	> 1
Gastrointestinal disorders	2	> 1
Other[a]	2	> 1

[a]Manifestation of advanced infection (hepatorenal syndrome $n = 1$, bleeding of oesophageal varices n = 1); *DAA* direct-acting antiviral agents, *LDV* ledipasvir, *SOF* sofosbuvir, *DCV* daclatasvir, *RBV* ribavirin, *RTV* ritonavir, *SMV* simeprevir, *DSV* dasabuvir, *OBV* ombitasvir, *PTV* paritaprevir, *PEG-IFN* pegylated interferon, *TVR* telaprevir, *ETR* end-of-treatment response, *SVR12* sustained virologic response twelve weeks after therapy

patients with treatment experience and without liver cirrhosis ($n = 2$) receiving DAA therapies in combination with ribavirin or PEG-IFN (SOF/RBV/PEG-IFN; dasabuvir (DSV)/ombitasvir (OBV)/paritaprevir (PTV)/ritonavir (RTV)/RBV). These were completed after the standard twelve weeks and led to SVR12 in the insured individuals.

Treatment results and summary statistics

The ETR rate was 97% and the SVR12 rate was 94% (Table 2). Virus RNA could still be detected in six individuals directly after the end of treatment. At the results monitoring twelve weeks after the end of treatment, six patients showed no change or a reduction in viral load, while four patients had a relapse (Additional file 1: Table S1). The results of univariate and logistic regression analysis regarding treatment response (SVR12) are described in Table 3. Prior experience of treatment resulted in no significant difference in terms of SVR12 (naive $n = 45$/experienced $n = 114$: SVR12 98% vs 94%, $p = 0.44$), while there was a statistically significant difference with regard to cirrhosis status. For individuals without cirrhosis ($n = 102$), the treatment was statistically significant more likely to be successful than for patients with diagnosed cirrhosis ($n = 50$) (SVR12 98% vs 86%, $p = 0.006$). For insured individuals with a RWA grading of ≤50% ($n = 139$), the DAA treatment was also statistically significant more likely to be successful than for patients with a higher RWA grading ($n = 36$) (SVR12 97% vs 86%, $p = 0.019$). It was somewhat more likely for women ($n = 133$) to reach SVR12 after therapy than men ($n = 47$) (SVR12 96% vs 89%, $p = 0.130$). The multivariate regression showed that cirrhosis was a statistically significant independent predictor of decrease odds of SVR12. Participants with cirrhosis were 10 percentage points less likely to reach SVR12 in comparison to patients without cirrhosis. This resulted in an adjusted OR of 0.098 (95% CI 0.01–0.75; $p = 0.03$). With an increase in age, there was also an increase in the probability of achieving SVR12 (OR 1.11; 95% CI 1.01–1.23, $p = 0.04$). The variables of prior treatment (OR 0.42; 95% CI 0.05–3.92; $p = 0.42$) and gender (OR 0.41; 95% CI 0.08–2.18; $p = 0.3$) showed no statistically significant correlation with the end-point SVR12 in the multivariate analysis. Nagelkerke's R-squared was 0.24, which corresponds to an f-value of 0.56, which Cohen classifies as a large effect size. The liver enzyme laboratory values (GOT, GPT, ɣGT) for 102 insured individuals at twelve weeks after the end of treatment were available at the time of the evaluation. For 90 (88%) of the individuals, the liver enzymes were in the normal range twelve weeks after the DAA therapy.

Evaluation of RWA after DAA therapy

Evaluation of RWA after DAA therapy was done for 115 (64%) of the insured individuals, on average nine months after the end of treatment. The RWA was adjusted for 87 (76%) of the insured individuals. The RWA determined before treatment lapsed for 56 individuals, 25 individuals had a decrease in the RWA after the evaluation and six increased their RWA (Table 4). Reasons for an increased RWA included liver transplant after successful DAA therapy, bleeding of the oesophageal varices and incipient hepatorenal syndrome. The correlation between age and RWA was low ($r = 0.16$, $p = 0.04$).

Table 3 Summary of univariate and logistic regression analysis for variables regarding treatment response SVR12 (n = 180)

Univariate analysis					
Variable	Missing values	n total	% SVR12 rates	OR (95% CI)	*p*-value
Cirrhosis (no/yes)	28	152 (102/50)	98% versus 86%	0.12 (0.03–0.62)	< 0.01
Treatment (naive/experienced)	21	159 (45/114)	97.8% versus 93.9%	0.35 (0.04–2.90)	NS
RWA (≤50%/> 50%)	5	175 (139/36)	97.1% versus 86.1%	0.18 (0.05–0.72)	< 0.05
Gender (women/men)	0	180 (133/47)	96.2% versus 87.5%	0.32 (0.09–1.19)	NS
Multivariate logistical regression model with SVR12 as end point					
Variable	Missing values	n total	OR (95% CI)	*p*-value	R^2
Cirrhosis (no/yes)	34	146 (98/48)	0.098 (0.01–0.75)	< 0.05	0.242
Treatment (naive/experienced)	34	146 (42/104)	0.42 (0.05–3.92)	NS	
Gender (women/men)	34	146 (112/34)	0.41 (0.08–2.18)	NS	
Age[a]	34	146	1.11 (1.01–1.23)	< 0.05	

SVR12 sustained virologic response twelve weeks after therapy, *RWA* reduced work ability; Dependent variables - the first category is established as a reference; [a]as a continuous variable; OR (odds ratio) for the primary end point of SVR12; *NS* non-significant

Discussion

Patients with and without experience of treatment who have a CHC infection achieved high SVR12 (94%) rates in the observed sample. Cirrhosis status (OR 0.098; 95% CI 0.01–0.75; p = 0.03) and age (OR 1.11; 95% CI 1.01–1.23; p = 0.04) had a significant correlation with treatment success. Significant independent predictor of decrease odds of SVR12 was liver cirrhosis. Even though, the correlation between age and SVR12 was statistically significant, advanced age is no barrier to DAA therapy. SVRs are associated with reducing morbidity and mortality resulting from a CHC infection, irrespective of individual cirrhosis status. They are also associated with an improvement in health-related quality of life [8, 9, 15, 16]. In the study population, positive effects on the patients' RWA were observed on average nine months after successful completion of therapy. An evaluation was carried out in 64% of the insured individuals after DAA therapy, showing an improvement in work ability for more than 70% of those being analysed. Hence we assume that pension payments will decrease as well.

In a study with patients with a genotype 1 HCV infection, Backus et al. [17] investigated predictors of achieving SVR (at least ten weeks after the end of treatment) to determine the efficacy of LDV/SOF ± RBV and OBV/PTV/RTV/DSV ± RBV. The variables included in the multivariate analysis were treatment status (naive/experienced), ethnic background, body mass index (BMI), cirrhosis status (FIB-4 > 3.25), age and gender. SVR rates of 94% were achieved in the patient collective (average age: 61, 96% male, 23% with experience of treatment, 30% with cirrhosis). Cirrhosis status (OR 0.60; 95% CI 0–49–0.72, p = 0.001), having an African-American background (OR 0.71; 95% CI 0.59–0.86, p = 0.001) and a BMI of ≥30 kg/m^2 (OR 0.73, 95% CI 0.60–0.89, p = 0.002) had a significant correlation with achieving SVR. In another study, no significant differences were found between treatment naive patients with and without cirrhosis in terms of SVR12 (97.9% vs 96.2%) [18]. Overall, the authors reported that no relapses were observed in patients once they had achieved SVR12. According to Zeuzem [19], the lack of evidence of HCV

Table 4 Reduced work ability before and after DAA therapy (n = 115)

RWA as %		After DAA therapy						Overall	
Before DAA therapy		0	20	30–40	50–60	70–80	90–100	n	%
	0	6	0	0	0	0	0	6	5.2
	20	38	7	1	0	0	0	46	40
	30–40	15	4	7	1	0	0	27	23.5
	50–60	2	2	10	6	0	0	20	17.4
	70–80	1	0	1	0	4	3	9	7.8
	90–100	0	0	0	0	4	3	7	6.1
Overall	n	62	13	19	7	8	6	115	
	%	53.9	11.3	16.5	6.1	7	5.2	100	100

RWA reduced work ability, *DAA* direct-acting antiviral agents

RNA twelve weeks after the end of DAA therapy signifies a permanent eradication of the virus. Relapses after this point are rare and generally take the form of a reinfection [19]. The most common DAA combination therapy administered in the observed sample was LDV/SOF (49%) and, according to Zimmermann et al. [20], was also the most commonly administered among patients with statutory health insurance in Germany (64%) in 2015. The frequency of the combination of DAA treatments with RBV was not quantified in that particular study. The authors stated a decrease in prescriptions of monthly PEG-IFN therapy regimes from around 2700 in January 2014 to around 650 in December 2015. In this study, a DAA therapy with RBV was administered in 36 cases (20%), and the combination with PEG-IFN and RBV was used in four cases (2%). Treatment was generally administered for twelve weeks (67%). Comparable treatment periods were also observed in the German Hepatitis Cohort (GECCO) [20]. The most commonly described side effects in our study, which were mainly described as mild, were nausea, headaches and sleep disorders, and were also listed by Zeuzem [19] for therapies with SOF and simeprevir (SMV). According to the author, photosensitivity reactions have also been observed during treatment using SMV. These were also observed in our study during combination treatment with SMV, without any consequences for the course of treatment. Decreased haemoglobin was observed in two DAA treatments with LDV/SOF in combination with RBV. The occurrence of haemolytic anaemia during treatment with RBV has been documented in the literature. The therapies were administered successfully (SVR12). In addition, side effects such as anxiety and depression were observed in two individuals with DAA treatments in combination with RBV or PEG-IFN (SOF/RBV/PEG-IFN, DSV/OBV/PTV/RTV/RBV). The treatments were successfully completed (SVR12). The occurrence of depression has been described in the literature both for PEG-IFN and RBV, and particularly when administered as a combination therapy [21, 22].

Cost effectiveness models analysed in the review by Nuno Solinis et al. [15] show that interferon-free DAA therapies are more cost effective than previous interferon-based therapies. The models also showed that early treatment is more cost-effective than therapy in later stages of the disease.

Data analyses showed an increase of costs associated with HCV as an OD in the period from 2000 to 2014 [12]. Despite lower OD HCV prevalence, the cost related to occupational exposure have increased in this period. About of € 87.9 million were spend by the statutory accident insurance for HCV as OD (n = 1.121), of which 60% were attributable to pension payments and around 15% to expenses for pharmaceuticals and other medicines. The cost of CHC are largely defined by the rising expenses for pensions due to increase in RWA. However, there was a strong rise in cost of drug therapy in 2012 to 2014 from € 1.7 to € 2.7 million. In 2015, the cost of antiviral drugs for CHC as OD increased to approximately € 11.9 million [23]. As reported by Zimmermann et al. [20], in 2014 about € 664 million were spent on HCV antivirals by the German statutory health insurance (SHI) and approximately € 1.3 billion in 2015. In Germany, more than 70 million persons are insured by the SHI, which represents about 85% of the German population. DAAs initially involve higher expenses, but as an effective treatment they may reduce long term treatment costs. Although the therapy success is convincing, and in Germany anyone with CHC has general access to DAA therapy, prescriptions have been showing a downward trend among patients with statutory health insurance since the end of 2015 [20]. Some possible reasons listed are insecurities regarding the authorisation of treatments and a lack of clarity in the reimbursement system. As a result of the unspecific course of the disease, researchers assume that around 100,000 people in Germany may have an HCV infection and not know about it [24, 25]. According to the WHO, less than 5% of people with chronic hepatitis worldwide (hepatitis B and C) are aware of their status [26]. The lack of compulsory screening strategies for at-risk groups (e.g. HP, intravenous drug users (IVD), men who have sex with men (MSM) and migrants from countries with high prevalence rates) has been criticised internationally [21, 25, 26]. The implementation of screening strategies to identify infected individuals and to interrupt the channels of infection is a major step in the prevention of the disease [24, 25]. There is no vaccine against HCV infection and a successfully treated infection does not offer protection against reinfection [19, 27]. To prevent reinfections (i.e. from needle-stick injuries) it is advisable to include employees with DAA therapy into regular check-up schemes.

The case figures presented here do not provide a complete picture for occupational HCV infections. The BGW only records notifications of occupational illness from employees of non-government institutions. This evaluation is based on register data with specific sociodemographic information, the data is not clinical in nature and not always complete (e.g. missing's in stage of liver disease (15.6%) and treatment experience (11.7%)). Information about co-infections with HBV or HIV could not be evaluated from this database in a statistically valid way because it has not been requested in a standardised form. However, we assume that there is a lower likelihood of co-infection with HBV or HIV because the individuals in the study were HP. These employees have regular check-ups from occupational healthcare practitioners, which include checking their HBV vaccination status. Three quarters of the sample size in the study are female. Men are more commonly affected by HCV infections than women. Men are more often in at-risk groups, such as the IVD and MSM groups, and are more often co-infected with HIV [25, 26]. Interim results from the GECCO study confirm that men are significantly more likely to have an HCV/HIV co-infection than women [4].

Only the occupational acquired HCV as insured event was taken into consideration in this study. We do not have information on co-morbidities not related to the CHC infection. If the working ability is reduced by several insured events, the RWA is determined separately for each insured event. As these co-morbidities are not considered when grading the RWA for CHC the confounding effect should be minor. We expected that with increasing age the RWA would also rise. However, we observed only a low positive correlation between age and RWA ($r = 0.16$, $p = 0.03$).

Our report is based on the experience of a major German statutory accident insurance with the treatment of Hep C carriers in HP with new antiviral drugs. It is a great achievement that HP with a CHC and failed treatments in the past can be successfully treated. The major outcome is the high therapeutic success (SVR12 94%), although the majority of insures had liver disease. Even if not all of them are still in employment and actively working as HP, a decrease in RWA signifies a reduction in individual disease burden and in pension's payments.

Conclusions

Patients with and without experience of treatment who have a CHC infection achieved high SVR rates in the observed sample. Early treatment is preferable in order to keep the individual disease burden as low as possible. It appears that early treatment is also indicated for cost reasons, e.g. as a result of the influence of cirrhosis on treatment success. DAA therapies make it possible to eradicate the HCV viruses, thus enabling early recovery from the chronic infection. SVRs are associated with substantial reductions in the individual disease burden and with the patient maintaining their ability to work. Over the long term, this will probably lead to cost savings for statutory accident insurers and also for other social security systems. However, we require long-term experiences with DAA therapies in order to be able to reliably interpret the results. Successful completion of treatment does not provide protection from reinfection. HCV screening programmes for at-risk groups are therefore essential, even after successful treatment.

Abbreviations

BGW: Berufsgenossenschaft für Gesundheitsdienst und Wohlfahrtspflege; CHC: Chronic hepatitis C; DAA: Direct-acting antiviral agent; DSV: Dasabuvir; ETR: End-of-treatment sustained virological response rate; GECCO: German Hepatitis Cohort; HBV: Viral hepatitis B; HCV: Viral hepatitis C; HIV: Human immunodeficiency virus; HP: Healthcare personnel; IVD: Intravenous drug users; LDV: Ledipasvir; MSM: Men who have sex with men; OBV: Ombitasvir; OD: Occupational disease; PEG-IFN: Pegylated interferon; PTV: Paritaprevir; RBV: Ribavirin; RNA: Ribonucleic acid; RTV: Ritonavir; RWA: Reduced work ability; SOF: Sofosbuvir; STROSA: A Consensus German Reporting Standard for Secondary Data Analyses; SVR: Sustained virological response rate; WHO: World Health Organisation

Acknowledgements

We would like to thank the Occupational Diseases working group (BGW) for their support.

Funding

No special funds were received for this study. However, the Institute for Health Services Research in Dermatology and Nursing of the University Medical Centre Hamburg-Eppendorf (UKE) receives an unrestricted fund from the Institution for Statutory Accident Insurance and Prevention in the Health and Welfare services (BGW) on an annual basis to maintain the working group at the UKE. The funds are provided by a non-profit organization that is part of the social security system in Germany. The funder had no role in study design, data collection and analysis, decision to publish, or preparation of the manuscript.

Authors' contributions

CW and AN developed the study design. DW and CW conducted the data collection, CW and AN conducted the data analysis. The interpretation of the data was made by DW, CW and AN. CW wrote the manuscript, with significant contribution from the other authors. Uncertainties were discussed between the authors regularly. AN revised the manuscript critically for important intellectual content and gave final approval for the version to be published. All authors read and approved the final manuscript and gave approval for publication.

Competing interests

The authors declare that they have no competing interests.

Author details

[1]Competence Centre for Epidemiology and Health Services Research for Healthcare Professionals (CVcare), Institute for Health Services Research in Dermatology and Nursing (IVDP), University Medical Centre Hamburg-Eppendorf (UKE), Martinistr. 52, 20146 Hamburg, Germany. [2]Department of Occupational Medicine, Hazardous Substances and Public Health, Institution for Statutory Accident Insurance and Prevention in the Health and Welfare Services (BGW), Pappelallee 33-37, 22089 Hamburg, Germany.

References

1. Askarian M, Yadollahi M, Kuochak F, Danaei M, Vakili V, Momeni M. Precautions for health care workers to avoid hepatitis B and C virus infection. The international journal of occupational and environmental medicine. 2011;2(4):191–8.
2. Global Hepatitis Report 2017. Geneva: World Health Organization; 2017. Licence: CC BY-NC-SA 3.0 IGO. http://www.who.int/hepatitis/publications/global-hepatitis-report2017/en/. Accessed 15 Sept 2017.
3. Sarrazin C, Berg T, Buggisch P, Dollinger MM, Hinrichsen H, Hofer DH, et al. Aktuelle Empfehlung zur Therapie der chronischen Hepatitis C S3 guideline hepatitis C addendum. Z Gastroenterol. 2015;53:320–34.
4. Ingiliz P, Christensen S, Kimhofer T, Hueppe D, Lutz T, Schewe K, Busch H, Schmutz G, Wehmeyer MH, Boesecke C, et al. Sofosbuvir and Ledipasvir for 8 weeks for the treatment of chronic hepatitis C virus (HCV) infection in HCV-Monoinfected and HIV-HCV-Coinfected individuals: results from the German hepatitis C cohort (GECCO-01). Clinical infectious diseases: an official publication of the Infectious Diseases Society of America. 2016; 63(10):1320–4.
5. Lubel J, Strasser S, Stuart KA, Dore G, Thompson A, Pianko S et al. Real-world efficacy and safety of ritonavir-boosted paritaprevir, ombitasvir, dasabuvir +/- ribavirin for hepatitis C genotype 1 - final results of the REV1TAL study. Antivir Ther. 2017;22(8):699–710. https://doi.org/10.3851/IMP3168.
6. Sarrazin C, Berg T, Ross RS, Schirmacher P, Wedemeyer H, Neumann U, et al. Prophylaxis, diagnosis and therapy of hepatitis C virus (HCV) infection: the German guidelines on the management of HCV infection. Zeitschrift fur Gastroenterologie. 2010;48(2):289–351.
7. Westbrook RH, Dusheiko G. Natural history of hepatitis C. J Hepatol. 2014; 61(1 Suppl):S58–68.
8. Gonzalez-Grande R, Jimenez-Perez M, Gonzalez Arjona C, Mostazo TJ. New approaches in the treatment of hepatitis C. World Journal of Gastroenterology : WJG. 2016;22(4):1421–32.
9. Tada T, Kumada T, Toyoda H, Kiriyama S, Tanikawa M, Hisanaga Y et al. Viral eradication reduces all-cause mortality in patients with chronic hepatitis C virus infection: a propensity score analysis. Liver Int. 2016;36:817–26. https://doi.org/10.1111/liv.13071.
10. Nienhaus A, Kesavachandran C, Wendeler D, Haamann F, Dulon M. Infectious diseases in healthcare workers - an analysis of the standardised data set of a German compensation board. J Occup Med Toxicol. 2012;7(1):8.
11. Dulon ML, Lisiak B, Wendeler D, Nienhaus A, Occupational infectious diseases in healthcare workers. Data from the institution for statutory accident insurance and prevention in the health and welfare services. Zbl Arbeitsmed. 2014;65:210–6.
12. Westermann C, Dulon M, Wendeler D, Nienhaus A. Hepatitis C among healthcare personnel: secondary data analyses of costs and trends for hepatitis C infections with occupational causes. J Occup Med Toxicol. 2016;11:52.
13. Swart E, Bitzer EM, Gothe H, Harling M, Hoffmann F, Horenkamp-Sonntag D et al. [A Consensus German Reporting Standard for Secondary Data Analyses, Version 2 (STROSA-STandardisierte BerichtsROutine fur SekundardatenAnalysen)]. Gesundheitswesen (Bundesverband der Ärzte des Öffentlichen Gesundheitsdienstes (Germany)). 2016.
14. Cohen J, Cohen P, West SG, Aiken LS. Applied multiple regression/correlation analysis for the behavioral sciences (3rd ed.). Mahwah: Lawrence Erlbaum; 2003.
15. Nuno Solinis R, Arratibel Ugarte P, Rojo A, Sanchez GY. Value of treating all stages of chronic hepatitis C: a comprehensive review of clinical and economic evidence. Infectious diseases and therapy. 2016;5(4):491–508.
16. Stahmeyer JT, Krauth C, Bert F, Pfeiffer-Vornkahl H, Alshuth U, Huppe D, et al. Costs and outcomes of treating chronic hepatitis C patients in routine care - results from a nationwide multicenter trial. J Viral Hepat. 2016;23(2): 105–15.
17. Backus LI, Belperio PS, Shahoumian TA, Loomis TP, Mole LA. Comparative effectiveness of ledipasvir/sofosbuvir +/– ribavirin vs. ombitasvir/paritaprevir/ritonavir + dasabuvir +/– ribavirin in 6961 genotype 1 patients treated in routine medical practice. Aliment Pharmacol Ther. 2016;44(4):400–10.
18. Lawitz E, Makara M, Akarca US, Thuluvath PJ, Preotescu LL, Varunok P, et al. Efficacy and safety of Ombitasvir, Paritaprevir, and ritonavir in an open-label study of patients with genotype 1b chronic hepatitis C virus infection with and without cirrhosis. Gastroenterology. 2015;149(4):971–80.e1.
19. Zeuzem S. Treatment options in hepatitis C. Dtsch Arztebl Int. 2017; 114(1–02):11–21.
20. Zimmermann R, Kollan C, Ingiliz P, Mauss S, Schmidt D, Bremer V. Real-world treatment for chronic hepatitis C infection in Germany: analyses from drug prescription data, 2010–2015. J Hepatol. 2017;67(1):15–22.
21. Schäfer M, Schwaiger M. Incidence, Pathoetiology and treatment of interferon-α induced neuro-psychiatric side Effetcs. Fortschr Neurol Psychiatr. 2003;71(09):469–76.
22. Slim J, Afridi MS. Managing adverse effects of interferon-alfa and ribavirin in combination therapy for HCV. Infect Dis Clin N Am. 2012;26(4):917–29.
23. 14th Congress for Hospital Hygiene 2018, Berlin, March 18–21, 2018. Lecture on March 19 at 2.45 p.m.: [Vision 'zero infections' - can this be achieved in view of the temporal trend in occupational infections? A contribution to the discussion from the perspective of BGW - A. Nienhaus (Hamburg)]. https://www.congress-compact.de/pdf/2018_03_18-21_DGKH_Jahreskongress_Hauptprogramm.pdf. Accessed 10 Apr 2018.
24. Ltd. LHP. THE ECO-HEP REPORT. A macroeconomic overview of viral hepatitis C in Germany https://www.leberhilfe-projekt.de/das-eco-hep-modell.html: Leberhilfe Projekt gUG (Liver Help Project Ltd.); Babette Herder and Achim Kautz; [2.8.2017]. Accssed 15 Sept 2017.
25. Warpakowski A. Hepatitis C: Elimination in Europa möglich. Dtsch Ärztebl International.113(21):-20-.
26. WHO. GLOBAL HEALTH SECTOR STRATEGY ON VIRAL HEPATITIS 2016–2021 [updated 2.8.2017; cited Juni 2016]. Available from: http://www.who.int/hepatitis/strategy2016-2021/ghss-hep/en/. Accessed 17 May 2018.
27. Webster DP, Klenerman P, Dusheiko GM. Hepatitis C. Lancet 2015;385(9973): 1124–1135.

Permissions

All chapters in this book were first published in JOMT, by BioMed Central; hereby published with permission under the Creative Commons Attribution License or equivalent. Every chapter published in this book has been scrutinized by our experts. Their significance has been extensively debated. The topics covered herein carry significant findings which will fuel the growth of the discipline. They may even be implemented as practical applications or may be referred to as a beginning point for another development.

The contributors of this book come from diverse backgrounds, making this book a truly international effort. This book will bring forth new frontiers with its revolutionizing research information and detailed analysis of the nascent developments around the world.

We would like to thank all the contributing authors for lending their expertise to make the book truly unique. They have played a crucial role in the development of this book. Without their invaluable contributions this book wouldn't have been possible. They have made vital efforts to compile up to date information on the varied aspects of this subject to make this book a valuable addition to the collection of many professionals and students.

This book was conceptualized with the vision of imparting up-to-date information and advanced data in this field. To ensure the same, a matchless editorial board was set up. Every individual on the board went through rigorous rounds of assessment to prove their worth. After which they invested a large part of their time researching and compiling the most relevant data for our readers.

The editorial board has been involved in producing this book since its inception. They have spent rigorous hours researching and exploring the diverse topics which have resulted in the successful publishing of this book. They have passed on their knowledge of decades through this book. To expedite this challenging task, the publisher supported the team at every step. A small team of assistant editors was also appointed to further simplify the editing procedure and attain best results for the readers.

Apart from the editorial board, the designing team has also invested a significant amount of their time in understanding the subject and creating the most relevant covers. They scrutinized every image to scout for the most suitable representation of the subject and create an appropriate cover for the book.

The publishing team has been an ardent support to the editorial, designing and production team. Their endless efforts to recruit the best for this project, has resulted in the accomplishment of this book. They are a veteran in the field of academics and their pool of knowledge is as vast as their experience in printing. Their expertise and guidance has proved useful at every step. Their uncompromising quality standards have made this book an exceptional effort. Their encouragement from time to time has been an inspiration for everyone.

The publisher and the editorial board hope that this book will prove to be a valuable piece of knowledge for researchers, students, practitioners and scholars across the globe.

List of Contributors

Hilde Marie Erøy Edvardsen, Asbjørg S. Christophersen and Hallvard Gjerde
Norwegian Institute of Public Health, Nydalen NO-0403 Oslo, Norway

Inger Synnøve Moan
Norwegian Institute for Alcohol and Drug Research (SIRUS), , Sentrum NO-0105 Oslo, Norway

Saara Taponen
Finla Occupational Health, Satakunnankatu 18 B, 33210 Tampere, Finland
Faculty of Medicine and Life Sciences, University of Tampere, 33014 Tampere, Finland

Lauri Lehtimäki
Allergy Centre, Tampere University Hospital, 33521 Tampere, Finland
Faculty of Medicine and Life Sciences, University of Tampere, 33014 Tampere, Finland

Jukka Uitti
Faculty of Medicine and Life Sciences, University of Tampere, 33014 Tampere, Finland
Finnish Institute of Occupational Health, 00251 Helsinki, Finland

Kirsi Karvala
Finnish Institute of Occupational Health, 00251 Helsinki, Finland

Ritva Luukkonen
Clinicum, Faculty of Medicine, University of Helsinki, 00014 Helsinki, Finland

Pirjo Hakkarainen, Jarmo Heikkinen and Kimmo Räsänen
School of Medicine, Institute of Public Health and Clinical Nutrition, University of Eastern Finland, Kuopio, Finland

Leena Moilanen
Department of Medicine, Kuopio University Hospital, Kuopio, Finland

Vilma Hänninen
Department of Social Sciences, University of Eastern Finland, Kuopio, Finland

Kristinn Tomasson
Department of Occupational Medicine, Administration of Occupational Safety and Health, Reykjavik, Iceland

Gunnar Gudmundsson
Faculty of Medicine, University of Iceland, Reykjavik, Iceland
Department of Respiratory Medicine and Sleep, Landspitali University Hospital, Fossvogur, 108 Reykjavik, Iceland

Haraldur Briem
Centre for Health Security and Communicable Disease Control, Directorate of Health, Reykjavik, Iceland

Vilhjalmur Rafnsson
Department of Preventive Medicine, University of Iceland, Stapi/ Hringbraut, Reykjavik, Iceland

Piotr Malara
Institute of Engineering Materials and Biomaterials, Silesian University of Technology, 18a Konarskiego str, 44-100 Gliwice, Poland

Agnieszka Fischer
Department of Toxicology, Medical University of Silesia, 4 Jagiellonska str, 41-200 Sosnowiec, Poland

Beata Malara
Institute of Medicine, Katowice School of Economics, 3 Harcerzy Wrzesnia str, 40-659 Katowice, Poland

Roberto Cappelletti and Justina Claudatus
International Society of Doctors for the Environment (ISDE Italy), via della Fioraia 17/19, 52100 Arezzo, Italy

Valerio Gennaro
International Society of Doctors for the Environment (ISDE Italy), via della Fioraia 17/19, 52100 Arezzo, Italy
Istituto di Ricovero e Cura a Carattere Scientifico (IRCCS) Azienda Ospedaliera Universitaria "San Martino" Istituto Nazionale per la Ricerca sul Cancro (IST), largo R. Benzi 10, 16132 Genoa, Italy

Marcello Ceppi
Istituto di Ricovero e Cura a Carattere Scientifico (IRCCS) Azienda Ospedaliera Universitaria "San Martino" Istituto Nazionale per la Ricerca sul Cancro (IST), largo R. Benzi 10, 16132 Genoa, Italy

Brankica Juranić, Jelena Jakab, Štefica Mikšić and Ivka Blažević
Faculty of Medicine, Josip Juraj Strossmayer University of Osijek, Cara Hadrijana 10/E, HR-31000 Osijek, Croatia

Željko Rakošec
Department of Culturology, Josip Juraj Strossmayer University of Osijek, Trg Svetog Trojstva 3, Osijek, Croatia

Suzana Vuletić
Catholic Faculty of Theology in Đakovo, Josip Juraj Strossmayer University of Osijek, Petra Preradovića 17, Đakovo, Croatia

Marul Ivandić
Public Health Centre Osijek, Park kralja Petra Krešimira IV. 6, HR-31000 Osijek, Croatia

Ove Björ, Håkan Jonsson and Lena Damber
Department of Radiation Sciences (Oncology), Umeå University, SE-901 85 Umeå, Sweden

Lage Burström and Tohr Nilsson
Department of Public Health and Clinical Medicine, Occupational and Environmental Medicine, Umeå University, SE-901 85 Umeå, Sweden

Andreas Seidler
Institute and Policlinic of Occupational and Social Medicine (IPAS), Faculty of Medicine, Technische Universität Dresden, Dresden, Germany

Anna Lene Seidler
Institute and Policlinic of Occupational and Social Medicine (IPAS), Faculty of Medicine, Technische Universität Dresden, Dresden, Germany
NHMRC Clinical Trials Centre, Systematic Reviews and Health Technology Assessment, University of Sydney, Sydney, Australia

Jochen Schmitt
Institute and Policlinic of Occupational and Social Medicine (IPAS), Faculty of Medicine, Technische Universität Dresden, Dresden, Germany
Center for Evidence-Based Healthcare, University Hospital and Medical Faculty Carl Gustav Carus, TU Dresden, Dresden, Germany

Constanze Rethberg
Center for Evidence-Based Healthcare, University Hospital and Medical Faculty Carl Gustav Carus, TU Dresden, Dresden, Germany

Albert Nienhaus
German Social Accident Insurance Institution for the Health and Welfare Service, Hamburg, Germany
Institute for Health Services Research in Dermatology and Nursing, University Medical Center Hamburg-Eppendorf, Hamburg, Germany

Raffaela Olivieri, Annalisa Ciabattini, Gianni Pozzi and Donata Medaglini
Laboratorio di Microbiologia Molecolare e Biotecnologia, Dipartimento di Biotecnologie Mediche, Università degli Studi di Siena, Siena, Italy

Sara Scarnera, Giulia De Vuono and Giuseppe Battista
Medicina Preventiva e Sorveglianza Sanitaria, Dipartimento di Biotecnologie Mediche, Universita' degli Studi di Siena, Siena, Italy

Pietro Manzi
Direzione Medica di Presidio, Azienda Ospedaliera Universitaria Senese, Siena, Italy

Birte Pantenburg, Melanie Luppa and Steffi G. Riedel-Heller
Institute of Social Medicine, Occupational Health and Public Health, University of Leipzig, Philipp-Rosenthal-Str. 55, 04103 Leipzig, Germany

Hans-Helmut König
Department of Health Economics and Health Services Research, University Medical Center Hamburg-Eppendorf, Martinistr. 52, 20246 Hamburg, Germany

Janika Mette, Marcial Velasco Garrido, Volker Harth, Alexandra M. Preisser and Stefanie Mache
Institute for Occupational and Maritime Medicine, University Medical Centre Hamburg-Eppendorf, Hamburg, Seewartenstr. 10, 20459 Hamburg, Germany

Enzo Emanuelli, Enrico Alexandre, Diego Cazzador, Tiziana Volo, Alessia Zanon and Alessandro Martini
Department of Otolaryngology and Endoscopic Surgery of the Upper Airways, University Hospital of Padua, Via Giustiniani 2, 35100 Padua, Italy

Vera Comiati, Maria Luisa Scapellato, Mariella Carrieri and Giuseppe Mastrangelo
Department of Occupational Medicine, University Hospital of Padua, Via Giustiniani 2, 35100 Padua, Italy

Sebsibe Tadesse and Yalemzewod Assefa
Institute of Public Health, The University of Gondar, Gondar, Ethiopia.

Temesgen Kelaye
Southern Nations Nationalities and People's Regional State Health Bureau, Hawassa, Ethiopia

Vanessa Neuhaus, Dirk Schaudien and Katherina Sewald
Fraunhofer Institute for Toxicology and Experimental Medicine, Hannover, Germany, Biomedical Research in Endstage and Obstructive Lung Disease Hannover (BREATH), Member of the German Centre for Lung Research (DZL), Member of the REBIRTH Cluster of Excellence, Hanover, Germany

Armin Braun
Fraunhofer Institute for Toxicology and Experimental Medicine, Hannover, Germany, Biomedical Research in Endstage and Obstructive Lung Disease Hannover (BREATH), Member of the German Centre for Lung Research (DZL), Member of the REBIRTH Cluster of Excellence, Hanover, Germany
Institute of Immunology, Hannover Medical School, Hanover, Germany

Tatiana Golovina, Ulla-Angela Temann, Carolann Thompson and Vidadi Yusibov
Fraunhofer USA Center for Molecular Biotechnology, Newark, DE, USA

Torsten Lippmann, Danny Jonigk and Peter Braubach
Institute for Pathology, Hannover Medical School, Hanover, Germany, Biomedical Research in Endstage and Obstructive Lung Disease Hannover (BREATH), Member of the German Centre for Lung Research (DZL), Hanover, Germany

Claus Bersch and Olaf Pfennig
Klinikum Region Hannover (KRH), Institute of Pathology, Hanover, Germany

Hans-Gerd Fieguth
Klinikum Region Hannover (KRH), Division of Thoracic and Vascular surgery, Hanover, Germany

Gregor Warnecke
Division of Cardiac, Thoracic, Transplantation, and Vascular Surgery, Hannover Medical School, Hanover, Germany, Biomedical Research in Endstage and Obstructive Lung DiseaseHannover (BREATH), Member of the German Centre for Lung Research (DZL), Hanover, Germany

Tom Loney, Anza Elias and Soha Ali
Institute of Public Health, College of Medicine and Health Sciences, United Arab Emirates University, Al Ain, United Arab Emirates

Tar-Ching Aw
Institute of Public Health, College of Medicine and Health Sciences, United Arab Emirates University, Al Ain, United Arab Emirates
PAPRSB Institute of Health Sciences, Universiti Brunei Darussalam, Japan Tungku Link, Gadong BE1410, Brunei Darussalam

Balázs Ádám
Department of Preventive Medicine, Faculty of Public Health, University of Debrecen, Debrecen H-4012, Hungary

Sylvia Jankowiak, Uwe Rose and Norbert Kersten
Division Work and Health, Federal Institute for Safety and Health (BAuA), Noeldnerstr. 40/42, D-10317 Berlin, Germany

Sabine Werner and Eberhard Nies
Institute for Occupational Safety and Health of the German Social Accident Insurance, Unit Toxicology of Industrial Chemicals, Alte Heerstrasse 111, 53757 Sankt Augustin, Germany

G. Jordakieva and J. Godnic-Cvar
University Department of Physical Medicine, Rehabilitation and Occupational Medicine, Medical University of Vienna, Waehringer Guertel 18-20, A-1090 Vienna, Austria

I. Grabovac
Department of Social and Preventive Medicine, Centre for Public Health, Medical University of Vienna, Kinderspitalgasse 15/1, A-1090 Vienna, Austria

E. Valic
Austrian Worker's Compensation Board (AUVA), HUB, Adalbert-Stifter-Straße 6, 1200 Vienna, Austria

E. Schmidt
University Clinic of Internal Medicine II, Institute of Occupational Medicine, Medical University of Vienna, Waehringer Guertel 18-20, A-1090 Vienna, Austria

A. Graff and A. Schuster
Austrian Dust-Silicosis Control Center (ÖSBS), Einödmayergasse 12, 8700 Leoben, Austria

K. Hoffmann-Sommergruber, C. Oberhuber and O. Scheiner
Department of Pathophysiology and Allergy Research, Medical University of Vienna, Waehringer Guertel 18-20, A-1090 Vienna, Austria

A. Goll
Section of Medical Statistics, Core Unit for Medical Statistics and Informatics, Medical University of Vienna, Waehringer Guertel 18-20, A-1090 Vienna, Austria

Daniel Mauss and Raphael M. Herr
Mannheim Institute of Public Health, Social and Preventive Medicine, Medical Faculty Mannheim, Heidelberg University, Ludolf-Krehl-Str. 7-11, D-68167 Mannheim, Germany

Töres Theorell
Institute for Stress Research, Stockholm University, Stockholm, Sweden

Peter Angerer and Jian Li
Institute of Occupational, Social and Environmental Medicine, Centre for Health and Society, Faculty of Medicine, University of Düsseldorf, Düsseldorf, Germany

Thomas Schettgen, Andrea Kaifie, Michael Felten, Thomas Kraus and André Esser
Institute for Occupational, Social and Environmental Medicine, University Hospital Aachen, RWTH University Aachen, Pauwelsstr 30, D-52074 Aachen, Germany

Sahar Eftekhari
School of Medicine- International Campus, Tehran University of Medical Sciences (TUMS), Tehran, Iran

Omid Aminian
Center for Research on Occupational Diseases, Tehran University of Medical Sciences (TUMS), Tehran, Iran

Zeinab Moinfar
Community and Preventive Medicine Department, Tehran University of Medical Sciences (TUMS), Tehran, Iran

M. J. Fröhlich and T. Welte
Department of Respiratory Medicine, Medizinische Hochschule Hannover, Carl-Neuberg Str. 1, 30625 Hannover, Germany

R. F. Kroidl
Stade, Germany

Oğuzhan Bol
Health Science University Kayseri Training and Research Hospital Emergency Medicine Department, Kayseri, Turkey

Serhat Koyuncu
Gaziosmanpasa University Emergency Medicine, Tokat, Turkey

Nurullah Günay
Erciyes University Emergency Medicine, Kayseri, Turkey

Claudia Westermann
Competence Centre for Epidemiology and Health Services Research for Healthcare Professionals (CVcare), Institute for Health Services Research in Dermatology and Nursing (IVDP), University Medical Centre Hamburg-Eppendorf (UKE), Martinistr. 52, 20146 Hamburg, Germany

Albert Nienhaus
Competence Centre for Epidemiology and Health Services Research for Healthcare Professionals (CVcare), Institute for Health Services Research in Dermatology and Nursing (IVDP), University Medical Centre Hamburg-Eppendorf (UKE), Martinistr. 52, 20146 Hamburg, Germany
Department of Occupational Medicine, Hazardous Substances and Public Health, Institution for Statutory Accident Insurance and Prevention in the Health and Welfare Services (BGW), Pappelallee 33-37, 22089 Hamburg, Germany

Dana Wendeler
Department of Occupational Medicine, Hazardous Substances and Public Health, Institution for Statutory Accident Insurance and Prevention in the Health and Welfare Services (BGW), Pappelallee 33-37, 22089 Hamburg, Germany

Index